Health in
Ruins

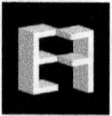

EXPERIMENTAL FUTURES
Technological Lives, Scientific Arts, Anthropological Voices

A series edited by Michael M. J. Fischer and Joseph Dumit

Health in *Ruins*

The Capitalist Destruction of
Medical Care at a Colombian
Maternity Hospital

CÉSAR ERNESTO
ABADÍA-BARRERO

Duke University Press
Durham and London   2022

© 2022 DUKE UNIVERSITY PRESS
All rights reserved
Designed by Courtney Leigh Richardson
Typeset in Franklin Gothic and Arno Pro
by Westchester Publishing Services

Library of Congress Cataloging-in-Publication Data
Names: Abadía-Barrero, César, author.
Title: Health in ruins : the capitalist destruction of medical care at a
Colombian maternity hospital / César Ernesto Abadía-Barrero.
Other titles: Experimental futures.
Description: Durham : Duke University Press, 2022. | Series: Experimental
futures | Includes bibliographical references and index.
Identifiers: LCCN 2022026369 (print)
LCCN 2022026370 (ebook)
ISBN 9781478016298 (hardcover)
ISBN 9781478018933 (paperback)
ISBN 9781478023562 (ebook)
Subjects: LCSH: Hospital San Juan de Dios (Bogotá, Colombia) | Medical
care—Colombia. | Public health—Colombia. | Privatization—Colombia. |
Hospitals—Maternity services—Colombia—Bogotá. | Maternal health
services—Colombia—Bogotá. | BISAC: SOCIAL SCIENCE / Anthropology /
Cultural & Social | HISTORY / Latin America / South America
Classification: LCC RA395.C7 A233 2022 (print) | LCC RA395.C7 (ebook) |
DDC 362.1109861—dc23/eng/20220628
LC record available at https://lccn.loc.gov/2022026369
LC ebook record available at https://lccn.loc.gov/2022026370

Cover art: *Shadow 2*, digital photography. © María Elvira Escallón.
From the series *Cultivos*, part of the project "In State of Coma."
Courtesy of the artist.

For Malena and Laila

For El Materno and all its people

ACKNOWLEDGMENTS

First of all, a big thanks to the El Materno family, professors and students from the Universidad Nacional Colombia, and El Materno's employees and patients. Whether named or not in this book, all of you have been a part of the history of this hospital and, by extension, of the history of medicine in Colombia. This book is a tribute to all of you and your wonderful Materno.

It was very difficult to decide how to name the many protagonists of this book since several of you are quoted extensively throughout. I discussed these issues at great length with the highly esteemed and respected professors, researchers, and workers who struggled for years to keep the hospital afloat and have their labor rights respected. I also asked the Press. For professors, hospital alumni, and professional nurses, we agreed on using first and last names the first time they appear in a given chapter and only first names afterward to privilege the personal experience over the public figure. In a few passages that could be compromising personally or politically, we use pseudonyms or altered content or context slightly. For most of the workers and patients, we do use pseudonyms throughout. Some workers have been very vocal and are recognized as public figures, and they decided to use their own names. For the majority, we agreed only to use a first name or a first name pseudonym. Those familiar with the history will very likely recognize who is narrating different aspects of the story. To facilitate following the history, a historical timeline with dramatis personae is included before the introduction. To all of you—those included in these acknowledgments by your real name, those who appear with pseudonyms, and those who are part of El Materno's history but not named here directly—we say thank you, with deep admiration for who you are, for your role in this history, and for creating a legacy of medical care for global health.

Thanks to Professors Odilio Méndez, Carlos Pacheco, Santiago Currea, Ignacio Méndez, Raúl Sastre, Lida Pinzón, Luis Carlos Méndez, Ariel Ruiz, Yolanda Cifuentes, Clara Arteaga, Astrid Olivar, and Gabriel Longi. Many thanks to all professional nurses at El Materno, especially Lucy Lucas, Patricia Farias, Rosa Bernal, Sonia Parra, and Elsa Myriam Pedraza. Thanks to alumni and students Matheo Martínez, Nicolas Martínez, the late Gabriel Lamus, Adriana Ardila, Yadira Borrero, and Elena Fino. Thanks to the El Materno workers, including Sor Maria Emma Muñoz, Esperanza Naranjo, Carmenza Acosta, Yaneth Castro, Washington Rosero, Irene Contreras, Gilma Carrión, Graciela del Salvador, Elsa Chaparro, Edelmira Castilblanco, José Gustavo Segura, Leo Vargas, Luisa Gutiérrez, Myriam Menjure, Luz Mery Roa, Margarita Silva, Marisol Martínez, Berónica Báez, Cecilia Araque, Dilma Díaz, Alejandrina Fitiquiva, Marlén García, Mélida Rincón, Mercedes Flórez, Ramiro Barbosa, Sandra Muñoz, Aurora Bernate, Gilma León, late Jesús María Montalvo, Constanza Ruíz, Alba Lucía Henao, Flor Aroca, Nelsy Gómez, Blanca Flor Villarraga, and Sandra Rodríguez. Thanks also to Jose Antonio, Rosa, Shirley, Verónica, Natalia, Maria, Jerson, and many other patients who shared their stories with us, including Juan David, the last patient of El Materno. For fighting for El San Juan, thanks to Blanca Flor Rivera and to professional nurses Margarita Castro and the late Janneth Damian. Thanks to all the professors and workers from El San Juan and El Materno for fighting for public hospitals, for the country's memory, and for labor rights. Thank you for sharing your experiences and wealth of knowledge, for caring for us, the research team, and for co-theorizing with us.

Other organizations did tremendous work in supporting the judicial fights for El San Juan, El Materno, their workers, and their legacy. Thanks to the Mesa de Trabajo Jurídico por el San Juan de Dios, the Instituto Latinoamericano para una Sociedad y un Derecho Alternativos (ILSA), Comité por el San Juan de Todos, Asociación de Pacientes del San Juan de Dios, the Grupo de Acciones Públicas (GAP) from Universidad del Rosario, and, especially, Salud al Derecho.

Over more than ten years of collaborative research, the following activist/researchers got involved at different moments in the fight to keep El Materno alive and helped create or consolidate the Critical Medical

Anthropology Research Group, where many of the discussions presented here unfolded. All of you, my dear friends, are part of the collective authorship of this book. Thanks to Maria Yaneth Pinilla, Camilo Ruíz, Adriana Martínez, Vanesa Giraldo, the late Marco Alejandro Melo, Adriana Ardila, Katerine Ariza, Emma Shaw Crane, Fabián Ardila, Levinson Niño, Fabián Betancourt, Indira Pinilla, Manuel González, Claudia Platarrueda, Maria Teresa Buitrago, Daniel Gallego, Amanda Abbott, Martha Bejarano, Andrés Góngora, César Tapias, Guillermo Sánchez, and Catalina Muñoz. Thanks to the Colombian anthropologists Myriam Jimeno and Maria Clemencia Ramírez for years of friendship and support. Other Latin American anthropologists have provided rich and nurturing intellectual discussions, including Susana Margulies, Rosana Gúber, Maria Epele, Maria de Lourdes Beldi de Alcantara, Ceres Vitora, Andrés Salcedo, Jaime Arocha, and Erica Quinaglia.

Thanks to the late historian of medicine, Estela Restrepo, for teaching us so much about the history of these hospitals and of modern medicine in Colombia. Along with Mario Hernández and Maria Yaneth Pinilla, we wanted to organize a lecture series and a museum exhibit around the living memory and struggle to keep the legendary university hospitals San Juan de Dios and El Instituto Materno Infantil alive. Thank you to all who participated in the exhibit and in the lecture series *Memoria Viva*: Mario Hernández, Carlos Pacheco, Estela Restrepo, Raúl Sastre, David Cristancho, Alvaro Casallas, Luis Carlos Méndez, Héctor Ulloque, Lida Pinzón, Luis Heber Ulloa, Myriam Gutierrez, Janneth Damián, John Harold Estrada, Fernando Sánchez Torres, Hugo Fajardo, Margarita Castro, Fernando Galván, Santiago Currea, Edmon Castell, Maria Elvira Escallón, Alberto Posada, Maria Yaneth Pinilla, and Jorge Arango. Thanks to the collective IMI en Espera and to Ingrid Morris for making it possible for El Materno to tell its history.

I am grateful to the following Colombian scholars who embody Latin American critical traditions and unapologetically embrace participatory action research: Mario Hernández, Yadira Borrero, Samuel Arias, the late Robert Dover, Claudia Puerta, Germán Cortés, Claudia García, Ernesto Valdés, Román Vega, Rafael Malagón, Amparo Hernández, Susana Ferguson, Claudia Rojas, Isabel Bedoya, John Harold Estrada, and the beloved professor of many of us, Lyla Piedad Velosa.

Thanks to Joanne Rappaport, Jean Jackson, Mary-Jo DelVecchio Good, Michael Fischer, Byron Good, and the late Paul Farmer for their unwavering support of my academic career in the United States. Thanks also to Joia Mukherjee, Salmaan Kevshavjee, David Jones, Scott Podolsky, João Bielh,

José Ricardo Ayres, Clara Han, Richard Parker, Lenore Manderson, Alejandro Cerón, Sarah Horton, Seth Hannah, Paloma Rodero, Iván Merino, David González, Dairo Marín, Angela Franco, Emilia Maria Ochoa, Gloria Alvarez, William Díaz, Alicia Yamin, Kim Fortun, Rodolfo Hernández, Claudia Lang, Dominik Mattes, and Janina Kehr who invited me to present aspects of this research or provided insightful feedback or suggestions at different moments and on different continents. For trust, inspiration, and friendship, my gratitude goes to Michael Knipper, Amalia Bueno, Pablo Simón Vicente, David González, and Guillermo Ros.

At the University of Connecticut's anthropology department, I have been fortunate to have the support of many esteemed colleagues, including Sarah Willen, Pamela Erickson, Merrill Singer, Richard Wilson, Samuel Martínez, Françoise Dussart, Eleanor Ouimet, and Natalie Munroe. Special thanks to all my colleagues at UConn's Human Rights Institute. You have provided an extraordinary interdisciplinary environment. Special thanks are due to the Institute's director, Kathy Libal, for her incredible leadership and resolute support for my scholarship and human rights in Colombia. UConn's Humanities Institute awarded me a fellowship that allowed me to write most of the manuscript. Thanks to many graduate and undergraduate students at the Universidad Nacional de Colombia and at UConn for being a source of intellectual engagement and inspiration. At *La Nacional*, the anthropology department, the Centro de Estudios Sociales (CES), and the Interdisciplinary Doctoral Program in Public Health were the intellectual homes of many discussions about El Materno and, more broadly, the privatization of health care.

Most of the collaborative research conducted at El Materno was unfunded. Nonetheless, some research efforts were partially supported by a small grant from CLASCO (Consejo Latinoamericano de Ciencias Sociales), three research grants from the research division of the Universidad Nacional de Colombia, and small research grants from UConn's Human Rights Institute and Office for the Vice President for Research.

While one never knows the exact moment when a collaborative research endeavor can be narrated and analyzed in a book format, in the case of *Health in Ruins*, it happened as I was sitting at a Harvard Friday morning seminar by Michael Fischer. Mike told me that I should write a book about the hospital and that, if I did, I should consider his Experimental Futures series at Duke. Thank you, Mike, for years of encouragement, for engaging so deeply with this work, and for helping me understand what Latin American scholarship and El Materno's history had to say with this book.

At Duke, Ken Wissoker's expertise was invaluable as I navigated reviewers' comments and refined the manuscript. To the two anonymous reviewers, thank you for helping bring this book to its current form. It was a privilege and pleasure to work with your feedback. Anna Ziering edited the whole manuscript, and Andy Klatz has provided invaluable editorial assistance, and friendship, at different points. Professor and documentalist Gustavo Fernández shared the image that comes before chapter 7, and artist María Elvira Escallón graciously authorized the use of her work for the cover of the book and for the image that comes before chapter 4.

Last, friends and families are our sources of support, joy, and life. Thank you to all my friends, most already mentioned, and families in Colombia and the United States. Thanks, Mom, brothers, cousins, in-laws, nieces, and nephews for constantly showing me how much I am loved. Thanks to my life partner, Maria, and our daughters, Malena and Laila, for such a wonderful ride.

August 1992

I made my way off a crowded bus close to downtown Bogotá, at the corner of 10th Avenue and 1st South Street. Even though I knew it was bad for my back, I carried a heavy bag by a strap on my right shoulder, blocking the zipper with my right arm and hand to protect its contents from potential pickpockets. I knew the area was not very safe, and I worried about my dental instruments. I was in my last year of dental school, arriving at a mandatory hospital rotation at Colombia's main public hospital, *Hospital San Juan de Dios (El San Juan)*, which was affiliated with the country's main public higher education institution, the *Universidad Nacional de Colombia (La Nacional)*. Clinic started at 7:00 a.m. and we (the students in the hospital rotation) had to arrive early, before 6:40 a.m., to deliver our dental instruments to the sterilization unit so that they would be ready for our first patients. Luckily, we didn't have to bring our own dental materials (amalgam, composite resin, and so on), as was the norm in many private universities' dental school programs. In fact, the previous year, the school administration had considered this as a possibility: forcing students to bring dental materials to treat the clinic's paying patients. But the dental school students, concluding that our role as public university students was not to subsidize the dental school, initiated a series of marches; joining forces with students from other schools in a university-wide strike, we protested the university's plans to raise tuition and the government's intentions to cut the already insufficient university budget even further.

At the hospital rotation, we had the opportunity to work on multidisciplinary teams overseeing the care of patients with different medical diagnoses. We were also on call at the hospital's emergency department, where a dental unit was housed in a small office. Despite our discontent with many aspects of the school's and university's policies, we felt privileged to be learning at El San Juan, as the hospital was most commonly known. We knew that we were part of the symbiotic history of two legendary institutions (El San Juan and La Nacional) that, together, had given rise to the country's most important advances in modern medicine. Their graduates had a reputation for being the country's best clinicians; the hospital developed medical knowledge, housed the most respected professors, and saw an unrelenting stream of patients.

That particular day, I was going to rotate at the hospital's maternity ward, known as *El Materno*, where professor of dentistry Astrid Olivar stubbornly insisted that dentists were fundamental to health care provider teams in child and maternity centers. She taught dental and medical students the importance of caring for the edentulous newborn mouth and of providing oral health care to pregnant women. The maternity ward was one of the many hospital pavilions built under French medical architectural influence at the beginning of the twentieth century. Corridors with massive windows led to infirmaries where small groups of poor women from all parts of the country shared stories and beds; the hospital was always running over capacity. The massive green quad, with its walking paths connecting the maternity hospital to the general hospital and specialty clinics, had succumbed to city development planners who saw a need for connecting the disjointed north and south 10th Avenue through the quad. A tunnel and a bridge were built to keep all the San Juan buildings connected with El Materno, which was now located on the east side of 10th Avenue.

On that particular August day in 1992, I had to bring a pregnant woman from El Materno to El San Juan's dental clinic, located in another beautiful French-style pavilion that greeted visitors with an impressive, marble staircase. Rather than using the bridge to cross the busy 10th Avenue, which by that time had grown into a busy, two-way, six-lane street, I did as everybody else did: pushed the patient in a wheelchair to the traffic light and waited for the signal. It was shorter and less tiring than using the bridge.

August 2005

I was now a newly appointed professor at an anthropology department in Bogotá. Sitting at my desk, I came across yet another piece of news about El Materno: the hospital's director was strongly opposing the government's claim that El Materno's closure would not affect the health of poor pregnant women and their babies, that the region's health care network could easily make up for the maternity and neonatal beds that El Materno provided. Aware that many public hospitals had already been shut down as a result of neoliberal health reforms, I thought to myself, "It is *El Materno*'s turn." I felt a sense of rage and an urgent need to get inside the hospital and record what the closing of a major public hospital looked like. I organized a small ethnographic research protocol to inquire as to how economic precarity and the threat of closure were affecting the hospital's provision of care.

A week later, I returned to El Materno to find out the required institutional steps for overseeing and approving research protocols. As I approached the hospital, walking up 1st South Street toward 10th Avenue, it seemed that the gate leading to San Juan Hospital's dental clinic was open. Only as I drew closer did I realize that the building was in fact closed; its parking spaces were now being used as a public parking lot. All the San Juan buildings (the eighth-floor general hospital and the several other buildings hosting clinical specialties and research institutes) had been shut down since 2000. Without patients, the legendary hospital complex now stood, a ghostly symbol, testifying to the calamitous situation of the country's health. Unkempt grass, layered dust, and city smoke were stuck to the layers of paint peeling off the buildings' brick walls. Surreally, a handful of security guards protected the abandoned buildings.

The following week, I experienced the same sense of intimidation I had felt as a student at the hospital thirteen years earlier as I presented my formal research protocol to El Materno's ethics committee: two prominent School of Medicine physicians/professors and the head nurse in charge of the hospital's education programs. This time, however, I was able to expound on issues they were less familiar with than I, such as ethnography as the prime method of anthropological research and the importance of applying social science to health scenarios. As the conversation went on and the formal task of approving the research proposal transitioned into a more casual conversation, the hospital committee members and I got to the political substance of my project. I said that I wanted to provide witness to the collapsing situation of the hospital and to understand what it was like for clinicians and patients to provide and receive care during economic uncertainty and under government threats of closure. I said that my purpose, more than anything, was to use research tools to register and synthesize data that might disrupt the deepening privatization of the country's health care network. The ethics committee shared my politicized research approach and assured me that they valued social sciences and that my work might help them with their main purpose: to remain open. I said that I was there to help them in any way I could, even if it just meant registering the hospital's evolving history.

1564	First religious hospital with private character, disputed as potential origin of Hospital San Juan de Dios (HSJD).
1635	Origin of HSJD as public hospital.
1810	Colombia's independence.
1828	First president, liberator Simón Bolívar, signs decree regulating El San Juan's budget reports and administerial functions.
1867	Creation of the Universidad Nacional, including its Medical School, Facultad de Medicina de la Universidad Nacional (FMUN). Law 66 elevated the medical school as the academic reagent of the Hospital San Juan de Dios.
1869	Beneficiencia de Cundinamarca (Main "Welfare Institution" of the State. Became the administrative unit in charge of hospitals). (ch. 2 and 4)
1944 (May 4)	El Materno is formally created as Instituto de Protección Materno Infantil.
1948–1958	La Violencia, decade of civil war between the liberal and conservative parties.

1953	El Materno is renamed as Instituto Materno Infantil "Concepción Villaveces de Acosta."
1955	Gabriel Lamus (ch. 2) starts pediatric residency at El Materno.
1969	Carlos Pacheco (ch. 1) passes the admission test for the FMUN.
1972	SINTRAHOSCLISAS (clinics and hospitals workers' union) is created.
1975	New Health Care System: Sistema Nacional de Salud (SNS).
1975 (May)	Medical School takes over the San Juan de Dios under Dean Guillermo Fergusson.
1976	The administration of HSJD is transferred to the Universidad Nacional.
1977	Santiago Currea starts working at El Materno. (ch. 2)
1978	President Julio César Turbay Ayala decrees the Estatuto de Seguridad (Security Statute) that unleashed a new wave of violence against leftist sectors of society.
1978/79–2005	Private Foundation San Juan de Dios administered the hospitals based on 1564 private origin of the hospital. In 2005 Colombian Council of State nullified the decrees that originated the Private Foundation and returned the public character to the hospital.
1978	Luis Carlos Méndez (ch. 1) takes admission test for FMUN.
1978	Kangaroo Care Program (KCP) is created by Edgar Rey Sanabria, director of El Materno.
1979	Carlos Pacheco starts residency in gynecology at El Materno. (ch. 4)
1979	Héctor Martínez starts to run the KCP.
1981	Gabriel Navarrete starts to run the KCP.

1982	Carlos Pacheco finishes residency and is hired as gynecologist at El Materno.
1983	Edgar Rey and Héctor Martínez publish the first results of KCP.
1982–1984	El Materno is remodeled.
1984	The Universidad Nacional is closed for a year.
1985	Luis Carlos Méndez (ch. 1) arrives at El Materno as a rural in medicine (one year of mandatory social service for recent graduates in health disciplines). (ch. 2)
1985	Rosalba Bernal (ch. 3) arrives at El Materno as a rural in nursing.
1985	Germán Sandoval, physician chief of surgery.
1985	Sister Emita (Sor María Emma Muñoz, ch. 3) is hired as nurse assistant.
1986	Rosalba Bernal is hired as head nurse chief of surgery. (ch. 4)
1986	Germán Sandoval, Director of Surgery.
1987	Rosalba Bernal becomes Chief of Pharmacy. (ch. 4)
1987	Elena Fino (ch. 1) passes the admission test for the FMUN.
1988–1992	Carlos Pacheco's first term as auditor/director of El Materno. (ch. 4)
1990	Mother Teresa Vecino retires as chief of El Materno's nursing department. Head nurse Rosalba Bernal becomes the new chief. (ch. 4)
1990	Law 10. Decentralization law.
1990	Law 50. Neoliberal labor reform.
1991	WHO's Sasakawa Health Prize awarded to Edgar Rey and Héctor Martínez.
1993	Law 100. Market-based/privatization of social security, including health and pension.

1995	Santiago Currea becomes auditor/director of El Materno (ch. 4). He finished his term early 1998.
1996	New collective agreement signed with El Materno workers.
1997	$3.6 million loan to El Materno and contract with Social Security Institute (*Instituto de Seguros Sociales—ISS*).
1997	Sonia Parra, head nurse chief of surgery, is designated as responsible for administrating admissions. (ch. 4)
1998	Ariel Ruiz becomes auditor/director of El Materno for a short term. (ch. 4)
1998	Verónica and Maria's miracle. (ch. 3)
1998–2001	Carlos Pacheco's second term as auditor/director of El Materno. (ch. 4)
2000	HSJD is closed down.
2001	Manuel Mercado becomes auditor/director for a short term.
2001–2005	The Ministry of Health brought external auditing firms, primarily McGregor, to oversee the hospital finances.
2002	Law 735. Declares HSJD and El Materno as National Patrimony and Centers for Education and for the treatment of the poor.
2003	Odilio Méndez, retired pathology professor, becomes interim director of El Materno. (ch. 4)
2004	Odilio Méndez, supported by El Materno Defense Committee, becomes auditor/director of El Materno.
2005	Threats of closure by Pablo Ardila, governor of Cundinamarca Department, as the government official responsible for the Beneficencia de Cundinamarca.
2005	Leidy and Yerson, Berenice, and Carmenza deliver their babies at the hospital in the middle of the economic crisis. (ch. 5)

2005	Rosaura, secretary, Raúl, nurse assistant, Lucía, secretary, Yamile, nurse assistant, Nancy, nurse assistant, Yolanda, X-ray technician, Amparo, secretary, Jefferson, porter. (ch. 5)
2006	Lida Pinzón is the director of KMC. (ch. 2 and 5)
2006 (June)	Final agreement to "save" El Materno.
2006 (July 1)	Liquidating agent Ana Karenina Gauna Palencia is appointed by Pablo Ardila, Governor of Cundinamarca.
2006 (August 1)	Police come into the hospital. La Cruz starts operations at the hospital.
2006 (October 23)	Agreement with La Cruz overseen by the Office of the Defense Attorney.
2006 (December 26)	Head Nurse Patricia Farías signs resignation letter. (ch. 5)
2006 (December 28)	Edict announcing the end of the working obligations for the remaining workers.
2006	Gustavo, nurse assistant, Yolanda, X-ray technician, Flor, general services, Marisol, secretary, La Carpa members, Camilo, member of the Critical Medical Anthropology research group. (ch. 6)
2006	Esperanza, nurse assistant, is rehired by La Cruz (ch. 7)
2007	KCP reopens under La Cruz's administration. Esperanza, nurse assistant, is appointed to the program. (ch. 7)
2007	Alcira Muñoz, La Nacional professor, collaborates with KCP. (ch. 7)
2008	Matheo, son of Patricia Farias, passes the admission test to the FMUN. (ch. 8)
2008	Agreement with Hospital San Carlos as training sites for students of FMUN.
2008	Constitutional Court Sentence (SU-484) recognizes workers' entitlements to all their benefits but sets up cutoff dates for the contractual obligation. (ch. 6)

2008	Head Nurse Sonia Parra rehired by La Cruz as chief of surgery. (ch. 7)
2011	José Antonio and Rosa had Oscar at El Materno and enrolled in the KCP. (ch. 2)
2011	Strike of Medical School students and residents from La Universidad Nacional. (ch. 8)
2013	Nicolás passes the admission test to the School of Medicine of Universidad del Valle. (ch. 8)
2015	Yadira Borrero's research on social mobilization around health. (ch. 8)
2015	New Hospital Universitario Nacional (HUN) opens.
2016	HUV (Hospital Universitario del Valle) invokes the bankruptcy law. (ch. 8)
2016–2020	New labor conditions, including interns and residents, Elena Fino, Lida Pinzón, Luis Carlos Méndez, Adriana Ardila, Guillermo Sánchez. (ch. 8)
2019	Final eviction of workers from La Carpa. (ch. 6)

When the Colombian government shut down the San Juan de Dios Hospital complex in 2000, it put an end to over 400 years of history of medical practice in Colombia and close to 150 years of the hospital's relationship with the country's most important public university, *Universidad Nacional de Colombia (La Nacional)*. Students from La Nacional's medical school and other health care schools were left without a university hospital, except for their training in gynecology and neonatology at El Materno, which had managed to remain open. When government officials announced in 2005 that El Materno was economically unviable and that a liquidation of the hospital assets would be the only way to pay off its accrued debts, the hospital's director, the workers, and the professors confronted this liquidation announcement and decided to remain at the hospital, fighting for its survival.

What happened? How did the country's main university hospital complex get shut down? How did government officials declare the country's most important maternal and child health care institution dispensable and threaten it with closure? The common answer in academic and public health circles is that these hospitals succumbed to the 1993 neoliberal health care reform that ordered the implementation of a market of insurance companies and providers. Many public hospitals were forced, under threat of closure, to adopt a clear market orientation. Others were closed down and reopened after a drastic for-profit administrative restructuring. Thus, the common answer sees think tanks and Colombian government officials and legislators as successfully turning neoliberal ideology into a full-fledged, market-based health care reform that destroyed many public institutions, including El San Juan and El Materno. But "What happened?" can also be a profound ethnographic question: one that demands a multilayered answer accounting for historical trends, legal maneuvering, people's experiences, and collective efforts to defend the hospital. Thoroughly answering this question destabilizes the commonly accepted idea of neoliberal health care policy reform as a linear, uncontested history that occurs equally in all places and results in the privatization of public health. In this book, the history of "what happened" illustrates how capitalism transformed (and continues to transform) the Colombian health care system during neoliberal times, and how this transformation is full of violence, conflict, hope, and uncertainty.

Logically, transforming a health care system implies the existence of a former structure and its replacement with a new one. This happened via the implementation of multiple pro-market reforms, at different moments in time. One could say that the main transformation happened when Law 100 (the law that privatized the Colombian health care system) was signed on December 23, 1993. Law 100, however, was both the culmination of a set of political fights and the beginning of a new series of confrontations under a new framework of action. Laws evolve over time, both legally, as regulatory decrees get implemented, and socially, as the decrees transform existing conditions and social interactions around the area of regulation: in this case, health. Thus, El Materno's history during the decades before and after the reform, the core of this book, serves as a case study of the social life of neoliberal health policy—what we might call a lawfare strategy implemented by market forces.[1]

When health is the area being restructured and market-based health care reform is the technique of power that capitalist sectors use to further their for-profit interests,[2] other relevant questions emerge. What is being transformed? Health care legislation? The operations of health care institutions? Or, more fundamentally, the practice of medicine and the essence of health care? A plethora of discussions have followed, concentrated on evaluating the reform through studies of coverage, pricing, availability, quality, affordability, equity, clinical indicators, and so on. Many critical perspectives analyzing the bourgeois notions that sustain public health and political economy have played an important role in refuting claims about the reforms' success. Nonetheless, *we*[3] aim to advance a different critical perspective here, one that emphasizes the substrate being transformed; in short, health and medical care.

In using El Materno's story to understand how health and medicine are transformed by neoliberal policies, we do not confine the analysis to how the transformation relates to profit increases in the health sector. Rather, we demonstrate how El Materno's history illustrates the sets of cultural norms and health care practices that must be established and those that had to be devalued and extinguished for the new for-profit health care structure to become hegemonic. In service of this project, we offer examples of the epistemic conflicts and contradictions that flourished as certain capitalist sectors (i.e., insurance companies) expanded into the health field in neoliberal times. Our objective is to align this ethnography not with debates around how neoliberal health policy affects public health or clinical outcomes, but rather with the conflicts that arise around transforming epistemologies of care.

Epistemologies of Care under Capitalism

By "epistemologies of care," we mean the ways in which medical care is created, practiced, taught, experienced, researched, validated, and confronted: processes that are embedded in particular historical frameworks and connect health care with affects, politics, and markets. The epistemological debates that we advance here are not those between ways of approaching and understanding reality; they deal, rather, with contestations about which reality one is studying, participating in, and creating. Boaventura de Sousa Santos clarifies that there is never a single epistemology. Instead, there are many ways of knowing that are in constant struggle, particularly in postcolonial settings.[4] Indeed, the kind of knowledge and praxis that emerges from social and political struggles in the Global South, such as those that happened at El Materno, "cannot be separated from those struggles."[5] Hence, we need to contextualize different intellectual, educational, and practice-oriented traditions within their particular historical contestations.

The main struggle faced by these epistemologies of the South is the dominant Western epistemology that credits value only to one kind of knowledge deemed universal and scientific, which emerges and is sustained through the forces of capitalism, colonialism, and patriarchy.[6] Hence, we can argue that there is a dominant epistemology of medical care that originated with Western colonialism and co-evolved with the forces of capitalism, modernity, patriarchy, and racism. Despite its dominance around the world, this epistemology of medical care, which is frequently called biomedicine, is in constant confrontation with other epistemologies of medical care from the Global South, including the one advanced by El Materno through its centuries of history, which this book will unveil.

In order to advance our analysis of the epistemology of care, it is important to understand one of the main characteristics of contemporary capitalism in its neoliberal phase. Neoliberal or market-based health care reforms speak to the commodification of health care service delivery through the institutionalization of individual rather than social insurance, which require the co-production of life, markets, and law around neoliberal principles of health care financing, delivery, and administration. Hence, the introduction of insurance companies in Colombia as a key capitalist health sector disrupted the existing hegemony of the medical industrial complex (MIC) as prime constitutive of biomedicine during the mid-twentieth century (i.e., the pharmaceutical industry, biotech companies, and for-profit physicians and hospitals), which was maintained by the limited social pact of the welfare era characteristic of Latin American countries after World War II.[7]

During the mid-twentieth century, more health-related products became available, and their prices continued increasing through patent protection mechanisms, regulated market competition, and tendencies toward consolidating oligopolies. Key economic and political challenges started to emerge: how to make sure that governments of developing countries continued purchasing new pharmaceuticals and biotechnologies from developed nations while ensuring that they paid their foreign debt obligations? How to respond to the demands of capitalists operating in the health sector (the MIC) to maintain and increase their profit rates? How to finance this increased consumption of health-related products around the world while acknowledging people's limited purchasing capacity and governments' limited budgets?

The capitalist solution proved to be very lucrative for a sector that had previously not been able to profit from health care, the financial sector. The model of individual and private health insurance had a long history in the United States but was virtually unknown in the rest of the world. Then, the questions were: how to shift regimes of capital accumulation from former welfare state configurations with significant government investment and control to a global neoliberal doctrine characterized by the financialization of the economy? What would it take to develop a new model of "deregulated" health insurance markets around the world?[8] As with other critical moments in capitalism's history, where violence had been a standard strategy, the imposition of neoliberal health policies has not been the exception.[9] Capitalist violence during neoliberalism has taken different forms. Even though it has been supported by dictatorships and authoritarian governments, with the associated political violence and repression, it has also included coercive shock doctrine strategies such as structural adjustment policies, or the conditioning of international loans to the implementation of neoliberal reforms in arenas including health care reform.[10] The end result of this overly simplified history of neoliberalism—that took place primarily during the 1980s and 1990s but is still ongoing—has been the expansion of insurance companies' global markets via policy reform.

In Latin America, neoliberal reform demanded the dismantling of whatever pension and health benefits of the insufficient and fragmented welfare state[11] to open the door for a market of insurers and providers. It required a new set of institutional practices and subjectivities that facilitated the circulation of money in different ways. If the main goal of the reform was the incorporation of an intermediary that administered health insurance policies, the reform had to put an end to government's direct funding of health care and transform bureaucratic mechanisms for affiliation, networks, billing, and payments.[12] Thus, this process demonstrates the development and implementation of a legal technology (health care reform) and aggressive and violent mechanisms of control that are necessary for maintaining power.[13] Control, in this case, refers to a reconfiguration of each capitalist sector's actions, transactions, and profits. Control also refers to the effective transformation of the social dynamics of health care, which include all the activities of those involved in the health service delivery sector, including patients, providers, and administrative staff. El Materno's case will illustrate how different power control mechanisms operate, more or less violently, and how they relate to students, patients, workers, and professors from the country's main public university.

Besides the profits generated directly out of medical care—whether commercialization of biotechnologies and pharmaceuticals, payments for appointments or hospitalizations, or labor exploitation of the health care workforce—it is the promise of new markets, its speculative characteristics that draws investments. Indeed, in order to expand their markets, transnational health insurance companies required countries to develop and pass market-based health care reforms[14] but, perhaps more importantly, needed the consolidation of a market mentality in these countries, meaning that life and health are acknowledged and accepted as individual risks that should be individually "insured."[15]

Investments into the future, Michael Fischer clarifies, are not only financial but also psychic, cultural, and political, and as such, require work and the construction of collective ideas as to what the future could be like. Such investments, still following Fischer, require a recalibration of life as a credible future, with anthropology being particularly well equipped to untangle what underlies those attempts to build the future.[16] Of course, capitalist investments and the social recalibrations they aspire to are contested, particularly when imposed on political projects that are trying to create alternative futures. El Materno's history will illustrate how the power play between two future-oriented investment projects is not simply a debate between public versus private/insurance-based health care systems. The historical, political, and cultural struggle is about instituting an epistemology of profits that relies on particular institutional structures[17] in which health and life are enabled as profitable insurable commodities. This process requires the displacement of an epistemology of care that profoundly believes in the public character of health care and in subaltern—and often feminized—practices of caring.

Hence, medical care here is not simply the neutral or ahistorical application of standardized biomedical interventions. Medical care, several studies have clarified, is a profoundly affective labor in which intersubjective relationships are constituted by the material and political histories of infrastructures, health care systems, patients, and, we will add, policy.[18] The affective practices, the "heart" that one pours in medical care settings,[19] speaks to the creation of communities of care that contest the colonial, scientific, capitalist, racist, and patriarchal aspects that continue to shape the epistemology of care that biomedicine represents.[20] Drawing from feminist scholarship, the affective labor of care disputes its devalued place in capitalist systems, while simultaneously emphasizing that it cannot be reduced to monetary transactions.[21]

Feminist perspectives and analyses of care help us understand how at different moments El Materno's team practiced attentive listening and acted in solidarity with women and their children even if their provision of health care services was still defined by biomedicine, patriarchy, racism, and capitalism.[22] While it is true that El Materno shared with other overcrowded public hospitals in Latin America "the lack of respect for birthing women and of sensitivity to their needs in assembly-line childbirth,"[23] with even two women in labor or postpartum sharing a stretcher,[24] there was also a deep awareness and acknowledgment that it was women themselves, and not the medical teams, who could offer the biological and psychoemotional tools to grant the best possible care for their children.

This ethic of care, which was constantly growing and changing, was also the result of a "clinical social medicine" approach (chapter 2) in which gender, class, and race inequalities were acknowledged as fundamental in order to provide the best possible care for women and their babies.[25] Hence, negotiations about the role of clinicians and biotechnologies in the care of women and their newborns were constant. While pathologies in gynecology and neonatology continued to be understood in biomedical terms, affective and effective forms of care were seen as a process of collaboration between the institution and the women and their families. Importantly, clinicians and medical teams debated how to best support the women and their families. In a complex mix of patriarchal and antipatriarchal narratives, clinicians would even instruct fathers and other relatives to make sure that domestic responsibilities did not fall on the recovering women and, quite the opposite, that they were treated as the "household queen." Since most women treated at El Materno were poor, the best standards of care demanded not only a full understanding of their living conditions but also the design of medical protocols that incorporated life challenges both at the hospital and at home. El Materno's epistemology of care, then, was a constant struggle between reproducing and dismantling well-known patriarchal, classist, and racist legacies of colonial medicine in obstetric care.[26] And this epistemology of care, always in the making, was institutionalized and passed on to new generations of students, workers, and families, who would start experiencing, witnessing, learning, and practicing it.

El Materno's history confirms that men are frequently, although not exclusively, the ones who reproduce many forms of symbolic, linguistic, psychological, and physical violence against pregnant women in medical settings, including obstetric violence.[27] However, El Materno's history also shows that men can be exemplars of how to embrace, perform, and teach an ethics of care that challenges patriarchy in women's care, even if with significant contradictions. As Carol Gilligan made clear in her groundbreaking work, the ethics of care is not feminine but feminist, meaning a more radical movement that moves away from the binary and hierarchical gender model and goes to the root, to humanity itself. Rather, feminism should liberate democracy from the patriarchal order.[28]

It would be a stretch to conclude that El Materno's team was in the process of liberating medical care from the patriarchal order. Nonetheless, less biomedical intervention and acting in solidarity with women and babies did mean that clinicians learned to control the urge to intervene with powerful biotechnologies to "save the women and their babies" (see chapter 2). Even the mechanical metaphors that biomedicine uses to describe and diminish women's bodies and reproductive capacities described by Emily Martin were not always assumed by El Materno's physicians and nurses to be universal or desirable. It is unclear if they thought of these metaphors as sexist and bad science,[29] but they would definitely argue that the disregard of women's bodies or their intellectual, emotional, and practical knowledge led to bad medical care. In this process, inspired by Gilligan's work, we can say that birthing and caring for newborns at El Materno was becoming more democratic than at other maternity hospitals.[30] El Materno's epistemology of medical care further contests the idea that acts of care and caring can be evaluated as either feminist or patriarchal, or totalities; that is, "fully feminist" or not.[31] Rather, in a single act, a male physician can be not only reenacting male superiority to the subordinate women that surround him (nurses who are mostly women and the pregnant woman who is subjected to the mandatory lying-down position) but also subordinating himself as he assumes a facilitator's role and elevates each woman as the most important person in the labor required to celebrate the arrival of the new life and, later, to take care of the newborn. It is in such acts and relationships that feminist and anticapitalist ethics of care can never appear as a totality but always as a creative struggle with oneself, with others, and with history.

Of course, women's solidarity and leadership were also paramount in shaping an epistemology of care that confronted existing patriarchal structures and practices at El Materno and later leading the fight to keep the hospital open. Such recognition of the role of women in shaping El Materno's history and the recognition of El Materno as an institution with the mission to care for women also resulted in an unequivocal acknowledgment of the stature of women as patients, workers, or leading medical scientists and care providers. Hence, beautiful exemplars of a liberating epistemology of medical care practiced by both men and women appear hand in hand with remnants of the colonial matrix that shape biomedical power and involve patriarchy, capitalism, and racism.

As market-based neoliberal reforms threatened and ruined the very existence of public hospitals, they also attacked specific "subaltern forms of care" that defied not only biomedicine but also its ingrained patriarchal and racist order. Hence, through El Materno's history it becomes evident that a capitalist destruction of these kinds of subaltern epistemologies of medical care implies an attack of all the aspects that made that care subversive, including, as we will see, challenging biotechnologies as the best standards of care, imposing medical knowledge over women's knowledge of their own bodies, acknowledging the need for stable and well-paid jobs for the worker's body, or deeply caring for students' needs that bridge a feminist ethics of medical care with a feminist ethics to medical pedagogy.

In this context, medical care becomes loving forms of caring in which what matters is not only a successful medical treatment or recovery but also a deep concern about the other's well-being and a plethora of medical and nonmedical actions that ensure that patients, families, students, and workers are well cared for. Such epistemology of medical care transcends clinical and scientific parameters to propose ways of seeing, knowing, and being with one another that are closer to feminist and anticolonial proposals that this book aims to convey.

Shifts in health care policies and funding facilitate certain kinds of care while negating or ruining others. The book title *Health in Ruins* is intended as a powerful metaphor for the current situation of the hospital and its workers and for the larger state of health care in Colombia. El San Juan's abandoned and collapsing buildings were declared national patrimony because of their beautiful colonial/European architecture. Unlike other material patrimonies, however, the buildings have received scant resources for maintenance and repair. Despite the official declaration, the hospital complex's buildings are not being preserved; rather, governmental neglect aids the decay process's strength and speed. Nonetheless, as Anne Stoler argues, all ruins, including these deteriorating buildings, are active and alive.[32] Workers go daily to the hospital to await final payment of their severance, meaning a dual process of time-related deterioration that affects infrastructure and workers. As time passes, buildings, people, and their epistemologies of care are becoming memories, legacies of the past.

The book title also aims to convey the purposeful process of ruination during neoliberalism: a politics of transforming buildings and people into ruins. This process of ruination uses political neglect as a major strategy; its violence resides in inaction.[33] Such ruination becomes "incarnated" in people and buildings.[34] Besides its physical and emotional destruction, ruination has a powerful symbolic role in that it transforms the social constructions of the hospital complex and its workers. If, before, the hospital and its workers were considered the epitome of modern medicine, the shift toward market-based practices required turning their public image into an obsolete, outdated, and undesirable wreck.[35] This destruction of symbols of particular social value opened up the possibility of colonizing new symbolic spaces, in this case around epistemologies of care. But we can never forget that ruins are always open for historical reinterpretation, even more so when ruins (buildings and people) continue to speak and produce "artifacts."[36] These specific health ruins are part of a larger political process of resignification, which depends on political proposals that pretend to speed up their destruction, convert them into museums, or recuperate them as university-based and public health care institutions.

A tension persists: the more the ruin is destroyed, the less symbolic power it has as a physical presence. And yet, the more it is destroyed, the more terrifying it looks and the more threatening its legacy can become for the interests working to consolidate a market hegemony around health care. Thus, *Health in Ruins* is intended both as a testament to capitalist acts of violence during neoliberalism (both active and passive destruction of material and immaterial elements) and as a legacy of a kind of care that can help defeat the growing influence of capitalist sectors in global health.

Struggles around the kinds of citizenry and epistemologies of care that are valued or devalued are more visible at public and maternity hospitals like El Materno.[37] What this book adds to the analysis of health and capitalism's coproduction is the interplay between the profit-driven epistemology of care advanced during neoliberal times and El Materno's, which finds creative ways to confront, contest, and survive, even if in alternative, precarious, partial, or broken forms.

This book aims to convey El Materno's epistemology of care in its rational, emotional, scientific, historical, and contestatory domains, how it is taught and learned by professors and students, how it is practiced by larger health care teams, how it is experienced and learned from patients, and how it has been transformed and ruined over time by shifts in capitalist accumulation in health care. And yet one of the book's main arguments is that as the hospital's ruination progressed, these subaltern forms of care found creative ways to continue existing, for history can never be silenced.[38] El Materno, in short, is an example of a very particular history of a subaltern epistemology of medical care that continues to exist even without infrastructure.

History and Hegemony: The Challenges to Ethnography

All ethnographies face a circular problem: how to incorporate history, given that they are in themselves historical accounts? Anthropologists are constrained by the specificities of time, region, and access that define their fieldwork. History usually makes its way into our ethnographies through a mix of oral history, secondary sources, and a deep immersion in what is known about the people, region, and topic we are studying.

For this ethnography, we have taken the challenges of history and anthropology in the opposite direction. Our task is not to convey how history informs the data or to coalesce history and fieldwork data in a meaningful explanatory and narrative way; rather, we want to make clear that this ethnography is part of a longer historical process that neither started with the field nor finished with the ending of this book. In this perspective, the question of "What happened?" takes a new form: "What is happening?" With this new question, we aim to represent fairly the many histories and experiences occurring at the hospital in particular moments while avoiding simple contextualization (i.e., this happened within the context of health care privatization) or a simplified consideration of history as directly causal (i.e., this happened because of neoliberalism). The question "What is happening?" then corresponds to a deep ethnographic inquiry within history, which requires profound attention to the details of individual and collective action and discourse and a critical understanding of the forces that are maintaining order *while* producing change.

Seen this way, history is never entirely of the past, a total rupture, nor is it a series of successive events. Structural forces—for example, the need of capital accumulation to expand across borders and into new domains such as health—did not originally come into being alongside neoliberal reforms. In other words, the coproduction of health and capitalism, as a system of economic production and social organization around health, did not begin with neoliberalism, even though neoliberalism did drastically change that relationship. This ethnography aims to contribute to the growing body of ethnographies of neoliberalism and health through a different understanding of what neoliberalism is and how it is enacting its power.[39] Neoliberalism, from an anthropological perspective, is neither a "historical moment" that we can encapsulate in set definitions or descriptions (deregulation, free market, privatization, fiscal austerity, and so on), nor a cultural trope that defines a new era.[40] Neoliberalism is a historic and dynamic process of class reconfigurations characterized by a new global pattern of capital accumulation with profound contradictions at local levels, in moments when capitalist hegemony, rather than being consolidated, is in fact destabilized.[41]

Hence, the concrete historical "moment" of this ethnography is not neoliberalism itself, but the period in which neoliberalism is trying to become hegemonic. This conveys both an ethnographic sense of spatiality that is no longer about enclosed communities or geographic boundaries and a sense of historical spatiality—of considering simultaneously the *where* and *when* of events. To focus on a particular locale allows us to connect ethnographic studies with the diverse development of capitalism around the world. Locale, in this case, includes both that idea of specific spatiality and the multiple influences and connections that form the locale. Thus, the locale under discussion here is both El Materno, and, as regards health and social security, Colombia more broadly. This book, then, focuses on the conflictual process of transforming epistemologies of medical care in a particular locale within a larger historical trend that illuminates what is at stake as capitalist sectors work to develop new regimes of accumulation and what the role of health is in that process.[42] This is why we have structured the book as an ethnography of hegemonies around health care epistemologies.

While the Gramscian notion of hegemony acknowledges the complex relationship between power, social praxis, and subjects, it is careful to negate any historical possibility of full conquest and, consequently, full transformation. Like Sherry Ortner, we find the Gramscian notion of hegemony "as strongly controlling but never complete or total to be the most useful."[43] Hegemony has characteristics of power and dominance, but it is never total nor absolute. Hegemonies "are never total in a historical sense, because in the flow of history, while one may talk of hegemonic formation(s) in the present, there are always also remnants of the past ('residual') hegemonies and the beginnings of future ('emergent') ones."[44]

The Gramscian concept of hegemony exceeds any exact definitions. Precisely because of its Marxist legacy, Gramsci used hegemony methodologically rather than theoretically, as a way to "explore relationships of power and the concrete ways in which these are lived."[45] Hence, with hegemony, Gramsci refuses to "privilege either ideas or material realities, but to see them as always entangled, always interacting with each other."[46] In Gramscian thinking, power relationships can take different forms in different contexts, on a continuum characterized by brute force, coercion, and domination at one pole and willing consent at the other.[47]

Such potential to understand why subaltern groups can consent to (and reproduce) those tacit and covert relations of power,[48] or advance different strategies for resistance and, eventually, subversion,[49] can explain why Gramsci was very influential to many prominent Latin American thinkers of the mid-twentieth century.[50] Within Cold War geopolitics and the many military, political, and economic aggressions of the United States in the region, Gramsci's uses of hegemony to link historical power with human action and political consciousness were indeed very appreciated. The possibility to understand the domination of subaltern cultures and articulate academic inquiry with emancipatory projects was echoed among many Latin American scholars who were already, by Gramsci's definition, organic intellectuals. Indeed, Gramsci's translated work transited from university centers to unions and social movement struggles, and people appropriated and redefined his categories in many creative and political ways.[51]

Contemporary Latin American scholars have expanded the historical reach of hegemony as an analytical category to explain the long-lasting effects of the social configurations of the colonial matrix of power that still influence ongoing struggles for liberation in the region.[52] As capital accumulation shifted during neoliberalism and expanded to areas such as health, the colonial matrix of power in Latin America was destabilized from above. Specific technologies of market power, such as Law 100 in Colombia, stir a range of changes in the political, economic, administrative, and everyday relationships happening at health care institutions. To create its new infrastructure and maintain power, neoliberalism in health needs new mechanisms of social control, including violence and coercion, that exhaust, devalue, co-opt, or transform specific epistemologies of medical care that contest the idea that health is an insurable commodity. Without people's acceptance of this new market mentality, however, neoliberalism will have a harder time gaining hegemony.

One specific action at El Materno clarifies the fruitful possibilities of using Gramsci's fluid and methodological take on hegemony for our analysis.[53] After the market-based health care reform, El Materno directors and administrators saw that their only chance of ensuring steady incomes— of survival—was improving their systems of billing insurance companies for medical activities. Nonetheless, they were not willing to compromise their standards of care and so invented many clinical, administrative, and economic strategies that allowed them to provide comprehensive care even to patients who could not be entered formally into the system. So, how are we to analyze their willingness to engage with the billing logics of the health care market? It is clear that they were coerced into seeking profits—an action of class power enforced through legislation that changed the administrative logic of the system. But they also implemented strategies for staying true to their standards of medical ethics and medical care, which prioritized medical needs over market-based administrative requirements. How is market power exerted here? How extensive is it? What does it accomplish?

Has it changed the ways medical care is practiced? Are resistance practices overcoming or subverting market power? Are El Materno workers being co-opted by the market, or are they inventing ingenious anti-market practices and planting seeds for a future subversion of market-based medicine? Obviously, we can offer no simple answers. But hegemony invites us to think about institutional actions (i.e., improving the billing system) and individual actions (i.e., correcting the code of a procedure in the billing system to ensure payments) as part of a larger set of power dynamics in which domination is occurring and, at the same time, resistance is taking place. Only by studying the specifics of these actions within the larger historical process of class conflict's evolution over time can we learn how dominant market forces are, how hegemonic they are becoming, and, quite importantly, what strategies are being orchestrated to challenge their hegemony. Thus, we understand Gramsci's invitation as opening up the field of power relationships around capital, class conflict, and subjectivity to history, rather than close it down by way of facile contextual or deterministic conclusions.

Hospitals such as El Materno run under a specific epistemology of the public and, as *Health in Ruins* will show, an epistemology of comprehensive and humane care characteristic of the mid-twentieth century welfare state in Latin America. Under this epistemology, patients, regardless of their ability to pay, would receive all necessary care. This benefited the medical industrial complex and kept its market hegemony strong; generally, profits flew to the medical industrial complex sectors, the state fulfilled its promise of providing care, practitioners provided the best available care based on their training and according to their oaths, and patients received the medical care they needed.[54] Often, as the book will show, the care provided departed from the biomedical model or was considered merely a complement to more important natural and social modes of care for Colombian women and their babies. Thus, biomedicine, as an expression of capitalism and modernity in health, was widespread in Colombia and practiced at El Materno before neoliberalism, but it was an epistemology of medical care that was not *entirely* hegemonic.

Ethnography as a Collective and Political Project

How does one conduct an ethnography of a hospital threatened by privatization? This ethnography belongs to the Latin American tradition in which ethnographic work is assumed as always political, with many anthropologists supporting counter-hegemonic struggles and subaltern ways of thinking about power and reality.[55] Colombian anthropologist Myriam Jimeno, for example, argues that Latin American anthropology has a "critical vocation" that reflects the anthropologists' "dual position as both researchers and fellow citizens of our subjects of study, as a result of which we are continually torn between our duty as scientists and our role as citizens."[56] The reflexivity involved in this kind of ethnographic work questions what is "ethically important" in anthropological research, which does not reside in ethics approvals or consent forms but in the deep questioning of how the researcher's political actions are advancing counter-hegemonic struggles or enhancing oppressive power structures.[57] As Brazilian Roberto Cardoso de Oliveira argues, the ethics of anthropological work in Latin America is about acting; in other words, a politics of participation.[58]

Hence, two relevant questions emerge for anthropological exercises that presume to be political or activist oriented. First, who conducts the ethnography? And second, what kinds of actions do ethnographers take while engaging with their fellow citizens in political struggles? This particular ethnography of El Materno must be understood as a group effort. While I (César) initially approached the hospital in 2005 and started Participatory Action Research with workers, patients, and professors, many members of the Critical Medical Anthropology Research Group acted in solidarity with hospital workers, patients, and professors and conducted other research and activist activities. Along with some friends, in 2006 I created this research group, which served as a training platform for students interested in activist-oriented research around health and a collective to discuss medical anthropology. Members of this group, primarily anthropologists and health professionals, engaged in different conversations regarding biopower and health care privatization. Importantly, while biomedical care and health care systems seemed to be a new area for anthropological studies in Colombia, several of us were familiar with how Latin American social medicine (LASM) scholars had been incorporating frameworks from social sciences into the understanding of health and capitalism in novel and important ways. Importantly, many of us had been trained at El San Juan and El Materno, and some had been born at the hospital or knew of relatives or friends who had been born or had delivered their babies at El Materno. The majority of us were suffering from the neoliberal transformation of labor; we shared family or personal histories in which the institutions where we worked were undergoing different levels of privatization that threatened job security, family economies, and future pension plans. El Materno, for many, was a personal history or a history that resonated with our experiences.

We engaged in different research projects, became members of nongovernmental organizations (NGOs) and social movements, and acted in solidarity with different social justice struggles, including those related to El Materno. Indeed, as years went by, many people from the research group participated and provided data and insights as to what was going on in the relationship between health, normalization, and capitalism in Colombia.[59] But also, each of us brought in networks of friends and activists to help with El Materno's efforts to resist and survive privatization. Over the years we came to understand that we were not only co-citizens but that it was impossible to define our subjectivities as activists or scholars since we were always engaging in action and, at the same time, conducting research. In a reflective piece, we concluded that at many moments we had failed to keep adequate and extensive field notes of what was going on, but we understood that this academic failure happened because much of our energy was dedicated to support whatever specific political action was more relevant at the moment.[60] To reconstruct notes and memories, we relied on other documents such as memos, recordings of meetings, emails, and shared conversations. As such, our collective ethnographic project assumed a collective "diary" with many members' field notes.

Furthermore, some specific actions and documents were planned, discussed, edited, or presented with members of El Materno; hence, creating a further blurring between activist-researchers and members of the El Materno community. We (the research team) admired the workers' analytical expertise and extensive legal, political, and historical knowledge about what was going on, which humbled the social scientists.[61] Since 2005 the workers at El Materno have explained the hospital's legal, administrative, and economic situation to us (researchers, journalists, and other visitors). It took us (workers and researchers) years of continuous analysis to understand what was going on and how the hospital's present and uncertain future resulted in so much pain and destruction. Acknowledging coparticipation and cotheorization has also been part of how Latin American Participatory Action Research supports subaltern struggles.[62]

Many undergraduate and graduate students, workers from El Materno, colleagues, friends, relatives, and friends of friends participated, collaborated, and coproduced in one way or another, this ethnography. It is impossible to put an end date of our collaborative relationship with El Materno, but, for the formal requirements of research, we can say that the bulk of the data were collected until 2015, with occasional follow-up conversations until 2019. While going to El Materno and formal interviews did take place, many people coordinated workshops, searched for important material in the fight to keep El Materno alive, produced a photographic registry for the legal protection of the hospital patrimony, drafted documents for public authorities or newspapers, or simply engaged in heated conversations about health care and the future of the hospitals. All these people—the majority being anthropologists and El Materno workers and professors, but also other health professionals, administrators, and artists—can be considered coauthors. This is why a politics of a collective authorship is symbolized in our use of *we* throughout the book.

In this collective endeavor, research in itself, or this book for that matter, was not the main goal but an instrument for larger political goals.[63] Thus, there are epistemic and political implications for the uses of *we* in anthropology—not necessarily as a nonspecific notion of collective subjectivity but as a political project with collective belonging, representation, and action. Collective subjectivities are a common way to represent efforts in Latin America to combine social activists, intellectuals, and political party leaders. By assuming collective subjectivities, we do not want to convey the incorrect idea that attention to individual experiences and biographic accounts was unimportant in this ethnography; in contrast, it was paramount. However, individual biography was important for connecting particular individual experiences with larger historical processes in a critical phenomenological sense, whether in order to identify the larger process's specific implications for a particular subject or the ways in which that particular subject's history and experience influenced the larger historical process.

The most frequent action-research activity at El Materno did not differ substantially in technique from what is known as participant observation. However, the fieldwork entailed being at the hospital *with* the workers and professors; this resulted in a politics of being with them, a deeply emotional process of exerting solidarity that Myriam Jimeno calls "emotional communities."[64] Often, the research team's visits were seen as extremely important—not only because, as the years accumulated, workers and professors felt isolated and unacknowledged but also because ideas about future actions often emerged from them. We were involved as confidants and recipients of harmful gossip about hospital colleagues and forced to take moral stances around those claims. We also felt compelled to intercede and explain the perspective or situation of different groups inside the hospital in tense moments, and we intentionally reoriented political efforts toward larger goals, such as keeping the hospital afloat or securing a fair termination of labor contracts. Frequently, we felt defeated and felt that our efforts, whether academic articles, legal documents, art activities, solidarity visits and conversations, or media denunciations, had little effect to transform the course of history. Thus, most activities, such as a workshop, a series of lectures about the hospital, the elaboration of a legal document, or the coordination of a guided visit, were not intended as fieldwork activities, even though they could later be converted into field notes through the reconstruction of the collective diary.

Understanding power and taking sides means acknowledging one's political positionality. Of course, issues of reflexivity and situated knowledge, discussed extensively in anthropological research,[65] are helpful for advancing a proposal for ethnography as a form of collective political action. An activist-researcher positionality in anthropology—rather than being harmed by a lack of the necessary scientific neutrality that is often advocated to generate rigorous scientific knowledge,[66] can produce deeper comprehensions of a specific social dynamic given that it invites researchers, research teams, and social groups to find connections between everyday life and violent coercion or willing consent. More importantly, by acting against dominant forces, we can see more clearly how power operates, what forces and strategies are being implemented by dominant groups and what actions accomplish better results and facilitate subversion, both in the short term and in later and better times.

We hope that this book itself offers a counterhegemonic force to neoliberalism by showing both its devastating effects and the many opportunities that the world has for overcoming biocapital, that is, the coproduction of health care and capitalism.[67]

Book Overview

In chapter 1, The National University Escuela, current professors of medicine and one alumna tell the story of what it was like to pass the admission test for the School of Medicine at the National University in Colombia in the 1960s and 1970s. Chapter 1 describes the political, economic, and intellectual challenges of the students during their preclinical and clinical years, during which they received practical training as medical students, interns, and residents at the most prominent public and university hospital in the country.[68]

Chapter 2, Clinical Social Medicine, paints a vivid picture of the imbricated relationship of El Materno and the rapidly growing city of Bogotá during the mid-twentieth century. In particular, we learn about "simple alternative solution[s] to complex medical problems," strategies that professors of pediatrics and neonatology created to confront the medical challenges poor pregnant women and babies brought to a chronically underfunded hospital.

Chapter 3, Religion and Caring in a Medical Setting, emphasizes the importance of the religious presence at the hospital and El Materno's fundamental politics of care. Patients and workers came to see El Materno as their second home; devotion to work duties, patients, and colleagues further blurred the boundaries between households and hospitals. A health miracle related to a virgin apparition connects care, healing, and faith.

Chapter 4, Hospital Budgets before and after Neoliberalism, deals with the hospital's administration through the narratives of several hospital directors and section chiefs. This chapter unveils the turning point in the hospital's economic viability with the full implementation of neoliberal reforms, when state funding was completely cut off and the hospital was forced to compete for resources within the new for-profit and insurance-based system. The chapter ends with the government declaring the hospital economically unviable and threatening to close it.

In chapter 5, Violence and Resistance, we read about how workers became "burned out" from the emotional toll of a lack of patients and close to eight months of unpaid salaries. The chapter describes what it was like for El Materno workers to experience a "liquidation process" and then wait years for their severance packages. Then, the chapter turns to workers' efforts to keep the hospital afloat, satisfy their patients' rights to health, and respond to continuous threats of closure and liquidation. It details the many strategies workers implemented over the course of many years to keep fighting for their labor rights and preserving the hospital's material and immaterial patrimony.

In chapter 6, Remaining amid Destruction, workers who were rehired by a new administration and professors of the National University narrate what it was like to work in the same building but under different management. They had new, temporary contracts without benefits and with reduced pay, but at least workers had salaries and were able to continue working at "their" hospital. Professors voiced their dissatisfaction with the way the hospital was run and with clinical services that had been reduced to what was successfully billable. Nonetheless, they remained determined and committed to staying and fighting for their roles in the university/hospital system.

Chapter 7, Learning and Practicing Medicine in a For-Profit System, integrates the voices of recent graduates from the National University, who explain what it is like to graduate from the School of Medicine without having received training in its legendary hospitals. Their voices and those of the professors who oversee medical students, interns, and residents illustrate many of the current problems of medical education and medical care in Colombia.

In the Final Remarks, Medicine as Political Imagination, we link the hospital's history with other processes of ruination of public health care and the protest they are generating around the world. This section helps us realize that other stories like El Materno's are happening in other places, as the neoliberal "health insurance logic" garners expanding influence around the world.

CHAPTER 1. The National University Escuela

This first chapter emphasizes that any study of medicine, medical care, or medical training must be embedded in larger political histories.[1] In particular, this chapter explains that becoming a Colombian physician is a political experience that extends beyond specific theoretical training in basic and social sciences or clinical training at the hospitals. As we will see, both the specific university and the specific hospital where one is trained contribute to the embodiment of particular professional praxes and political subjectivities that shape the way one sees, thinks, and feels about one's professional obligations. Not only does one become part of the history of these institutions, but one continues that history by enacting a particular epistemology of care.[2]

That larger sense of being part of a tradition is as powerful emotionally as it is politically. We call this tradition the National University Escuela, or La Nacional Escuela, meaning an institutional legacy of knowledge, training, and praxis of medical care. And becoming part of an *escuela* happens in the middle of the contentious relationship between politics and health that defines the very future of these institutions. The stakes, as we will see throughout this book, could not be higher. Political action in the defense of the public universities and hospitals is essential: it shapes the actions and imagination of physicians and helps define the course of history.[3] At the same time, internalizing the standards of care exemplified by the professors also means that the students feel a responsibility to provide the

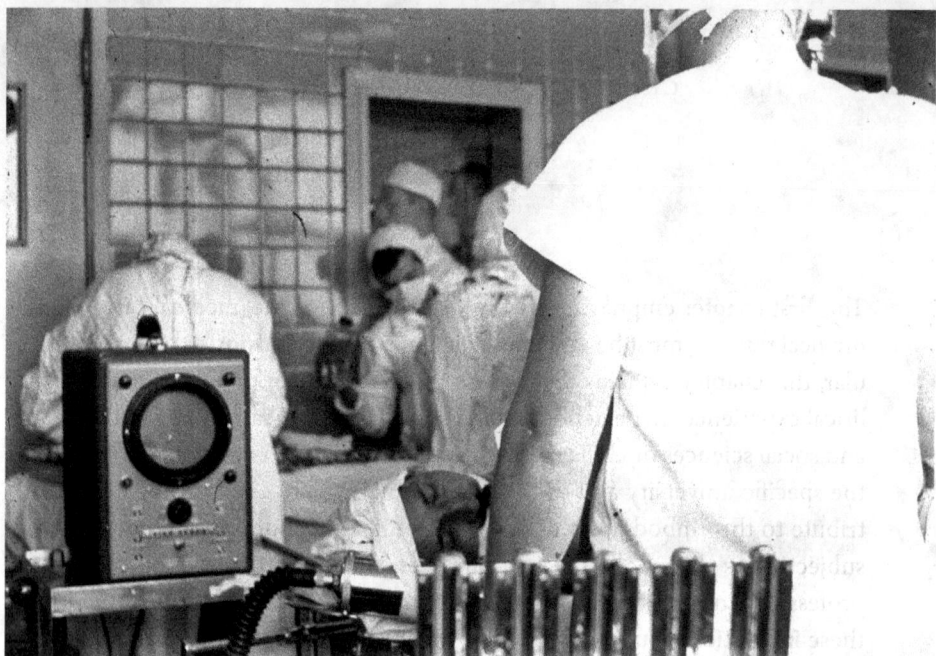

FIGURE 1.1. Operating room, 1950s. (Photo by Father Hernán, courtesy of Constanza Ruíz.)

best care—thereby demonstrating the ongoing excellence of La Nacional Escuela. To be the best, this chapter conveys, is a political, emotional, and clinical exigency.

Grasping the history of an escuela means reaching back in time to colonial legacies in order to understand contemporary dynamics that could otherwise be misinterpreted. Public hospitals like El San Juan de Dios and public universities such as La Nacional were at the epicenter of Colombia's efforts to gain intellectual and administrative autonomy after independence. Nonetheless, the elite characteristics of medicine, including its hierarchies and patriarchal structures, mean that medical care was still haunted by its colonial beginnings. We will see how, besides the knowledge and gender hierarchies that students, interns, residents, and faculty experienced, the colonial legacies of charity-based care were enacted in the way poor patients were seen and treated at the hospital. Although this chapter challenges the easy association between charity care and poor care, discourses around human dignity as a social and economic right and health as a human right, had not, in the 1960s to 1980s, been incorporated into hospital or university debates.[4] Perhaps, because of the new wave of violence against leftist sectors, intellectuals, and civic society leaders, the basic right to life was already enough to think about. Poverty was understood either as a problem of lack of development on the part of the government, or as a main component of leftist political and subversive platforms, which, for threatening the elites' power, were faced with state repression and political violence. Within the fragmented health care system of Colombia (i.e., public, social security, and private facilities and networks), however, public hospitals and public universities were seen as the institutions through which the state duties of education and health care were discharged. This chapter, then, will help us understand how the particular tradition in medical care of La Nacional Escuela was perpetuated and why, later on, with the rise of neoliberalism, it was violently attacked.

Medicine within Politics: A Combined History before Neoliberalism

I was in doubt as to what to study all the way to the very last months of high school. My father had once mentioned that he wanted me to study medicine. I remember I liked math, but I just don't know why I wasn't thinking seriously about it. One day, I was playing basketball with a classmate of mine and he asked me, "Did you ask for the registration form to apply to University?" I said no, and he told me: "You better wise up because registration is open and it will close soon." He had brothers who were already in college and had sent him the registration forms from different universities, but my oldest brother didn't go to college so I didn't have contacts or any way of knowing about applications. My friend ended up with some extra forms for three universities, which he handed over to me. La Nacional required two admission tests. The first test was done in the coast, where I lived, and for the second I had to go to the capital [Bogotá]. Fortunately, before the test for Antioquia University, the admission results of La Nacional came out and I had gotten in. Three of my uncles lived in Bogotá and I liked the city, I liked the weather, I liked everything. So, I landed in Bogotá from the coast, really young, to study medicine. I was alone; I arrived at the student residencies and remained there for the entirety of my studies.

Carlos Pacheco would go on to graduate from La Nacional as a physician specializing in gynecology. He became an attending physician at El Materno and a well-known expert in reversing tube ligations laparoscopically. He also became a professor of La Nacional's School of Medicine and a two-time director of El Materno and ended his professional career as the dean of the School of Medicine.

Back in the late 1960s when Carlos passed the admission test to enter La Nacional, medicine was the most socially prestigious career; graduating with a degree in medicine assured students of good professional options. Even today, the number of applicants far exceeds the university's institutional capacity, and only those who score at the very top on the admission test are accepted. Many students who do not get in reapply because of the university's prestige. Most significantly, for many families without economic resources—from the capital and across the country—studying at a public university is the only way to obtain higher education. At the time Carlos was admitted, students had access to residences and cafeteria and paid no tuition.[5]

Thus, getting into La Nacional was a common dream for many students and families. For poorer families, it meant financial security and class mobility; for elite members of society, it meant status maintenance. Nonetheless, as in other Latin American countries, public universities have always reflected the country's tensions around class and politics. Luis Carlos

Méndez's first memories of Bogotá and La Nacional were not as pleasant as Carlos's. Luis Carlos finished high school very young, at sixteen. He came from a humble household and had never been to Bogotá. The day he took the admission test to get into medical school, in 1978, "*hubo desalojo, hubo pedrea, hubo metralla, no, eso fue retenaz.*" A literal translation of this phrase would fail to capture the historical meaning of these words. "Hubo desalojo" means that the university was evacuated, which usually happens when there are "disturbances," or heated confrontations between people from inside the university and police who stand with guns and tanks outside of the campus. "Hubo pedrea" means that the people from inside the university were throwing rocks at the police. "Hubo metralla" means that gunshots were being fired. Such days are quite difficult, and when Luis Carlos said, "eso fue retenaz," he implied that the conditions were over the usual level of difficulty: something like "over-the-top tough."

Political conflict is a distinctive characteristic of Latin American public universities. The legacy of civilized intellectual debate of European academic traditions was central to the origins of Latin American academia. Nevertheless, the derived modern ideals of intellectual thinking and participation in politics through "rational" means have historically coexisted with belligerence, mobilization, organization, and revolt. During much of the nineteenth and early twentieth centuries, the state's promotion of public education and national scientific institutions was seen as a pillar for the consolidation of independent republics.[6] However, the mid-twentieth century reorganization of state budgets around "development"—characterized by promotion of national industries, increased productivity, and urbanization—started to put pressure on the state to be careful and strategic about social spending, a category into which both public education and public health fell. At this time, a growing gap between radicalizing conservative and liberal political sectors resulted in direct confrontations across society, from Congress all the way to small towns where neighbors and relatives committed heinous crimes against one another. This period (1948–1958), which was precipitated by the murder of popular leader and presidential candidate Jorge Eliécer Gaitán, is known in Colombian history as La Violencia (The Violence).

Thus, an "over-the-top tough" situation for Luis Carlos's father, who had suffered firsthand the effects of La Violencia in El Tolima (perhaps the area of the country with the highest death toll), raised unbearable concern over his son's safety. "My father had lived through very difficult times in one of the toughest areas at the time [of *La Violencia*], and with the situation that day . . . the day of the admission test, we were both running, he was holding my hand, and we didn't even know in what direction to go. That was tough. It affected him so much and he relived so many things he had gone through with his family that it was too much. . . . Fortunately," Luis Carlos concluded, "I did not get in La Nacional." La Nacional, then, was a microcosm of the country's political turmoil. In fact, political violence and instability are important aspects of the experiences that students, staff, and faculty live through. La Nacional and, to a lesser extent, other regional public universities are described as a reflection of the country—a place where people from all different geographic, class, and political sectors come together, where whatever is going on in the country seeps into the everyday dynamics of the institution.

Luis Carlos's father's fears were not simply an unfounded result of his first-hand experience of La Violencia. By the late 1970s the state's mid-twentieth-century developmentalist agenda had strained the social welfare pact badly enough that the country was experiencing another peak in its chronic history of violence. President Julio César Turbay Ayala (1978–1982) decreed the *Estatuto de Seguridad* (Statute of Security), which brought about a new wave of state repression of leftist sectors of society. As the center of intellectual thinking, La Nacional was a clear target for the state security apparatus, as were political parties, social movements, and labor unions.

It was not only leftist civic organizations and parties that fueled many of the academic debates inside and outside the classrooms. Guerrilla organizations—which emerged as a legacy of La Violencia during the 1960s and 1970s—would also have an important presence at the university, either by embodying the ideals of student organizations or by directly recruiting students.[7] On days of "confrontation," people inside the university would cover their faces with scarves to avoid being recognized and later detained or executed. A mix of members of student organizations and members of organizations from outside the university would take part in the confrontation. The military would also infiltrate the university, using students, workers, or other frequent visitors to identify "subversive" agents. As in other Latin American countries, the detention and disappearance of students were expressions of the country's political violence at the university level. As political repression worsened and governmental policies departed more and more from the welfare pact, confrontations escalated both inside and outside the university.

"Over-the-top tough" days at public universities started to be very common during the late 1970s and early 1980s. If heavy confrontations occurred on a Thursday or Friday, La Nacional would be evacuated and closed down until the following Monday. The gated "white city," as La Nacional's campus is known, would be guarded by the army, which would conduct thorough inspections of the campus, opening student lockers and residences, in order to find subversive material or guns. Leftist sectors claimed that the university's militarization was a clear violation of its institutional autonomy and that during military inspections the government was in fact planting evidence to target important political leaders.

Student protests, however, were not limited to direct confrontations. They also included pacific strategies such as public announcements and discussions of the university's situation in public spaces, such as squares or buses, during which they explained issues like insufficient budgets and government restrictions of academic autonomy and student freedom. At times, students would take over certain areas of the university or the city (such as churches or the Red Cross) in order to attract public attention and present their demands to the administration. These demands might include reversing students' expulsions and freeing others who had been detained. When the situation did escalate to *pedreas*, the administration responded with *desalojo* and threats of militarization and expulsion.[8]

In 1982 an economics professor was murdered; in 1983 five students disappeared. On May 9, 1984, Jesús Humberto León Patiño, a dental student and leader of the student movement, was found tortured and murdered.[9] On May 16, 1984, mourning and rage caused another "over-the-top tough" day. The university administration[10] responded with *desalojo*, including the arrests that had become common military practice after the Statute of Security, and decided to close down the university for almost a year. When it reopened in 1985, the university changed its student welfare strategies from residences and cafeterias, like the ones Carlos benefited from, to loans and partial scholarships, in which students' total debt depended on their academic performance. The reopening included strategies to put an end to the university's radical politics, including new security in all buildings and academic reforms that introduced economic principles like efficiency in higher education. Neoliberalism in education was on the rise, and La Nacional started to experience some of its effects.[11]

STUDYING AT LA NACIONAL meant both academic distinction and intellectual and political engagement. How was being trained as a health professional (physician, nurse, therapist, or dentist) at La Nacional and other regional public universities influenced by that environment of political activism vis-à-vis state repression, growing social inequalities, and the shift from a rural to a rapidly industrializing country?[12] Héctor Abad Gómez was a famous physician, university professor, and scholar of social medicine. He helped in the efforts to build the country's only National Public Health School, based in Medellín, which is now named after him.[13] In the late 1940s he proposed a mandatory social service year, in which recent graduates from health care programs were placed in rural areas to provide care to poor populations who did not have access to health care services. He also implemented health care promoters (a type of community health worker) as an integral component of the health care labor force and was a key figure in promoting and implementing countrywide vaccination campaigns. But his ideas, which linked health with poverty, were considered too radical. He received life threats and, on several occasions, was forced into exile. On August 25, 1987, while Goméz was on his way to attend the funeral of another professor and union leader after teaching at the campus of University of Antioquia in Medellín, a *sicario* (a gunman hired by a paramilitary organization) ended his life.[14]

We do not include the stories of Abad Gómez's and León Patiño's murders here in order to propose a direct link between political violence and health scholars. Instead, we hope to illustrate how both political consciousness and excellence in clinical medicine were distinct outcomes of training as a health professional at public universities in Colombia. This does not mean that all graduates shared leftist beliefs, worked exclusively in public settings, or defended social medicine or socialist ideas about health. In fact, many graduates—usually those coming from higher-income backgrounds—looked for lucrative careers in medicine or ended up working, if often unwillingly, in for-profit health sectors (see chapter 7).

However, during medical school, all students did gain firsthand experience discussing critical issues, whether by participating directly in some of the debates as student representatives, by enrolling in student organizations, or simply by interacting with more-involved peers and professors. The general professional profile of graduates from La Nacional and other public universities was very different from that of private institutions—not necessarily because of the content of their education, but because the university environment and the kinds of debates and interactions that went on produced different medical subjects. A common slogan on La Nacional's medical school documents is "We train the physician that the country needs."[15] Thus, it could be argued that, in general, La Nacional graduates had a commitment to social issues generated by the university's position at the epicenter of heated political debates about the country's construction of democracy.

Elena Fino passed the admission test for La Nacional medical school in 1987. Just like Carlos, she came from a provincial area and would go on to graduate from medical school and complete residency training in gynecology at El Materno. But unlike Carlos, Elena did not benefit from student residences and cafeteria; they had been shut down. She thinks it was fortunate that her grandmother lived in Bogotá and she could stay with her but remembers that for other students the economic situation in Bogotá was much harder. Many students were forced to work in order to fulfill family obligations or even to be able to afford to live in the city. The government did offer student loans,[16] which Elena took, but they were often insufficient. Either families helped or students worked. Some students opted for reducing their coursework to a minimum in order to balance on-campus and off-campus lives. Elena remembers classmates who had to leave school for economic reasons. And there were those who obviously came from money: "those with cars and those by bus," as Elena jokingly put it.

Combining studies and work in certain majors, such as medicine, was particularly challenging. Coursework was intense. Nevertheless, Elena remembers the school as a very hospitable and caring environment. "During the first semester the school divided us into 3 groups—A, B, and C [based on an alphabetical list]—and that created a sort of fraternal link among mates that remained throughout the whole career." Besides the importance of peer study groups, she remembers that peers and their families offered much-needed emotional support, like the parents of one of her peers from group A "who welcomed all of us as if we were their kids." This support was particularly important for those coming from the countryside.

But more than anything, Elena remembers key professors who instilled in their students a sense of respect for the others, of appreciation for life, humility, passion, work ethics, and commitment. "Like Profe Rubiano,[17] besides engraining in you [anatomy, which was his first-semester subject,] he was such an exceptional teacher, a true educator. But it was not just him; all professors insisted endlessly on the importance of humanity and of treating others with dignity." Coursework during the preclinical years at the medical school included what is generally known as basic science and laboratories. Students had to study and cover large amounts of information, and the school made a point of differentiating students' performance through the public display of exam scores. Lectures, tests, and labs made up the core of preclinical years. Importantly, the country's most recognized figures of medicine, who were also the most experienced and respected clinicians and researchers, took part in the preclinical theoretical training. The most common instruction occurred in large auditoriums with a prominent professor providing explanations on a chalkboard and, in later years, with the help of acetates or slides.

For some students renowned professors were not merely exemplars of what a physician should be, but of what a human being should be. Hence, they did not want to miss any possibility to learn from them. Other students, however, did not show much interest in the professors or their lectures. Students who did not meet performance expectations failed courses during the preclinical (also called basic, theoretical, or foundational) years or failed hospital rotations during their clinical years. They were required to repeat the courses or clinical rotations; some were expelled when they failed to get minimum scores after repeating a subject. Frequently, students took much longer than intended to complete their education, either because disruptions (protests, strikes, *desalojos*) extended the semesters to the point that it was impossible to make up enough classes in a calendar year, or because economic needs forced them to split one semester's coursework across two or three terms. If a student failed or was unable to register for a prerequisite course or hospital rotation, their entire plan of study would have to be rearranged. This would result in students exceeding the structured six-year plan of studies in the medical school template.

Once they had gotten into La Nacional—itself a very difficult task—students then found a diverse student body in terms of class, regions, interests, and academic performance. Nonetheless, the dual legacy of critical thinking and academic excellence became part of the collective experience of medical school students; in general, both alumni and professors recognized that despite differences, all graduates came out with very good training. A combination of endless hours of coursework around basic science in the preclinical years and hospital rotations at El San Juan, El Materno, and La Misericordia (the children's hospital) composed the core of the physician's training. Medical students would participate in all university activities and experience the university in full during their preclinical years. When they moved on to the clinical years, they were less in touch with what was going on in the campus, but faced firsthand the reality experienced by many poor Colombians. At the clinics, they integrated a knowledge based on basic science, social medicine, and clinical medicine, or what we call in chapter 2 "clinical social medicine."

Over the medical school's more than 150 years of existence,[18] social aspects of health have included coursework in public health, epidemiology, the history of medicine, and bioethics. Given that medicine, like other health fields in Colombia, is a professional undergraduate degree, students also have some coursework in the liberal arts, the natural and basic sciences (such as physics, chemistry, and statistics), and the social sciences and humanities. Depending on the year of matriculation, medical students at La Nacional take courses offered in history, sociology, anthropology, psychology, and so on. Clinical departments, basic science departments, and social aspects of health departments compete for how many hours, courses, and credits students have to take during their training. Such debates are heated in times of curricular reform. Departments that house deans or academic directors tend to have more power in curriculum construction. Over the years, the different medical school curricula have reflected more or less emphasis on each of the different components (i.e., basic science, clinics, or social aspects of health), and the development of new courses or areas of national or international interest have resulted in the restructuring, renaming, or disappearance of some items from the curriculum.

LUIS CARLOS MÉNDEZ WAS not able to study medicine at La Nacional but did study medicine at a regional public university, in a much calmer setting and surrounded by family. Luis Carlos's father was pleased with this decision, and Luis Carlos thought that he received an excellent education as part of the first cohort of physicians graduating from the Universidad del Quindío. In fact, as was common in many other newly funded universities, public and private, the professoriate was composed primarily of La Nacional graduates. At Universidad del Quindío, the same partnership between the university and the region's main public hospital (also called San Juan de Dios)[19] was the backbone of medical education. Luis Carlos was a particularly devoted student, but he is quick to acknowledge that he received so much support and help from professors, family, friends, and other students that his many successes should not be understood solely as the result of his individual merit.

"But I always dreamed about la Universidad Nacional de Colombia, because in my mind being part of it was something marvelous. Fortunately, as I was finishing medical school I met Dr. José Joaquín Bernal. He was an orthopedic surgeon and had many contacts. Since we were the first cohort, he was very invested in having us well placed for the *rural* (the one-year mandatory social service that health professionals are required to complete to get their professional license in Colombia)." Dr. Bernal got to place some of Luis Carlos's classmates at La Nacional–affiliated hospitals and research centers in intensive care, immunology, and physiology. He connected Luis Carlos with Dr. Santiago Currea Guerrero, one of the country's most distinguished neonatologists, professor at La Nacional, and attending physician at El Materno.

Arriving at El San Juan in Bogotá was another shocking experience. Luis Carlos comments how in El Quindío province, as it happens in smaller cities and rural areas, "people are closer, people are kind, people are tranquil, people are fresh, they touch you. For us, physical contact is important, to shake hands, to give a hug. And as soon as you get into Bogotá, you notice the difference in people's faces. Different weather, different rain, and people put their masks on. There are more buildings and less green, and people become rude." The city—a fast-growing metropolis that jumped from around one million inhabitants in 1960 to over four million in 1985—and its main hospital were, in fact, rough places. Many times, El San Juan was called a "war hospital" or a hospital in a "war zone."[20] The emergency and surgery departments became emblematic as places that saved lives. Not surprisingly, since El San Juan experienced the many peaks of the country's violence, many of the hospital's developments and advances were in trauma care. Whether from civil war, urban crime, or political violence, friends, relatives, the police, and ambulances transported severely injured people to El San Juan. The heliport helped with the transport of the far away and very wounded or very sick, whose chance of survival depended on getting to El San Juan as fast as possible. On top of that, health care networks from Bogotá and all of the Colombian provinces would refer their most complex patients to El San Juan, which served as the country's main referral unit. Thus, it was not just the emergency and surgery departments that ran at full speed; all the other specialty units also offered a powerful combination of state-of-the-art care aligned with international standards and unbeatable clinical expertise.

For the students, El San Juan was the place to see all kinds of complex patients and learn from the most distinguished professors. "You end up learning even if you are very dumb"; common jokes like this allude to the effects the intense training at El San Juan had on La Nacional students. Elena put it this way: at El San Juan, "you either learn or you learn, the same as at El Materno. This happens because you see so much variety, so much diversity. What patients teach you is just unbelievable; just an expression, a smell [is enough for a diagnosis]. It is not just what patients tell you; they teach you through all sorts of nonverbal cues and you have to awaken those perceptions within yourself." Developing a clinical gaze was not simply a matter of studying and identifying patterns of disease in patients but being attentive to subtleties and letting certain instincts flourish.[21] Like the social interactions between professors, students, and patients, medical training involved an essential rational, experiential, and emotional effort to synchronize the clinician's perceptions with what the patients said and showed. The best answers around a patient, El San Juan taught, are not found exclusively in books. Now, as a professor, Luis Carlos encourages his own students of medicine, pediatrics, and neonatology at El Materno to think creatively, beyond the books. Academic knowledge is vital, but becoming a good clinician demands a sensitivity to the wide range of patients' bodily cues. The most impressive professors had such finely tuned clinical gazes that they would know exactly what condition or disease a person had just by glancing at them.

This clinical gaze was developed over the years at hospitals like El San Juan and El Materno, which offered everything a student needed to become a good clinician. It was not a matter of a moment of revelation, but the result of intense work. Students would see a patient, gather all the clinical information from the exam (including physical, verbal, and nonverbal cues), and go back to the books and journal articles and study. The first task for medical students at the hospital during the semiology course was getting all the medical information from the patient. "When you start as a student at the hospital you are very scared," Elena remembered, "what a pity for the patients because you learn with them. You have to do your first medical histories. Some patients had been hospitalized for a long time, and some had pity on us and even helped us, telling us what to do, like, 'Dear, you forgot to ask me [such and such].' Some patients would help you but others didn't like you and didn't cooperate. Some would complain, 'Nobody touches me,' but others assisted us and we would thank them."

Only after learning to perform thorough medical histories would students master clinical exams and practice differentiating between normal and abnormal presentations. Later, as students advanced through their clinical rotations, they began to put medical histories and clinical exams together to offer a differential diagnosis and a *conducta*, or path of action. Paths of action could include some combination of tests, exams, *interconsultas* (evaluations by other departments), prescriptions, and a plan for new assessments—which would have to consider everything that happened from the patient's first visit on, and would conclude with a new conducta.

Each step in the process required impeccable knowledge of the patient, even if that meant asking the same questions again and again in case something was missing or had changed. Then students needed to conduct a new and extensive review of the relevant literature around the differential diagnosis, from the most to the least likely, and assess carefully all possible pathophysiological interactions and effects of the plan of action. Each step of the way became a new opportunity to learn and a chance to gain recognition. In the end, the students in each hospital rotation had to respond to these questions: What does the patient have? Is he/she improving? Why or why not? And, last, what is the new conducta?

Carlos, Luis Carlos, Elena, and many other graduates commented that, up until neoliberal times, the environment at El San Juan and El Materno was largely one of camaraderie. Older residents would teach younger residents, younger residents would teach interns, and interns would teach undergraduates. Professors would take any opportunity to teach them all, whether individually, in small groups, or during formal seminars and lectures. Other graduates, however, experienced instead a sense of hierarchy and top-down power that mimicked the structure of military institutions. Some alumni remembered a hospital environment in which relationships among peers, across groups, and patients and doctors could be inspirational but also recalled social dynamics that were rude, unfriendly, or even abusive. Clinical expertise and impeccable bedside manners did not necessarily go hand in hand; the tone was set by the professor or senior residents and by the specific configuration of each student cohort. Elena explained, "The person with the biggest responsibility is the 'big R' [the resident in his or her last year of training], but the one who ends up doing most of the work is the R1 [first-year resident]." The R1 assigned patients to interns, who "have more responsibility [than medical students.]" A hierarchy of responsibility does not necessarily mean that each person is responsible for one aspect of the patient but that the responsibility is passed down from a senior to a junior member of the training ladder. But lower-rung members are carefully supervised, because the most senior person is responsible for the actions of the supervised and, in the end, for the patient's outcome. So, the responsibility goes up and down the hierarchy, with everyone keeping an eye on everyone else. Each prescription, each evolución (annotation in the clinical record), and each procedure is supervised and corrected. As residents move on in their training, they make decisions more autonomously and the type or amount of supervision from senior residents or professors depends on the complexity of the case and procedure.

The interns were also responsible for ensuring that everything that was ordered was done. Elena explained, "The exams had to be updated, everything that the person needed. At that point, it was just how we were trained, it became your obligation to be thorough and to make sure everything was in place and nothing was pending. You would not feel like resting until you finished with everything. As students, we would be *'patinando'* (skating) all around the hospital." Part of this "skating" was due to the students' role as messengers. Before computer technology arrived, orders had to be written down on paper and handed in to the department responsible for their execution. Students were also responsible for following up with their assigned patients and entering all the information in the clinical records, *evolucionando*. Elena explained how the values transmitted from their professors since the very first semester quickly became a constitutive part of who the students were and how they enacted their professionalism. Having patients was very meaningful; students would see them day after day and learn how they were responding to treatment. But, more importantly, it nurtured in the students an emotional connection and a sense of professional responsibility. Graduates trained at El San Juan ended up knowing their patients very well and caring for them deeply; "It was not just any patient," they frequently said, "it was *my* patient."

The internship makes up the last of the six-year plan of studies and is the students' last opportunity to learn how to perform complex procedures and handle patients on their own. In Elena's experience, "You try to take advantage of each week at the hospital intensely. Internship is really tough. You end up living at El San Juan and El Materno and you rarely go home. You would be on call every other day or every third day, but you cannot just leave and go home. You have to leave everything in order, so you end up staying until 7 p.m. When I rotated in gynecology [at El Materno as an intern], I was so lucky that the attendings had so much experience and they would teach you so much. So, I would be glued to them, learning. Paying close attention to how a caesarean [C-section] is conducted, learning very well how everything is done." For Elena, as was very common, internship meant staying at the hospital as many hours as possible because that was where you learned, whether by helping another doctor's patient, watching a procedure for the first time, or revisiting a procedure in order to master it.

The epitome of the clinical work was "rounds." Rounds occur at all hospitals, but at university hospitals they are a space for constant and rigorous evaluation as professors assess how students are integrating real patients with academic literature. Morning rounds were both exciting and stressful.

The esteemed professor would enter the hospital ward assigned to his or her specialty, where patients rested in two rows of beds that faced each other and offered no privacy. The professor would be standing by the bedside of the first patient at exactly 7:00 a.m. After greeting the patient and the assembled students, interns, and doctors, the student responsible for that patient was expected to begin the presentation of the clinical summary, carefully balancing thoroughness with concreteness. Not only did the information have to be exact, but all the test results, consultations with other specialists, and patient's progress notes had to be available. This meant that if the afternoons were busy with students skating around the hospital, early mornings were tense; the last results had to be compiled and the clinical charts updated before 7:00 a.m. The aura of wisdom that some professors had was such that students, patients, nurses, and paramedical staff treated them as demigods. Just before 7:00 a.m., when someone spotted the professor's car entering into the parking lot, they would warn everybody: "Dr. So-and-so is arriving." Then the last-minute arrangements were performed as everyone awaited his (in this male-dominated profession, it was usually *his*) arrival.[22]

Depending on the specific condition of the patient and the students' training needs, professors would end rounds for a particular patient by demonstrating how to translate all that medical knowledge to patients and relatives in lay terms. Then everybody would move on to the next bed, where the process started again. "If there was a mistake, then . . . reprimands for everybody," Elena laughed. "Well," she amended, "not reprimands, but corrections, because [the professors] had very strong pedagogical skills." Elena's adjustment reminds us that many students considered professors to be excellent in all aspects, including but not limited to their clinical knowledge. She remembered how during rounds students would also learn by example, watching how professors interacted with the patients humbly and respectfully. This contradicts the memory of other alumni and professors who remembered some professors and residents as rude and arrogant.

The best clinical discussions around patients happened when several professors were interacting. Having multiple specialties and subspecialties allowed for exchanges of specific information and the opportunity to put together many methods around the diagnosis and plan of action for a single patient. On these occasions, a larger crowd surrounded the patient's bedside, including multiple residents, interns, students, paramedical staff and, at times, relatives. The clinical activities at the hospital were supplemented by programmed lectures, clinical-case presentations, and sessions to discuss journals' latest publications. If by the patient's bed it was mandatory to use the patient's name, in clinical-case presentations this was not required. Clinical "cases" usually started with "XX-year-old male/female who presented with . . ."

The environment of constant exposure and years of experience led to situations in which even paramedical staff, like a porter in charge of navigating stretchers and wheelchairs, would develop a clinical gaze and call out, "This patient is '*taponado*' (in cardiac and respiratory arrest usually as a result of a thoracic injury)! Call the OR [operating room]!" Professional nurses and nurse assistants became so skilled over the years both in terms of their clinical expertise and in terms of medical knowledge that they would be asked their opinion by residents and even by professors. Experienced nurses would often supervise students and even residents, who over time learned to defer to them and respect their knowledge and expertise. Nurses, Elena recalled, "helped us tremendously, they taught us tons. They managed very complex patients and were very skilled. . . . And they were not going around asking for recognition, they simply did what needed to get done." Experienced nurses would sometimes be called "R5," one step above the usual end of the most extensive, four-year residency training (R4). Besides helping with diagnoses, dosages, and procedures, nurses kept everything organized during the hectic daily routines.

If the preclinical years taught students how to see, speak, and, in general, relate to the human body in particular anatomical and pathophysiological ways,[23] the hospital years consolidated their clinical gazes and ethos of commitment and humility. Thus, the years at El San Juan, El Materno, and La Misericordia brought preclinical and clinical years together and ended up shaping a particular way of being for La Nacional doctors.

EL SAN JUAN HOSPITAL complex (including the main eight-story general hospital and the many colonial-style pavilions that hosted specialty clinics) treated primarily the poor and dispossessed. Everyday life at the hospital was tough. An overflow of complex patients and intense trauma led to a sense of working under fire; people were always tense and in a rush. And because the hospital cared mostly for the "wretched," there was a complex mix of class differentials stemming from the colonial legacy of charity-based care.[24] Tension existed between prioritizing excellence in care and a historically informed instinctive understanding of the patients as second-class citizens. Even though patients would always receive the best medical care, depending on the opinions of professors, residents, nurses, and paramedical staff, they would be treated with more or less respect and dignity.

The volume of patients was such that even undergraduates quickly learned to perform certain activities traditionally done by interns, residents, or professors. Of course, Carlos commented, there was always supervision. "I was also a good student and very dedicated so a resident let me [drain] abscesses and once he even let me insert a chest tube, a procedure for residents. . . . I even did an appendectomy." Was supervised medical students conducting upper-level procedures an unjustified risk for patients and a sign that second-class care was provided to these patients because they were poor? There is no easy answer to that question. The many interacting factors defy simplification: a university teaching hospital that carried the legacies of colonial charity-based care, an overflow of patients that strained the hospital's capacity, and the ways in which medicine was learned and practiced at the time. But careful expert supervision in an environment where any complications could be adequately addressed put the patients at a lower risk, perhaps, than in other hospital environments that offered fewer infrastructural and human resources. And the fact that El San Juan was simultaneously the only option for the poor and the best hospital in the country undermines the idea that patients were treated as second-class citizens. Moreover, health care graduates would go on to practice medicine in different parts of the country, both during their year-long rural and after they were officially licensed. Many graduates ended up working in remote areas that lacked specialists or robust health care networks; often, they would be the only physicians available, and they needed to be able to attend to all cases, from the simplest to the most complex. *Rurales* (those doing the *rural*), in the absence of surgeons and anesthesiologists, would end up performing emergency surgical procedures like appendectomies and C-sections because transferring patients could compromise their lives. Thus, La Nacional students' extra training and exposure to different complex cases and procedures would prove very handy after graduation—particularly in a country in which the coexistence of poverty, tropics, and violence translated into a complex population health profile.[25]

Nonetheless, even with so much training, new graduates had to face unexpected and unfamiliar cases. When Carlos finished his studies at La Nacional, he moved back to his natal region in the north coast for his mandatory rural. "And then one weekend, I found myself with a snake bite—and do you think that we saw any snake bites in Bogotá? We did read about them, but nothing in terms of clinical practice. Thank goodness that when I was looking into getting the serum, two workmates [who did have experience with snake bites] showed up."

Even the best training cannot expose students to all potential cases. But it can prepare them with strong basic science and social and clinical foundations to face complex and unexpected cases. The goal of medical training is to become embodied as a professional habitus,[26] a predisposition to see, think, and act in particular ways. Over time, different medical schools in the country build different kinds of professional profiles. Even though all medical school graduates have the same degree, each school imposes on its students a particular clinical gaze, a particular ethics around their professional practice, and a particular politics around their role in society. This transmission of school-specific traditions is known to create different "Escuelas de Medicina." While La Nacional was considered the most legendary and "the best" escuela, many public universities were understood as the regional equivalents of La Nacional, with strong faculty bodies and regional hospitals that provided excellent training—like the Universidad del Quindío, where Luis Carlos Méndez was first trained. Differences between the training received at public and private universities were modest during most of the twentieth century but became more pronounced as market mentalities took over health and education (an aspect that will be explored in chapters 6 and 7).

MEDICAL GRADUATES FROM La Nacional, regional public universities, and private universities populated the larger health care networks in the country. They also took academic positions at their own medical alma maters, which perpetuated the idea of different "Escuelas de Medicina." Professors from La Nacional would be appointed at El San Juan, and graduates were frequently hired by the hospital or the city's secretary of health. When a professor's position opened at La Nacional, teaching-inclined graduates and attending physicians would apply for the job, and whoever scored first in the evaluative hiring process would become the new professor. If La Nacional was the center of intellectual thinking, its medical school and El San Juan were the center of intellectual thinking in health. It was common for professors to be part of national discussions around specific health problems, giving lectures both in the city and around the country and joining scientific societies, often serving as presidents. Regardless of several shortcomings, up until neoliberal reforms began, El San Juan held an unchallenged public image as a place of excellence, where the best physicians provided the best available medical care in the country, and where medical students received the best training.

The prestige of this hospital complex was such that high-profile national and international figures would be treated at El San Juan (including presidents, other politicians, and important religious and business figures), even though there were different options for the working class and the elites. The health care system diversified during the first half of the twentieth century into a three-tier system called fragmented: public hospitals for the poor, social security institutions for the working class, and private institutions (called clinics) for the elites.[27] La Nacional and El San Juan graduates worked in all three sectors. As the country became more industrialized, the three-tier system consolidated itself. *El Instituto de Seguros Sociales* (The Social Security Institute, or El Seguro) developed a network of services for private sector workers almost as extensive as that of public health care secretariats. Before its collapse during neoliberalism, the El Seguro health care network treated over 30 percent of the Colombian population (including workers and their families).[28]

"When I finished my residency," Carlos told us, "El Materno hired me. The same day I was receiving the diploma, another physician from our working group who was working at El Seguro told me, I am not going to continue working there and we need someone who can cover. So, I started with '*turnos*' [shift work, which is paid independently]. I worked doing shifts [at El Seguro] for about two years. But it became really tough because I had already gotten into La Nacional [as a professor]. So, I moved to working night shifts at El Materno and during the day at La Nacional. So, I had to do the shifts at El Seguro at nights and on weekends."

In this part of Carlos's narrative, he shows the ways in which institutions from all three sectors were connected—not only public, private, and social security health care institutions but also educational and service delivery institutions. One single institution, such as El Materno, could function as both an educational institution (during the day) and as a health institution where he worked (during the night). In particular, his comments also show how there was a natural relationship that ended up with graduates being appointed at the hospitals (public sector) and at El Seguro (social insurance sector).

El Seguro had, besides the state-of-the-art San Pedro Claver clinic, a network of health posts and dispensaries both in Bogotá and around the country. In fact, La San Pedro and El San Juan were considered the top health institutions in the country. Their importance was demonstrated by the fact that, as the main referral centers, they treated the most complex cases among, respectively, the laboring population and the dispossessed. La San Pedro had, perhaps, as good a reputation as El San Juan, but it was not a teaching facility. Carlos continued,

And so I was waiting for a *concurso* [an official opening] at El Seguro, because it was the gold mine for health professionals in the country. El Seguro meant prestige, stability, and a very good salary. I took the test when they opened the concurso at La San Pedro, and I scored in first place. So, the directors asked me, "Where do you want to go, to La San Pedro or to a different unit?" I said, "To la San Pedro." But as I was about to sign the contract, they told me, "We cannot guarantee that you are only going to work nights and weekends. You will have to start with the opposite working hours." So, I had a dilemma, because they were offering a very good salary. And then I remembered the words of one of my professors, I remember so clearly, Laura Rojas. So, she told me, "Look, Carlos, if you go to work at El Seguro, you will earn a good salary but you are going to be just another gynecologist. If you stay at the university, you have a very good chance of climbing the ladder and getting into good positions; because of your work ethic, you will climb up. Money comes in life. Think about it. Perhaps you won't secure a salary like the one they are offering, but I think you will do better here." And that was it, I stayed. I told them [El Seguro] that I was very sorry but that I couldn't accept. They felt betrayed.

Managing the boundaries between public, social security, and private health institutions was complex. As Carlos commented, people knew each other and often worked shifts at different centers. Former classmates or professors would meet frequently, and the standards of care among institutions were not different. The most salient differences were the salaries (much lower at public places), the prestige (with good but different reputations depending on the institutions), and the social networks and accommodations needed to meet the expectations of the different patient populations. The nicest setup was found at private clinics. El Seguro had medium-level amenities, and public hospitals were run with minimal but sufficient infrastructure. In terms of populations and resources, there were also marked differences. Private clinics depended on their own resources and offered mostly fee-for-service care; El Seguro was funded in a typical social insurance way, with worker's wages and contributions from companies and the government.[29] Public hospitals received direct funding from the government. Depending on the region and the capacity of each network, El Seguro would contract services with the public network, and elite patients would end up being treated at El San Juan, because it was the most specialized center. Some El San Juan professors also worked in private clinics, and if they were unhappy with the clinics' equipment, they would "bring" their patients to El San Juan. In order to meet the different expectations of higher-status patients, the top floor of El San Juan's main general hospital was transformed. This floor, called *pensionados* (retired), offered all the paramedical care and hotel-like conditions that higher-status patients expected, including private or semiprivate rooms with bathrooms and TV, better furniture, and better food.

THE PHYSICAL SEPARATION BETWEEN El Materno and El San Juan, first by a quad and then by 10th Avenue, came to symbolize a difference in the ways in which people perceived them, particularly the kinds of care practiced at each hospital. Luis Carlos remembered the contrast between the urban coldness and the "marvelously conceived, European-style buildings" of El San Juan and El Materno.

> When I saw El Materno for the first time, I saw it as so grandiose. And as soon as I got in, I noticed the difference. People were different, people smiled at you, they were kind, they greeted you, they allowed you to be physically close; then, you see the mothers, you see the families, you hear the babies crying, you see that mothers are also crying. And so, I felt that I was in a totally different environment. And then, I went into the different clinical services, and I saw the murals and everything looked pretty and special. The best part of it all was the ways in which people interacted with one another. People were warmer, they greeted you with a smile, just like what I had gotten used to at my university. And then, I saw a newborn in the incubator and I saw the mom right by her. And that really impacted me tremendously. I felt something really deep inside me. And I said, this is it. I will stay here.

"And so," Luis Carlos continued, "I arrived at El Materno to do my rural. And they [the hospital administration] clarified, 'Look, you are being accepted as a rural, that is clear, and because of your high recommendation.'" A recommendation from Dr. Santiago Currea Guerrero practically assured Luis Carlos his spot. "'But,' they continued, 'you are welcome but you will not receive any salary.' And so, that meant that I had to continue being an adolescent because, imagine how embarrassing, being a rural [meaning having officially graduated from medical school] and having to keep on receiving money from my mom, my dad, my family. I had to live in my Aunt Rosa's apartment and keep on receiving money from my home. On top of that I had the ambition of helping my folks with the education of my younger sisters."

At this point, Luis Carlos's recollection is illustrative of the ways in which first-generation college graduates, especially medical doctors, finished their studies thanks to many family sacrifices and investments that families hoped would be repaid once their "children" graduated. And his decision to stay at the hospital, just like Carlos's decision to let go of the Seguro Social contract, represents the powerful magnet that these institutions (hospital and university) had to attract and keep certain people. Workers, graduates, and professors frequently commented, "El Materno is a place that draws you in," or "there is something in it." Imagine, Luis Carlos would say, "It smells like women, it smells like placenta, it smells like amniotic fluid, it smells like breasts, it smells like breast milk. So, it is a combination of feelings, once you get there you see images, you see human beings, laughs, smells. . . ." The fact that the hospital is centered on maternity brings powerful sensory experiences of the marvels of the beginning of life. The magnetic force of the hospital offered a perfect intellectual and spiritual match between finding one's personal call and an emotional connection with building, workers, and patients. Luis Carlos took the exam to be admitted to the three-year residency program in pediatrics and then to the two-year subspecialty program in neonatology, at the time called pediatric-perinatology and neonatology but currently known as perinatology and neonatology. He started as a rural and never left the hospital.

Staying at the hospital, or remaining even when the economic crisis hit bottom (see chapter 6), resulted in many challenges but also in many rewards. For Luis Carlos, back in the 1980s, doing the rural at El Materno was a wonderful experience. "I started to be in close contact with my 'maestros,' like Dr. Héctor Agustín Ulloque Germán, such a wonderful man. He became practically my godfather at the time because, as I understood later on, we had similar histories and he kept a certain Caribbean sensibility." The way Luis Carlos talks about his "maestros" (and he listed many, including "el gran maestro Santiago Currea Guerrero") is very telling. The word maestros, for all graduates and especially for those who go on to pursue academic careers, does not just mean teachers or mentors; the word carries a sense of prestige and admiration, not only for the extreme knowledge they have come to acquire over the years but, as Elena noted, because of their humility. They are exemplars of what their students aspire to be. Students refer to their maestros and most esteemed colleagues using their full names, including first, middle, and both paternal and maternal last names. This sense of specific identification is also a way of paying tribute. While people in the world of neonatology would clearly know who Héctor

Ulloque and Santiago Currea are, by stressing their full names, students bring credit to their families and celebrate their own connections with such incredible people. As their mentees, they become part of their maestros' prestigious lineages.

Of course, maestros do have their favorites—usually those who show the strongest commitment and dedication. Luis Carlos explained that hard work brought recognition, to the point where he was asked to cover shifts when other physicians could not. "So, I sometimes would get to the hospital and come out two, three, four, or five days later. I would live, sleep, and eat at the hospital." This extra work improved not only his clinical experience but also his finances. "At the end of the rural year I ended up earning more than what I would have in a different place, and I was finally able to tell my family, now I can help." Just like with Carlos, Luis Carlos's maestros and other physicians at the hospital demonstrated their trust in him by giving him shifts. Even though it was a risky business—nonspecialists were covering for specialists—this sort of demonstrated trust in mentees had immense emotional implications. Mentors received salaries and extra pay for shifts done outside of their contracted hours; then they would pass their mentees the money corresponding to the shifts they had covered.

Dedicated students, interns, and residents also participated in different research activities, on their own time and without pay. The environment at El Materno was very energetic. The clinical experience was intense because the pregnant patients often had high-risk pregnancies marked by a whole array of social problems. The women were not just poor. Many of them were homeless, sex workers, teenagers, or indigenous women who did not speak Spanish. Many of their babies would be very sick, born preterm or with very low birth weights, and had many medical complications. Treatment and research needed to respond to their clinical and social needs. El Materno, which started at the beginning of the twentieth century with a few hospital beds, expanded over the decades until it took over that whole marvelous colonial-style building on the east side of 10th Avenue, with different sections and subspecialties for gynecology, perinatology, and neonatology.

CHAPTER 2. Clinical Social Medicine

While chapter 1 invited us to think about medicine within politics, or medicine subsumed by politics,[1] this chapter explains how clinical practice unfolds in that context. Social medicine is often presented as a sort of radical understanding of the role of social, economic, and political factors in health that competes with public health approaches dominated by epidemiology and the risk paradigm. Clinical medicine is often thought of as the realm of the clinician's experience, which has been eclipsed by evidence-based medicine's many problematic conflicts of interest. These conflicts of interest are often due to the influence of the medical industrial complex, primarily the pharmaceutical industries, on basic science, clinical trials, and publications that serve as the basis of clinical guidelines. The other conflict of interest that we want to discuss is the hegemony of a particular "ethics of intervention," in which scientific technologies are assumed to be better, more powerful, and more ethical than noninterventionist approaches—which, unforgivably, can decrease profits. Indeed, fewer interventions mean less use of technologies, equipment, and medication, all of which hurt the health industries' profits.[2]

An additional discussion included in this chapter is how to regard socially minded clinicians who advance a critical understanding of the role of society in health outcomes. There are some biographical examples of such clinicians, who are presented as models to the medical community, "medical idols."[3] Their biographical narratives describe how they incorporated an

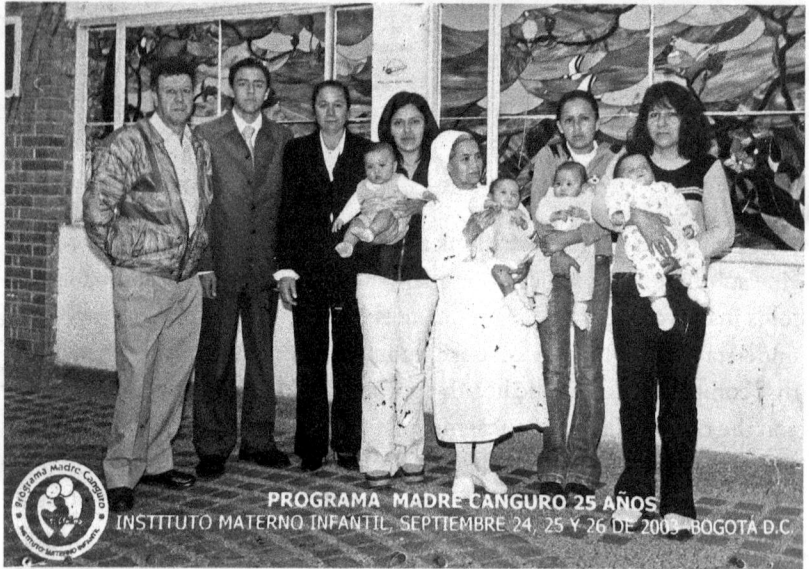

FIGURE 2.1. Kangaroo Care. (Photo by César Ernesto Abadía-Barrero.)

"ethos of care," which translated into a combined approach, in which excellence in clinical care goes hand in hand with advocacy and action-based projects and initiatives to tackle the structural inequalities that affect their patients' health. Rather than presenting these individuals as remarkable and unique, El Materno's history demonstrates that all professors there embody this powerful merging of clinical excellence and political advocacy.

What is special about this escuela that virtually all of its professors, and many alumni, reach such levels of expertise, knowledge, and political commitment? We think of them all as practicing a kind of "clinical social medicine." The whole escuela is indeed the historical force in which people grow a professional ethos characterized by a deep understanding of the social, economic, and political context in which medicine is practiced, paired with a careful study of biomedicine. Furthermore, people's "clinical social medicine" skills invite them not only to think of adaptations of international protocols but also to create native forms of care that respond to the country's clinical and social realities.

In this chapter, we will see not only how El Materno physicians practice a kind of medicine that responds to a particular epistemology of care but also how that epistemology of care creates its own collective history. This is a history in which the Kangaroo Mother Program and the delayed clamping of the umbilical cord, among other practices, are "subaltern health innovations," or strategies that are truthful to the role they advocate for medicine: helping nature along in times of need. Such subaltern health innovations refuse the power hierarchy of markets and technologies and center clinical questions on the collective effort to implement the best strategies for babies and families. In such powerful proposals, medicine is thought of as extra help for nature, supplementing the babies, mothers, and fathers' own tools for healing and thriving.

Simple Solutions to Complex Problems

In 1955 Gabriel Lamus started his residency in pediatrics at El Materno. He remembers that El Materno residents were required to attend clinical case presentations at El San Juan on Wednesdays at 11 a.m. A classmate of his was bitter about the chasm between the kind of knowledge professors discussed in these presentations and the conditions of care at the hospital. His classmate would complain, "Why should we go there if you know that there, inside [the hospital], you swim in an ocean of knowledge, but just two centimeters below it everything you step on is shit." Gabriel explained his classmate's words: "That was his short and cynical analysis of the situation. He meant that there were some wise people at El San Juan, very good physicians, who studied a lot and talked about proteins and all kinds of things, but you could never order any of that [because it was too expensive and had not become the standard of care at the hospitals]. So you had to know all about it, but you couldn't do anything with that information."

Gabriel's and his classmate's frustrations reflected the harsh realities of the hospitals and the city. Hospitals were administered and founded by the *Beneficencia de Cundinamarca* (Beneficence of the Cundinamarca Province, where Bogotá is located), which for many centuries served as the largest social welfare institution of the country.[4] Even though professors and attending physicians at the hospitals were excellent, they were dependent upon the Beneficencia's approval of budgets for operating expenditures, repairs, and new purchases. This dependence was a central organizing factor, throughout most of the nineteenth and twentieth centuries, for public institutions that were charged with caring for the poor and the destitute: institutions like hospitals and asylums for the homeless, the elderly, and those with disabilities.[5] Hospital directors had to ask constantly for resources, and their requests were usually after-the-fact petitions (e.g., "We have run out of X"). Hospital directors also had to convince the Beneficencia directors of the importance of specific requests that would require increasing the hospital budget (e.g., "We need more incubators" or "We need to get this new piece of equipment"). Consequently, the flow of money and supplies was slow and insufficient. Gabriel Lamus recalls, "Everything would take so long. It was never simply that you ordered a medication and it was there, that you ordered labs and they were done." Adding to all this, there was tension between the workers' union and the Beneficencia, which constantly resulted in each blaming the other for problems inside the hospital. According to the workers, the Beneficencia did not provide enough funding to run the hospital as it should; according to the Beneficencia, the workers' excessive demands stymied any efforts to improve the conditions of the hospital. Professors and students of La Nacional often found themselves trapped in the middle.

Even though the Beneficencia's wealth was public knowledge, thanks to numerous donations and inheritances received during both colonial and independent periods, its hospitals (including El San Juan and El Materno) constantly struggled with scarcity. Not only were medical supplies lacking but, according to Gabriel, "when you entered the labor and delivery rooms you would see the paint and plaster falling off the walls; [in the wards you would find] two patients sharing a single bed because there were not enough beds. You would notice the poverty [inside the hospital]."

Outside hospital walls, Bogotá was growing in a disorderly fashion. Squatter settlements of self-made houses often lacked proper infrastructure, like water and sewage. Such settlements would develop into more organized neighborhoods, which would be engulfed by the expanding city. Even as neighborhoods were incorporated, roads lagged behind. Authorities would improve transportation in more populated areas before fixing or paving makeshift dirt roads. In the mid-twentieth century, Bogotá, a city in the middle of the Andes, 2,640 meters (8,660 feet) above sea level, was mistier and colder than it is today. European-style overcoats, gloves, hats, scarves, and umbrellas were common cold weather attire in offices and public spaces in the city's multiple commercial hubs,[6] while *ruanas* (handmade wool ponchos) and other *campesino* (peasant) attires were preferred in the surrounding areas. Even though many people farmed, food was scarce and malnutrition and epidemics abounded. Gabriel recalls another classmate of his who served in a public health campaign in one of the poorer neighborhoods of the city. "When he arrived [back to the hospital] he had to be hospitalized because he could not deal with the impact of poverty, of neglect, of hunger.... We would tell him, 'Man, don't be a fool, that is all very usual,' but he just couldn't stand it. He said, 'Let me sleep, a day or two, I just don't want to see anybody.' Who knows what reality he had to face. There were some neighborhoods that were really doomed. It had to be really tough."

Gabriel had the chance to go with Francisco Millán, a newly appointed director of El Materno, to the Beneficencia, when Millán had to respond to growing complaints about El Materno's high reported mortality rates. When they arrived at the meeting at the Beneficencia offices, Gabriel remembered Millán's words: "I can see that you have called us to tell you what is going on, why there are so many deaths. Well, I do have to tell you, and please do not get alarmed, that we are indeed signing off more death certificates here [at El Materno] than Sangre Negra is [killing] in El Tolima." Sangre Negra was one of the most brutal killers during La Violencia, and El Tolima was the region with the highest death toll. With this reference, Millán admitted that the women arriving at the hospital were very sick, and in spite of their efforts too many died. Modern tools of medicine were just starting to be effective in combating the most serious diseases, and it was still common, not only in Colombia but around the world, for very sick people to come to hospitals to die. But Millán's allusion to La Violencia was also a political budgetary maneuver. By linking the harsh reality of the hospital (both in terms of insufficient budget and patients needing the most complex care) with very troubling and emotional times, directors hoped to secure funds and improve the relationship between the Beneficencia and the hospital.

In a country undergoing civil war and a growing city with poor infrastructure, the limited success of existing medicinal tools resulted in a bleak outlook for physicians. Employees at child and maternity hospitals like El Materno had to deal with very sick pregnant women and their children—deeply emotional work, given the potential rewards and devastations. Without birth control, unwanted pregnancies and unattended complications, both as a result of lack of prenatal care and complications from unattended births, were common. Some women would resort to abortions, considered an illegal practice at the time, which could lead to severe hemorrhage and infection. Penicillin, which would change dramatically the prospects for survival, was just arriving at the hospitals. Gabriel remembered that, before it became standard, penicillin was difficult to obtain. Gabriel was part of the first cohort of residents who learned how to prescribe penicillin and saw how infected women and newborns treated with it started to survive infections.

Other significant advancements slowly improved the care that women and newborns received at the hospital. Significant progress, Gabriel remembered, happened during those years: "There was still the intraosseous [into the bone] application of serum [fluids or blood]. Oh! That was a criminal act, so inhumane. Imagine, injecting directly in the medulla of the femur. Children would just cry their lungs out. Then it was changed to subcutaneous injections [under the skin]; we would apply the serum subcutaneously and make a pool of about 100 ml in the little leg of the infant until it got reabsorbed." But even with this improvement, "the children wouldn't survive, but that was what we did. And mothers asked for it because there weren't any other [alternative treatments]. We just didn't make any promises. Then, IV [intravenous] arrived and that was it. In our cohort, we totally moved on from the intraosseous and subcutaneous application of serum. We never did it again."

Problems with the functioning of the hospital, the lack of effective medical tools, and the interactions of poverty and illness did result in elevated mortality. Besides, Gabriel reminded us, "We are talking about the referral unit," which meant a problem of both quality and quantity: sicker patients, and more of them. Just as in other places around the world and before the invention of the incubators, premature and low-birth-weight newborns usually died. Bogotá's very cold weather and frequent rain did not help. Babies who were born during the winter months and had very low birth weight (VLBW) or were premature generally succumbed to hypothermia because, European research claimed, of their "lack of energy or vitality."[7]

In Bogotá, however, the "natural lack of energy" explanation was contested. Families and health care workers knew that poverty and lack of adequate care had to be considered as significant, if not sufficient, reasons. For Gabriel, "With all the social conditions I am telling you about, many of them came breech. Prenatal care was unheard of, nutrition was unheard of, and so if contractions started at seven months, women would deliver very tiny little creatures." Children's and mothers' deaths, though tragic, were common experiences and families, Gabriel remembered, "accepted them calmly. You would arrive at 7:00 [a.m.] to sign death certificates because there were so many deaths [every night]."

When incubators arrived at El Materno, they improved survival rates significantly. However, "incubators didn't work that well. They didn't provide enough heat; they didn't provide enough oxygen." Some incubators worked by using regular bulbs, and some nurse assistants remembered stories of babies being burned. One remembered an incubator that caught fire and killed the baby inside. Besides, Gabriel recalled, the hospital did not have enough incubators to match the demand: "We had to put two or even three babies inside a single incubator." And such technology did not respond to the needs of families who delivered babies at home or could not stay at the hospital with their sick babies. According to Gabriel, this difficult reality sparked creative thinking about solutions.[8]

DURING THE 1960S, AROUND 35 percent of all births in Bogotá happened at El Materno, and the progressive and severe shortage in hospital beds resulted in close to 70 percent of women without adequate hospital care.[9] In the late 1970s twenty-one thousand deliveries happened at El Materno annually.[10] It was common to see women in labor on stretchers or chairs in the hallway and, just as Gabriel remembered for the 1950s, one single hospital bed would serve two mothers, and one incubator would keep two or three babies warm at a given time. As medical care expanded and the country's health care services became more organized, El Materno became the national referral unit for high-risk pregnancies and severely compromised newborns. According to Lida Pinzón, a graduate from La Nacional and El Materno who became the director of the pediatrics department at El Materno and a professor at La Nacional, the neonatology service at El Materno had, at one point in the late 1970s, "120 newborn beds, over 20 babies in intensive care units and 80 incubators. It was a hospital inside another hospital."[11]

Despite the fact that low-risk deliveries began to be transferred to other facilities and El Materno started to receive primarily high-risk pregnancies and severely compromised newborns, lack of adequate funding and personnel continued to mean that El Materno, though aiming for excellence, was constrained by lack of resources. An article reports the situation this way: "The special care baby unit (SCBU) has always been very overcrowded, underequipped, and understaffed. Not surprisingly, cross-infection is common and survival of VLBW infants has been poor. Moreover, a failure of bonding was suggested by the disturbing number of babies abandoned by their mothers. Partially because of cost, most mothers do not receive antenatal care, and consequently uncontrolled toxemia, anemia, and infection add to the neonatal problem."[12]

At that time, Edgar Rey Sanabria, another La Nacional/El Materno graduate, was avidly reading European and North American reports in scientific journals. He took great strides to bring modern tools of pediatrics to the hospital. In 1978, when he was appointed as director of El Materno, he

> asked himself if there wasn't anything that could be done to stop caring for children under such conditions of overcrowding. The hospital couldn't afford more incubators and ventilators, so he tried to initiate an outpatient program for premature and low-birth-weight babies based on his observation of kangaroos and other marsupials—the vertebrate mammals with the most premature births.[13] [After a very short gestational period of about 4 to 5 weeks,] a newborn kangaroo is just a little mass of two centimeters, whose hands are the only well-developed parts of her body. [Baby joeys are born blind and furless, in a fetal-like stage.] Then, the kangaroo mother replaces any older children in her pouch with the baby joey. She marks the path [from the vaginal canal to the pouch] very well with her saliva and when the baby joey is born, it grabs the hair of the mother and starts climbing up [for several minutes][14] until it reaches the pouch, finds a nipple [and starts feeding immediately]. It finishes its growth there and becomes a mature kangaroo, without the need of the placenta, just benefiting from the mom's milk and the heat that she provides.[15]

The extrauterine growth from a fetal-like stage to a fully formed marsupial continues over several months in part because the lack of hair renders the immature joey unable to regulate its own body temperature. Thus, the survival of marsupial joeys depends on the food and temperature control provided by the mother's pouch. "When Dr. Rey saw this," Lida Pinzón explained, "he wondered if human mothers could do something similar. First to avoid the overcrowding [inside the hospital] and second to discharge the babies sooner and open up a place for those who were waiting [for an incubator]. In 1978, he started the preliminary implementation of the Kangaroo Care Program."

Obviously, Lida said emphatically, clinical parameters were taken into account to separate babies who needed medical interventions from those who did not. In 1979 "after Dr. Edgar Rey conceived the program, Dr. Héctor Martínez was appointed as attending physician and started running the program with the residents and other pediatricians at the hospital. In 1981 Dr. Gabriel Navarrete retired from the hospital as an attending physician [i.e., reached his age for retirement] but started to run the program, and he developed the concept of early discharge." The first results of what came to be known as Kangaroo Care Program (KCP) or Kangaroo Mother Care (KMC), as reported by Edgar Rey and Héctor Martínez in 1983, showed infant survival rates similar to those found in developed nations with the use of incubators. Between 72 percent and 75 percent of babies who weighed less than 1000 grams and had usually died in previous care conditions now survived, thanks to KMC. Survival rates of babies weighing between 1001 and 1500 grams increased from 27 percent to 81 to 89 percent with KMC. KMC even reduced the number of abandoned babies. Such survival rates were seen as "miraculous" and were received with a mixture of interest and skepticism, as exemplified in an article titled "The Myth of the Marsupial Mother."[16]

The World Health Organization (WHO) and the United Nations Children's Fund (UNICEF) endorsed with enthusiasm such wonderful results. UNICEF titled the Colombian chapter "Small is Saveable" in its 1984 annual report. In this report, UNICEF considered KMC a revolutionary technique that offered "life-saving intensive care to all low-birth-weight babies who need it whether they are born in a hospital or not."[17] According to UNICEF, KMC consists of "packing" babies close to their mothers, right next to the breast, which addresses two major problems of low-birth-weight babies (LBWB): temperature and feeding. "The baby thus gains all the advantages that breast feeding can provide—the best nutrition, immunity from infection, freedom from both diarrhea and constipation, and the affection fostered by the closeness between mother and child. . . . The Colombian team then took an even more unconventional step. As long as the baby is healthy, mother and child are sent home from the hospital as soon as possible, regardless of the baby's weight. . . . Because it is based not on expensive technology but on empowering mothers to save lives, it is a breakthrough with the potential to reach out and save children's lives in the poor communities of Bogotá, and beyond."[18]

Indeed, prospects for expansion both in Colombia and around the world followed. With the help of funds from UNICEF, the little pink house (*la casita rosada*) was built inside the inner quad of El Materno to house an outpatient clinic devoted exclusively to KMC care. UNICEF also funded Edgar Rey's and Héctor Martínez's travel around the world, sharing their knowledge of KMC. In addition, nurses and physicians from different parts of the world arrived at El Materno to learn the technique firsthand and start KMC programs in their countries.[19] The program expanded rapidly and in 1991 WHO awarded Edgar Rey and Héctor Martínez the prestigious Sasakawa Health Prize, awarded yearly for "outstanding innovative work in health development."[20] It was the first time this award was given to a Latin American country.

The initial "miraculous" results lauded by WHO and UNICEF were met with skepticism and concern by some neonatologists in the international community. Lida explained that the international scientific community

> thought that we [El Materno physicians who proposed and ran KMC] were claiming that the babies did not need ventilators or intensive care, which is totally inaccurate. Timely discharge [her way of updating and reconceptualizing Dr. Gabriel Navarrete's concept of early discharge] means that the baby is ready to go home; that is to say that the baby was premature, was hospitalized, we applied surfactant, the baby was ventilated, was discharged from the perinatal care unit, moved on to the nutritional recuperation component until she reached a particular weight, could keep a set temperature, and did not need any intrahospital medication, and the mother learned how to care for the baby at home.

Lida's extensive explanation of the path and progress of babies enrolled in the program rebuffs the discrediting claims of lack of scientific rigor and merit that some representatives of hegemonic academia (i.e., that coming from Europe and the United States) made while discussing El Materno's KMC.[21] Most likely, these prominent figures of neonatology saw in KMC a different epistemology of care toward low-birth-weight and premature babies, one that questions the primacy of modern technology (i.e., the incubator) over nature (i.e., the mother's body). Lida's explanations, however, make clear that KMC does not negate modern medicine; all the care of the baby follows the same parameters developed by hegemonic medi-

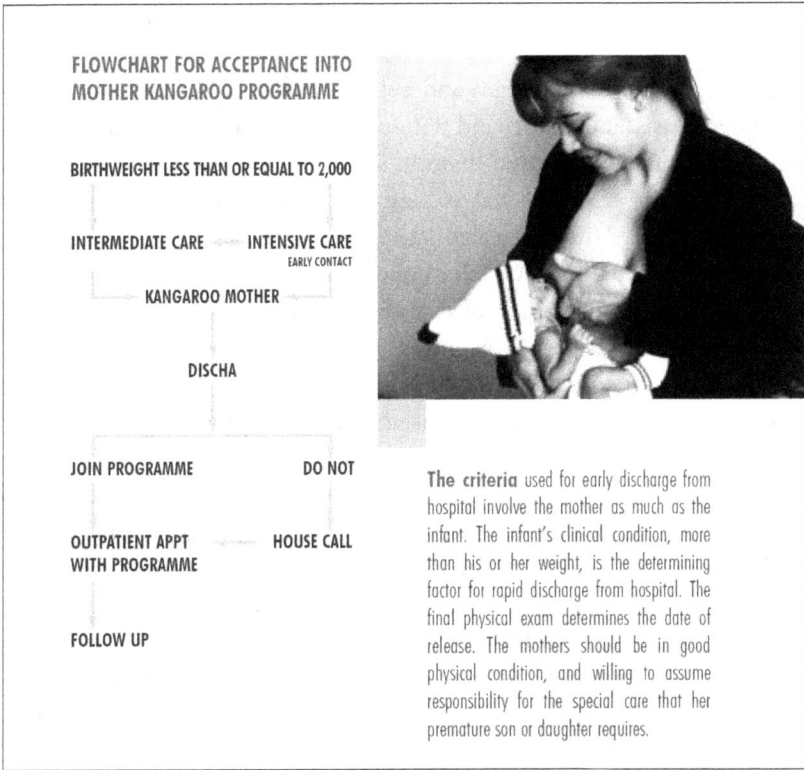

FLOWCHART FOR ACCEPTANCE INTO
MOTHER KANGAROO PROGRAMME

BIRTHWEIGHT LESS THAN OR EQUAL TO 2,000

INTERMEDIATE CARE --- INTENSIVE CARE
                          EARLY CONTACT

└─── KANGAROO MOTHER ───┘

DISCHA

JOIN PROGRAMME   DO NOT

OUTPATIENT APPT --- HOUSE CALL
WITH PROGRAMME

FOLLOW UP

The criteria used for early discharge from hospital involve the mother as much as the infant. The infant's clinical condition, more than his or her weight, is the determining factor for rapid discharge from hospital. The final physical exam determines the date of release. The mothers should be in good physical condition, and willing to assume responsibility for the special care that her premature son or daughter requires.

FIGURE 2.2. Kangaroo Care flowchart. (IDEASS n.d.)

cine furiously studied and implemented by professors to the extent that economic constraints permitted. However, the professors did not embrace hegemonic medicine blindly. If medical intervention was not needed (if the child had no other complications besides low weight and could feed vigorously), using incubators was not only wasteful but, they thought, detrimental for the well-being of the child, the mother, and the family.[22]

The need to prove the effectiveness of KMC in scientific terms, starting with the first reports of survival rates and continuing through today, speaks to an epistemological battle between different conceptions of care and health that translate into different practices of health care. On the one hand, hegemonic medicine embraces "science" as the leading force of care: in this case, the scientific technology represented by the incubator.[23] On the other hand, counter-hegemonic medicine like KMC uses science and technology but also includes "natural" approaches to provide medical care that can be more practical, humane, and economically sound.

Like the other neonatologists at El Materno, Lida insists that biomedical practices of prenatal care were not abandoned; the doctors were trained under a biomedical paradigm and believed in its importance. KMC neonatologists used incubators and state-of-the-art medical interventions and protocols, but they adapted them to local realities, treating them as one component of a larger arsenal of clinical, affective, and bodily practices of care. They created their own algorithms of clinical care that allowed for the integration of scientific technology and a natural approach.

This algorithm for the care of very-low-birth-weight and premature babies (figure 2.2., previous page) recognizes the interaction of the technoscientific and natural worlds.[24] Thus, KMC is not for or against technology, as some critics claimed. A mix of medical needs, the baby's gestational age and weight, psychoemotional aspects, and social conditions dictate how fast or slow a child can move from incubator to human chest inside the hospital, from being kangaroos at the hospital to being kangaroos at home and finally to leaving the pouch, which usually happens when the baby reaches a weight of around 2000 or 2200 grams and/or 37 weeks of gestational age. Nonetheless, the description in figure 2.2 is telling in that it speaks to the nonmedical conditions necessary for babies and mothers to be part of the KMC outpatient program.

JOSÉ ANTONIO'S MOTHER ABANDONED him when he was four or five. He lived mostly with his father and, for about four years when José Antonio was in his teens, his father's girlfriend. Ever since he was young, he wanted to explore the world, to move around. He lived in different parts of Colombia and had two stable relationships with women who helped him emotionally and economically. Because, he claims, of some bike accidents and their after-effects, he had a major psychotic crisis in his twenties. Since then, he sometimes feels "like someone is following me" and hears voices that intimidate him and cause paranoia. When he landed in Bogotá, after leaving college twice and living in different parts of the country, he developed his personal talent and business: he creates and sells sand clocks, jewelry, and kaleidoscopes.

After breaking up with one of his stable partners in Bogotá, he took down the sand clock studio that she had helped him build and went back to his native city, Medellín. While there, he felt he was living in exile. He said that this feeling had to do with his psychosis; he wanted to "break free" and got the idea that he had to leave Colombia. "And so, I traveled around South America." Despite the distance he put between his present and his past, "I felt [the psychosis] in Buenos Aires, I felt it in Florianópolis, I felt it in Manaus, I felt it in Lima, but given my stubbornness, I have always wanted to not let it dominate me—to keep on moving forward." He always had reservations as to what antipsychotic medications could do to his brain and preferred to self-manage rather than to ask for professional help.

"And then, a random day I went to Iquitos [in Peru] and met Rosa," the youngest and only daughter in a family with eight siblings. She had studied nursing and spent all her time between hospital work and studies. "I am not going to say that I didn't go out and have fun sometimes," she acknowledged, but she asserted that she hadn't been serious with anyone until she met José Antonio.

I fell for him, I think since the first day I saw him. On September 15th, people from Iquitos celebrate [a special town fair] and there were painting exhibitions and handcrafts from different countries. And so I went. There is a very big hotel over there [in Iquitos], it is called El Dorado, and there he was. His hair was down to here [long, shoulder level] and his eyebrows were very thick; and here, in Peru, men do not have such thick eyebrows. And since he is tall and I was wearing high heels, I caught his eyes and I told myself, "Oh my God, that man has such huge eyebrows," and I turned to see him again and the eyebrows caught my attention again. At that time they were black [now they are turning gray]. So, I can't deny that I have always liked his eyebrows, his hair. And so I went back and he was also looking at me. So he started to offer me all kinds of jewelry. And that day we just talked for a couple of minutes, chitchat like "I can offer you a discount," and so on, and then he asked if I had email. I told him my email but I never imagined that [he was learning it] because he didn't even write it, but he did memorize it and that was that. Sometime later, I went to check my email [at an internet café] to communicate with my brother who lives in Lima, and there were tons of messages from him [José Antonio]. And that is how everything started. He would travel and come back, and that is how we started to fall in love and then we started to live together.

Once they were in Bogotá, a friend of José Antonio lent him some money, "money that I still owe him today." In the backyard of his friend's house, José Antonio built the "bottle house," hoping to start his sand clock business again and to offer Rosa a house to live in. Rosa remembered that

the cottage was so pretty. It had a loft [with the bedroom] and the workshop downstairs. It was small but very well designed. It had shelves for the sand clocks and the kaleidoscopes—you need a storage place so that clients come and if they like one design or something special, they can see [different options] and place the order. It was very pretty because he made a design with bottles. I had never seen that in Peru. He put bottles of different colors, I am not sure how, but he put them in between the cement and the bricks. And at night, when you turned on the light, everything lit up so beautifully.

One day, Rosa discovered that she was pregnant. According to José Antonio, the pregnancy went on "with love, with affection. Everything I got went to provide good food to Rosa." When Rosa was six months pregnant, "she was very stressed, because she didn't know if it was a girl or a boy." So, José Antonio got in touch with a friend who was a physician, who helped them make a prenatal care appointment at a nonprofit clinic specializing in sexual and reproductive health. "Usually it is just fifteen minutes per patient, but she was there for a half hour. That really calmed her down because she got to see the baby and saw that the baby had no abnormalities or anything like that." However, Rosa kept worrying about her pregnancy because in another prenatal appointment, she had tested positive for cytomegalovirus and toxoplasmosis. "It was a big surprise for me," Rosa commented, wondering if her upbringing in the Peruvian jungle had anything to do with these test results.

Once assigned to a prenatal care program close to the bottle house, she began to have regular prenatal care. In one dental appointment José Antonio arranged through another friend, they discovered she had pre-eclampsia. She ended up hospitalized for a day at one of the city hospitals. "Fortunately," José Antonio remembered, "they gave her the right shots in time." They also confirmed that the baby's gestational age was seven months. Around that time, conflicts with the friend who was "renting" them the backyard escalated; he told them that because they had not paid their agreed-upon rent, his own finances were strained and he needed to sell the house. As José Antonio and Rosa understood it, the agreement was that they owned the backyard and the bottle house because they were paying for them, but they never signed anything. "I paid him parts of the rent, but the situation was unmanageable." Finally, the friend traveled, and the couple had to move out. "We lost all that," Rosa concluded.

José Antonio found an apartment attached to a larger house in the downtown area for a very good price. It had two bedrooms but no running water. "The house was fine," according to José Antonio, "it was only dirty, so we cleaned it up. We didn't worry about the water because I would get it from the viaduct [in buckets for cleaning], plus twenty liters [of potable water] that some friends and a store gave me for cooking." They would wash clothes at friends' places and sometimes bathe in public fountains. One Sunday night the electricity was cut off, "so besides water we had no electricity. The fuses went off or—I am not sure what happened." At around 7:30 p.m. that night, Rosa remembered, "I didn't have nausea or pain or anything, the only thing I had was that my blood pressure was elevated. The symptoms started as blood in my urine, no pain or anything, but a tiny bit of blood." José Antonio left immediately "to buy candles and a fuse. I didn't find the fuse but did find the candles and bought a bag with water. I came home and hugged her [and fell asleep]. It was as if we had slept the whole night. But at around 12 or 12:30 that was it. 'Oh no, I am still bleeding and now we do have to go to the hospital. Call an ambulance,' she told me." José Antonio had barely any money left as credit in his cellphone—280 pesos (around 25 cents in USD)—but it was enough to call emergency. He said, "'My wife is about to have a baby, her water broke, an ambulance please.' Ten minutes later the ambulance arrived. Then I said, 'Look, we have to take her to the Suba hospital [in the northwest part of the city where she had been hospitalized a week before and where she was registered before they moved to the downtown area]. But the paramedics [a man and a woman] explained that we were assigned a destination by proximity and that the closest hospital was El Materno."

"When we arrived," José Antonio continued, "we found those large corridors and second floors, and ramps and very few people." He still had bouts of paranoia, and, at that moment, it manifested as he wondered, "Did we arrive at a state medical institution or at a place where people get 'disappeared'?[25] So, I gave in, I told myself, it has to be God's will where a child is born. And then I realized that it was a state hospital and I thought, 'What a shame, very pretty and very big but very poorly painted. This has to be very old.' I had never been inside. And then, they told me to sign a document, and a doctor told me to go home and come back the next day, but I stayed in the waiting area." He did not have any money for a cab, and so he preferred to stay until early in the morning to be able to go home by bus, rest, and come back.

Rosa remembered,

> The doctor came and examined me, and I said that I wanted my baby to complete his nine months inside of me.... He explained that it wasn't possible, that they had to get the baby out because of other risks. They had me sign some papers and everything was so fast. Oscar

was born at 4:00, I think, 4:00 in the morning.... When the baby was born the doctor showed Oscar to me, a boy. I heard his cries and all I could say was, "God bless you, my love," and they put him by my side and I gave him a kiss [on his forehead]. Then they put a band over [his wrist with his identification] and they took him. Then they told me, "We are going to finish taking care of you and you can see your baby tomorrow and you can start breastfeeding him." But they explained to me that since the baby was born premature, my breast milk would come in more slowly than for women whose babies are born via natural delivery.

Rosa continued, "And so, I was worried, I was upset, 'Why don't I have as much milk as the others?' Then, the doctor explained, 'No, don't worry, that is normal in all women who undergo caesarean section, you will start having more and more milk slowly.' But I would start crying because I would think, 'Oh my son,' and I would hear the medical team talking, and they said that he was born with teeth . . . and I would ask myself, 'My son with teeth? Could I be hearing wrong?' And so I would start crying and the doctor would say, 'But why are you crying so much, '*Mamita*' [mommy]?' I felt really awful, just the thought of my son being premature and having teeth." For Rosa, babies being born with teeth brought images of monstrosity and deformity.

So, I told the doctor [that I was crying] because my son is premature and has teeth and I am perhaps the only one [meaning the only woman with a newborn like that]. "No, mom, you are not the only one. . . ." I thought he was telling me all those things just to cheer me up and I didn't believe him. And he would insist, "Don't cry anymore mommy, don't worry, you are not the only mom with a premature child." And I was also thinking that it was because of my age. [She was about to turn thirty.] "It is not because of your age. . . . Babies here are born even at five months and we mature their lungs, their brains," he would tell me all sorts of things. "Your son is practically fully formed, he will be running errands in no time, don't cry," he would tell me.

Rosa recounted the very emotional moments right after Oscar's birth. An unexpected delivery of a premature child brought in a cascade of worries and a mix of feelings in which guilt featured prominently. Bleeding at home, the ambulance ride, the caesarean section, the concerns about her breast milk and the baby's teeth: all this abruptly contradicted her ideas about what a normal child should look like and what a normal mother's body should do and left her without time to process. She explained how, in such an intense moment, the physician offered comfort and explanations intended to support her and help her cope, as the image she had of herself as a mother and her son as her perfect child collapsed.

And so, the next day, I went up to see the baby. Of course, it was a bit uncomfortable because of the caesarean. I asked again—I asked both the female physician who was there, in charge, as well as the nurses who were there [about her worries]. And it was true, the baby had two teeth. They put gloves on me so that I could touch him and they explained everything . . . that it wasn't weird that he was born like that [premature], that many babies are. And really I was not the only mom with a premature son, it was packed with babies, and there were mothers who were fifteen, forty-five, thirty-five years old.

Seeing many babies and mothers and talking to them started to comfort Rosa and offered a sense of normalcy to her experience as a new mother.

Oscar was hospitalized for twenty-eight days, because "he could not regulate his sugar," Rosa explained. She appreciated all the care she received at El Materno. As a nurse assistant, she admired the skills of pediatricians and nurses. About phlebotomy, for example, she said, "I do phlebotomies in Peru but starting with five-year-olds and up. . . . But there, at El Materno, phlebotomy is excellent . . . such anatomical skills, I admire that hospital tremendously. They would say we have to do these tests and I would be concerned because he was such a tiny baby and so much was going on but [the nurses] were very precise when they took the sample. Really good."

She only had one negative experience. Rosa shares her second last name with José Antonio. Because one of the causes for problems in sugar regulation can be genetic, physicians wondered if Rosa and José Antonio could be cousins. Added to the suspicion, some genetic tests showed markers consistent with shared genes. The two were questioned endlessly, even though Rosa constantly reassured them that it was impossible that they were related. At some point, after many days of hospitalization, "I would ask, 'But when is my child going to be okay?' and [one male physician] told me, 'If you had had your child with another man you might not have this problem, you might not be in this situation right now.' Of course, that was so hurtful." That was, she insisted, her only negative experience.

Rosa also explained how kangaroo care started while Oscar was hospitalized, since day one. "When I breast fed him, [the hospital staff] asked me to put him against my chest. The doctor also explained that the father's body heat is better for kangaroo babies."

"I did carry him but only the third day, not before, once he was progressing," José Antonio said. "They helped me, taught me how to do it. I carried him and talked to him. He would calm down. I think the first thing he saw when we took him out of the incubator was the sun. One day I brought him to the window, or was it Rosa? I think it was her and she said he smiled for the first time." Rosa and José Antonio took turns at the hospital putting Oscar against their chests, although José Antonio noticed that at the hospital he didn't carry him as much as Rosa did. At the hospital, workers sold special clothes for the kangaroo baby (shirts that open in the front, hats, and socks) and very soft, cheap, elastic girdles that facilitate keeping the baby secure and warm. Like all the other parents, Rosa and José Antonio bought the clothes and the girdle.

But kangaroo care was not just putting the baby skin to skin, José Antonio and Rosa explained. They had to learn many things. "Since the first day I went," José Antonio remembered, "I think it was the social worker who asked me, 'Are you the baby's father?' Yes. 'Since he is a kangaroo baby you need to go through a training program.' So I went and asked when the course was offered and it was every day at 11 a.m., one hour for eight or nine days. And it was really good. A nurse would teach us everything with a doll. I did the course first and then Rosa."

Rosa was discharged three days after the caesarean section and then came back every day to the hospital from very early in the morning until very late at night to be with Oscar. "Since I was breastfeeding him every so often [every two or three hours], I would stay at the hospital just to avoid going back and forth. . . . And José Antonio would leave and do his sales and would come back [to the hospital] to see me." Rosa noted the importance of José Antonio's emotional support but also of being at the hospital and receiving training and support from the staff of the neonatal unit and the Kangaroo Care Program. "I didn't have any relatives and neither did José Antonio, not even an aunt or uncle to ask for advice. I didn't even know how to change a diaper." In terms of breastfeeding after her discharge, Rosa explained, "There was a room [lactario] where mothers go and pump their milk and leave it for their babies when they are hospitalized, so that they can drink breast milk, which is the best for the babies." The lactario was indeed a key component of care; nurses would give the labeled milk to the babies at night, when the mothers were resting. When mothers were not able to pump or babies were abandoned, extra breast milk was always at hand.

Besides the technical aspects of keeping the babies warm, feeding them, and changing their diapers, the program taught parents how to take temperatures, provide stimulation, and identify signs of distress or sickness. Also, parents and other relatives learned about expected challenges and milestones. As José Antonio remembered it, the course was about

all the love one needs to give to a child when he is a kangaroo. They do emphasize that. That they are children that for some reason needed help from the incubator and special care and observation, and that the most important aspect is to keep them on the chest as much as possible, whether with the mom, the dad, or another relative. But the most important part was to give them tons of love, to talk to them, to be affectionate, to rub their little hands and feet, to tell them I love you, because some babies don't feel that kind of love. They might feel rejected, they might feel that they were not embraced immediately.

When Oscar was discharged, twenty-eight days after he was born, José Antonio remembered that they "brought him straight to San Agustin church and offered him to the Virgin of Consolation." And after that, Rosa recalled that what they said at the kangaroo course was true, that everything would be centered around the baby and that everybody has to care for the baby. "Caring for a baby kangaroo is definitely a hard task. Your day starts and you have to wash diapers, bathe [the baby], put under the sun for fifteen to twenty minutes, first the back, then the chest. Then, it is time for the massage, they taught us to use almond oil or sunflower oil. And it goes on the whole morning and you spend practically all of your time [caring for the baby]. Well, that is if you follow the instructions as you should." Besides that, "I would go to the hospital three times a week. That was my job, my obligation, because he had his vaccinations, he had controls for weight and height, then it was speech therapy, and then it was physical therapy . . . so I would divide my days in between one thing and another, until he was a year old."

The first year of Oscar's life, they lived in the downtown house without running water. This was no problem for the kinds of care he needed. Rosa explained,

I like cleanliness, and the owner bought a big barrel and we collected rain water. If it didn't rain, José Antonio had some friends that would give him water from some tanks. There was always water to clean the baby's clothes or for us to take a bath. Of course, you couldn't take a long shower . . . we tried to save. For example, if we washed clothes, we would reuse that water for the bathrooms or for mopping. I would reuse it, I wouldn't waste it. . . . Whenever we had time, José Antonio's job was to bring water. . . . He bought one of those cans for watering the plants and we used it as a showerhead. Or before that, we would take big [plastic] bottles and we would make holes in them to make showerheads. I would warm up water and then I would bring the tub and bathe my child with warm water.

José Antonio did get to put Oscar on his chest at home for long periods of time and usually every night, following the program's instructions to let the mother rest and because the father produces more heat. Oscar was in kangaroo care until he achieved the expected weight of about 2700 grams. Rosa affirmed what they heard at the KMC program: "[The babies are the ones who] ask you to take them out when they are ready." However, program workers and other parents also said that a kangaroo baby will always be a kangaroo. "For years Oscar loved to sleep on José Antonio's chest. Whenever he wanted, José Antonio let him. And he asked for it, he said, 'Quiero cariñito' (I want lovie),'" which is the word they developed for this special physical and emotional connection.

WHAT CAN WE LEARN from Rosa, José Antonio, and Oscar's illness narrative? An illness narrative attempts to place the personal experience of illness at the center of the analytical process, rather than centering the biomedical interpretations of what diseases are and how they manifest in the body. Because the illness narrative moves away from strictly medical interpretations, it reveals the interconnections between biology, emotions, and social, economic, cultural, and political orders. Rosa, José Antonio, and Oscar's account is necessarily a multivocal narrative. In order to understand a child's life, we need to understand the lives of their parents and social network. Further, multiple health-related conditions are interacting and influencing each person's lived experience. José Antonio's paranoid auditory hallucinations shaped the way he saw life and well-being and how he aimed to integrate his free spirit with his role as provider and caretaker. Rosa's preeclampsia was very much contingent upon her worries around seeking prenatal care as a foreign woman and having no relatives to seek for help. However, thanks to José Antonio's extensive social network,[26] which included several health professionals, she accessed important prenatal care services. Once the preeclampsia brought clinical complications, the health care system entered into their lives in a more formal way, both at the first hospital close to the bottle house and then at El Materno, where the emergency caesarean section was performed and where Oscar remained for twenty-eight days. Once Oscar was born, Rosa's training and work in nursing and her ingrained ideas about the "normal" child, the "normal" pregnancy, and the "normal" mother, all added to her worries. She searched for explanations and required comfort and reassurance in both clinical and emotional terms.

Remarkably, however, this multivocal illness narrative indicates several crossing points between the ways in which the hospital addresses the social, emotional, and historical realities of families and the ways in which the families experience them. Clearly, Rosa and José Antonio's precarious economic situation presented them with many difficulties that influenced their practices of care around food, shelter, and cleanliness. And yet their story challenges fixed ideas of poverty as a condition that impedes families' access to adequate care, even in complex situations such as caring for a kangaroo baby. Their story also highlights the importance of health care networks in providing families with support, confidence, and training.

In addition, their narrative conveys other emotional strategies that the hospital implemented in order to offer a sense of normalcy and to help mothers, fathers, and other relatives take care of their babies. Families learn that their role is important and that they can manage their responsibilities. They are encouraged to begin breastfeeding as soon as possible and to put the babies skin-to-skin. From the very first moments, the idea that the father's heat makes babies thrive more than the mother's shifts traditional gender roles around the kinds of responsibilities and tasks for each member of the family. José Antonio commented how at El Materno, "I learned the words *papito* and *mamita* [daddy and mommy] and I understood that . . . it was about solidarity and practicality. They help parents become more autonomous. They provide great help and build your trust so that you can take care of your baby."

The use of the diminutives *mommy* and *daddy* as terms of address can be criticized as subordinating and infantilizing; it might be understood as a subtle way of establishing differences between a more privileged and knowledgeable community (the health care team) and their inferiors, whose names do not matter (the patients' parents).[27] According to this line of analysis, all poor people can be grouped under generic words such as *mommy* and *daddy*. Such lack of recognition and the language of difference might be seen as stemming from the hospital's long tradition of charity care. Rosa's negative experience of the doctor accusing her of having a child with a relative can also be interpreted as a result of this pervasive patriarchal construct in which poor women treated at public hospitals were considered inferior and treated with disrespect or disgust. The pervasiveness of a colonial mentality indicates that a structured social order is created around power differentials that mix class status, gender, and race.

And yet the terms *mommy* and *daddy* are charged with an emotional language, because many families use them affectionately at home. Using this language at the hospital can also provide families with a sense of comfort and intimacy that makes them part of an "emotional community" that blurs the boundaries between home and hospital.[28] *Mommy* and *daddy*, in this reading, are words of affection but also words that connote status and respect inside the household. By referring to them in their roles as the most important members of the household, this hospital practice can result in feelings of importance rather than of inferiority or subordination. In fact, for families with babies that remain hospitalized for long periods of time, house and hospital become familiar places where their lives evolve in particularly difficult moments. The difficulties experienced by families at the hospital are physical as the health condition of baby and mother improve, emotional as they ride a tense and expectant roller coaster of healing and survival,[29] and economic, given the extra expenses that families are forced to incur in their new roles as parents of a hospitalized child and the extra time demands that impede labor-related activities. In addition, the use of *mommy* and *daddy* might also be a practical decision, given that the number of women and families in the hospital at any given time makes it very difficult to learn all their names. Over time, as children grow and develop, the KMC team does learn the names of babies, mothers, and fathers.

One of the most significant aspects in Rosa, José Antonio, and Oscar's experience is the overlap between their love story and the hospital's use of love as the most important aspect for the care of a kangaroo baby. According to their narrative, Rosa left her job, her country, and her family to follow a man she loved. José Antonio gave up much of his desire for mobility to settle with and care for Rosa and Oscar. Oscar felt this medically fundamental love from the first moment he was placed on his parents' chests. Oscar now demands "lovies" (*cariñitos*) when he wants to sleep on José Antonio's chest and José Antonio gladly accepts; like José Antonio, kangaroo parents more broadly recognize that having babies sleep on their chests is tiring but feels wonderful.

According to "El Gran Maestro" Santiago Currea Guerrero, perhaps the most prominent neonatologist of the country, love's power resides in its relational nature: love is transmitted and received, and in that interaction it transforms bodies and communities both physically and emotionally. According to Santiago, love has social and historical implications in addition to its clinical effects. In his words, "Breastfeeding is an act of love between generations in which babies receive from their mothers the impulse to continue existing outside the womb." Breastfeeding, then, besides the known clinical benefits, also represents a bioemotional connection between babies and mothers; it carries histories of generations coming together in the simple act of offering and being nourished by milk.

El Gran Maestro is well known for his poetic language. His words encapsulate an epistemology of care, the ways in which El Materno and La Nacional think about medicine as part of life. In terms of KMC, Santiago said, "Thanks to the knowledge created at El Materno, the Kangaroo Mother Program has saved the lives of thousands of premature children. KMC has contributed to make Colombia visible around the whole world not for violence or drug dealing, but for this methodology that is based on love among human beings."[30] In their illness narrative, Rosa and José Antonio agreed with the idea that love was the most important factor in allowing Oscar to thrive. So, does love work? And if so, how?

DR. HÉCTOR MARTÍNEZ, who developed KMC's core concepts, explained why KMC works:

"Mother kangaroo" is an innovative method for the treatment and outpatient care of premature and low birth weight children. Warmth, lactation and the kangaroo position are the basic foundations of the method. But more than anything, it is the loving and close relationship established between mother and child that allows the little ones to survive. The important and ongoing stimuli, affectionate as much as physical, improve and guarantee the respiratory and cardiac rhythms. The mother's voice, her cooing, the surrounding family, all serve as enriching triggers from the neurological and cognitive perspectives. It is the mother, and not the doctors or the hospital, who is in charge of and responsible for the care of her baby.[31]

Interestingly, the incubator has been seen as representing a transition in the kinds of knowledge and technology considered ideal for the survival of premature newborns. With the development of incubators, neonatal care was distanced from mothers in favor of primarily male medical professionals; the incubators were operated by obstetricians and, later, by pediatricians and neonatologists. KMC, according to Dr. Martínez, proposes to reverse this process. The philosophy of kangaroo care argues that, instead of technology and male medical expertise, women and their families can best take care of their children, using their emotions and their bodies rather than advanced technology. KMC thus challenges core constructs of modern biomedicine: not only modern ideas around efficacy and technology but also issues of prestige and power around gender, and, ultimately, market.[32] As UNICEF said when it first supported KMC in its 1984 state of the world's children, kangaroo care–associated costs are zero.[33]

At a public presentation in 2006, Lida Pinzón, who was then KMC's program director, explained the relevance of KMC's core principles as developed by Héctor Martínez—love, warmth, and breast milk—and the challenges that they pose to modern biomedicine, currently represented by evidence-based medicine (EBM) (figure 2.3).[34]

Love

From the perspective of evidence-based medicine, each treatment should have scientific proof. Love, the way we have seen it, is very hard to explain scientifically. We are intrigued as to why we have to prove something that is so evident.

Notice how we, physicians, don't use the word love. It is very hard for us to mention it because we want to explain everything through a blood test or an X-ray result. So, you find in the scientific literature the term "attachment" to explain what happens to babies when mothers caress them or are affectionate with them and establish early contact. In the mother's case, the term used is "bonding," meaning the emotional experience of mothers.

Warmth

Warmth does not connote just temperature; it is much more than that. Warmth is to be able to hold one's baby, to let my baby know my smell, for me to know what my baby smells like, for her to listen to my heart rhythm, to get to know her cries, to search for the breast whenever she wants. Scientifically, however, warmth has been defined as the maintenance of a constant temperature by transferring temperature from a warmer body to a colder body. We know now that the baby's temperature increases 0.3 degrees centigrade when she is taken out of the incubator and stays with the mother. When the baby stays with the father, the temperature goes up a whole degree centigrade, which is why we talk about kangaroo fathers and kangaroo families. . . . We had once triplets and the older siblings were kangaroos for the little ones.

Breast Milk

We are leaders in the promotion of breastfeeding and we strongly believe that there is nothing better than breast milk to feed a neonate. Formula could not

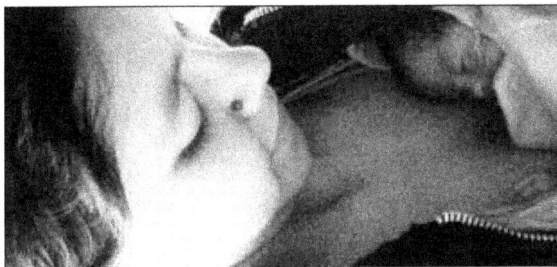

BASIC PRINCIPLES OF THE MOTHER KANGAROO METHOD

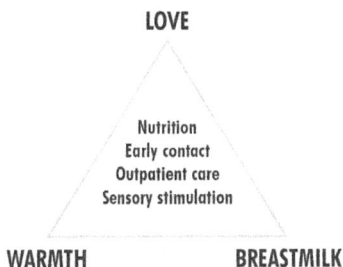

LOVE

Nutrition
Early contact
Outpatient care
Sensory stimulation

WARMTH   BREASTMILK

FIGURE 2.3. Kangaroo Care principles. (IDEASS n.d.)

compete with breast milk because it ... does not have the adequate defenses. The quality of premature breast milk is excellent. We now know that it has more carbohydrates, proteins and higher levels of immunoglobulins in comparison to mature breast milk. It is true that it has less fat and that is why babies don't put on weight as rapidly. There are now several controversial studies as to how much breast milk vs. formula premature babies should take and we are reviewing all that evidence-based literature to adjust our protocols.

Lida's explanations contain a kind of language that represents the epistemological tension between accredited knowledge based on scientific standards and credible results that cannot be fully proven in spite of their practical logic and obvious positive outcomes. She showed how some KMC results could be explained in biological and psychological terms but that the "nature" of human care, what makes KMC effective, could not be translated—that is, reduced—to science. While the importance of breast milk can be argued using nutritional terminology, a profound philosophy around breastfeeding, such as Santiago Currea's, resymbolizes its biological, emotional, historical, and political importance. KMC's principles come across as a direct confrontation to biomedicine, as a contradiction to its epistemology, and, consequently, as a menace to its hegemony. Warmth is more than body temperature, love cannot be reduced to attachment or bonding, and breast milk is not just nutrients and immune defenses. All three are undeniably biological, and yet they largely exceed the biomedical conceptions that can make them "scientific enough."

The epistemology of medical care at El Materno, as represented in KMC and evinced in the hospital's practices of care, the explanation of the program's founders and professors, and the experiences of families, represents a careful balance between "innate" and "hegemonic" understandings of health conditions and therapeutics. Medical hegemony,[35] in this case, reflects the global scientific understanding around perinatology and the care of very-low-birth-weight babies. And yet, as we have seen, KMC does not stand in direct opposition: it is a powerful alternative that challenges but also includes hegemonic knowledge.[36] At El Materno, physicians follow international guidelines and scientific reports. But they challenge and adapt them when they disagree or feel that the local social conditions and the patients they see require it. The KMC algorithm also reflects a balance between respecting existing knowledge and adapting it to each patient based on his or her needs. Nevertheless, KMC principles do represent a drastic threat to hegemonic medicine's conceptions of health, disease, and treatment. Rather than more technology, KMC puts its trust in mothers, babies, and other relatives. Many aspects of KMC cannot be measured and yet they are logical, effective, and simple. According to Santiago, KMC represents the importance of creating "simple alternative solutions to complex problems."[37]

KMC IS NOT THE only one of such "subaltern health innovations" to originate in postcolonies. Another simple "medical innovation" for a complex problem originated at El Materno in 1975, when gynecologist and professor Alvaro Velasco decided to break the hinge of traditional forceps to avoid compressing babies' heads during birth.[38] This and other changes to protocol—changes as simple as advocating for the use of street clothes rather than hospital clothes—have resulted in significant improvements in the care of pregnant women and children. This last change is now considered an adequate standard of practice given that clothes that remain at hospitals can carry more resistant strains of microbes. But when El Materno proposed it many decades ago, it received harsh criticism.

Luis Carlos Méndez, who through his recollections in chapter 1 helped us understand what the symbiosis between El Materno and La Nacional meant for physicians in training, stresses that these remarkably simple and powerful strategies, rather than being the result of isolated ideas, also belong to the larger history of that relationship. Through the kinds of teaching and care activities at the hospital, "You create a model that is not based on evidence but based on reality. You end up demonstrating that the anecdote or the experience has as much validity, if not more, than evidence. It is not that we do not respect evidence, but as opposed to the 'evidentologists' [a word Luis Carlos coined to mix evidence and the expert in a given technique or method], I have never mistrusted experience, I have never mistrusted the anecdote. They [evidentologists] have, we have not."

Indeed, in meta-analyses or studies that result in guidelines, the ranking of knowledge gives much less weight to anecdotes, qualitative material, observations, or expert opinions and, conversely, gives the highest weight to randomized clinical trials (RCTs) with large samples. However, Luis Carlos clarified, evidence does not have all the answers for all the problems. Along with a team of neonatologists he created the national guidelines for healthy newborns, and "Where is the evidence?" he intelligently asked. With this question, he indicated that evidence and medicine are a powerful pair when tackling diseases and when treatments find support through scientific studies, such as in RCTs. But the coevolution of clinical care and scientific experimentation has little to say about processes around caring (such as in guidelines for the healthy newborn) that are based not on testing treatments but on attention to clinicians' expertise and the experiences of patients and families. In the end, the guidelines for healthy newborns are intended to help clinicians find unique answers to the question of what is best for each specific baby.

Luis Carlos's reflections further clarified this tension between the holistic approach and EBM: "We know what the evidence tells, we know what the guidelines and protocols say and whatever is valid we use; whatever is not, we don't." Validity, here, does not refer to scientific assessments. Valid results at El Materno are the end result of a process of interacting with the data and contextualizing the clinical information of each patient with experience, local knowledge, and local conditions, a kind of clinical social medicine.

Even if there are aspects made unchallengeable by the "strong evidence" supporting them, Luis Carlos further explained, there is room to negotiate, to pick and choose. For example, he said, "Iron and breast milk. According to evidence, everybody [every child from a developing nation] needs iron. The studies say that, the labs say that, the sponsors say that, the pharmaceutical companies say that. Given that, we are all malnourished, right?" Luis Carlos was talking about how guideline parameters are not neutral; they follow interests, for example of pharmaceutical companies. And as the interests gain power, people end up transforming social parameters from guidelines into universals. Luis Carlos continued, "So, what is the deal then? Is breast milk the only food and is it sufficient for the child or isn't it? Imagine the absurdity and the violence if I tell a mother that I need to enrich her milk [by giving supplements such as powder milk rich in iron]." Here, he powerfully adopts a feminist position and applies the concept of symbolic violence by which a mother might feel biologically unfit to care for her own child. Of course, "if the mother is malnourished, we accept [that the iron supplement is important] but we do even that with caution. You have to prove to me that human milk is iron-deficient because [we know] that breast milk draws from wherever it needs to [from the women's body] to give [iron] to the baby." According to several guidelines on iron supplementation, all babies require iron after the second month, "all of them regardless of the kind of diet that people are consuming, which might be enough as a source of iron. So, we disagree and we mention that. We include it [iron supplementation] because there is evidence that supports it, but we do not always use it."

Luis Carlos's and Lida's explanations about treating each birth, each baby, each mother, and each family individually challenge protocols and standards in which the mean has been pushed, rather than as a guideline, as the universal standard of care that must be applied to everybody equally. Alongside these El Materno physicians, we can argue that decontextualized and passive understandings of evidence have become a form of oppression in clinical practice.[39] Certain escuelas, such as El Materno, are aware and critical of this fact, and that is why they study evidence cautiously, incorporating only the aspects that they consider "valid." Luis Carlos also argues for a kind of knowledge that incorporates the context of each patient (not all Colombian women are poor and not all Colombian poor women are malnourished) and the context of the specific practices that physicians at the hospital have established as ideal standards of care. Luis Carlos continued,

> We don't use iron in all cases, in part because we have another great advantage, which is that we respect the umbilical cord. In other escuelas they don't give much importance to the cord, they just clamp it and cut it right away, saying that it has nothing to do with anything. We do not. We respect the cord up to a certain point [given the post-delivery conditions of both baby and cord]. The conditions are very peculiar, very particular to each birth. Each birth is different because

all human beings are different. So, you have to respect that difference, understand it, and tolerate it. How can you tell me that all deliveries are the same if each birth is unique [both as a biological and emotional experience]?

RESPECTING THE UMBILICAL CORD is an example of the advances in neonatal adaptation made by El Materno/La Nacional professors over the decades, which have resulted in many simple but extraordinarily important practices of care. Santiago Currea is the professor whose expertise has been fundamental to this La Nacional/El Materno Escuela, helping people learn to respect nature, in this case symbolized by the protection of the umbilical cord. El Gran Maestro explained, "In adaptation there is no conflict [with international approaches] in reanimation . . . we have been very careful in recognizing the importance of protecting the umbilical cord at birth. Imagine, they [the hegemonic medical community] talk about physiological anemia of the newborn. [That is often] the consequence of errors in the timing of clamping the cord, because the baby can lose 30 or 40 percent of her blood volume [in the process]." Santiago cannot think of when exactly he started to advocate for delayed clamping, "since I was in training [in Pediatrics], I guess [in the mid-1970s]. They would clamp the cord automatically and I didn't agree with that practice." At that time he was thinking about two important issues that argued against immediate clamping:

First you observe the animal world, animal behavior. Mammals don't cut the cord immediately. They only do it after the placenta is delivered, then they chew on the cord. Second, I would ask myself "Physiological anemia of the newborn?" If it is anemia it is not physiological [i.e., normal] if it is physiological it is not anemia. . . . So, some old references were very important, nineteenth century books, a French author Budin who mentioned that he taught [clamping] after three or four minutes [after delivery]. . . . I started with a sort of case by case observation and then, later, I conducted a more systematic observation when I started to work at El Materno [in 1977].

"The umbilical cord has suffered from an amazing silencing, clinically and culturally. You do not see a painting about the cord, a sculpture about the cord. There is a very beautiful one at the Instituto de Perinatología de México, but it is the only one I have found. It is a mystery, something marvelous, transcendental, monumental." Santiago's passion for the umbilical cord is not to be read as a "clinical obsession" with a part of the body, but as a marvel at the role that any part of the human body has, even one as apparently insignificant as the cord, if doctors allow nature to take its course. Even in cases when babies are born compromised, as we will see, El Materno/ La Nacional Escuela advocates for using the umbilical cord to help the baby, rather than performing the traditional clamping and invasion of the baby's body that will be explained next.

Santiago's philosophy for that intersection between medicine and life is to try as much as possible to abstain from intervening, to minimize "invading" the body, and to let nature take its course. Neonatologists' role is not to stand by passively but to adopt a feminist ethics of care, to "aid," to "support" the process of beginning life outside the womb. "We had years when we were very invasive, in [my 2004] book we were still very invasive. . . . It is really rare that I invade a child nowadays [only in exceptional cases when they are severely compromised and his clinical judgment indicates that the child needs more than noninvasive maneuvers.] I don't invade them [with catheters] through the umbilicus or the airway. For airways, I do the 'fuente nariz' and the child ventilates beautifully." Here, he is referring to another simple solution he created for a complex problem; he closes one nostril with one finger, holds the chin and tongue, and provides a flow of oxygen with any catheter at hand into the other nostril until the child expands its thorax. "Fuente nariz" avoids inserting a catheter through the nose and fulfills the same function as expensive, invasive, and sometimes unavailable commercial equipment.[40] It allows doctors to perform effective ventilation anywhere—an important ability for physicians and residents who need to assist newborns in regions across the country where they might lack resources and equipment. The minimal requirement is a flow of oxygen.

> I don't insert a catheter in the stomach either [for suctioning], which is important because the stomach can fill with air. Another thing that irritates [other escuelas] immensely is that we have not used suction for 30 years. [The baby expels extra fluids] and can reabsorb the rest if the lungs are perfused. I take the students to the babies half an hour or an hour later [after the delivery] so that they can see them sleeping peacefully [without having been subjected to suction]. Another aspect we abandoned was the use of adrenaline in reanimation. It has very important effects for the heart but it is bad for the lungs; it closes the vessels, and we need the lungs to be perfused. So, we started reducing its use until we stopped using it completely. . . . It was very long ago that we stopped hitting or shaking a child to activate her. We

don't hit them, don't shake them, don't suction them, don't clamp the cord, don't apply adrenaline in cases of depression. It is an approach to protect them from potentially harmful interventions and in that context you see a very peaceful and comfortable adaptation when they are born healthy, and a recuperation when they are born compromised.

Such avoidance of intervention should not be taken as an unconscientious approach or a simple political refusal. On the contrary, it has required years of careful and systematic observation—a fundamental aspect of medicine that, unfortunately, has been underutilized in the wake of the forced application of universals to clinical medicine. In contrast to that passivity, Santiago reminds us, "It is about daring to believe that you can think on your own." That process of thinking, however, does not only involve biomedical and scientific thinking, not because they are unhelpful, but because "mother nature has all the tools you need." Thus, it is about thinking with and supporting nature.[41]

The debate at this point—whether to suction, to clamp, to use adrenaline and catheters, to avoid "invasions"—is clearly not a life-or-death issue nor an issue in which one can design studies to get outcomes that conclusively prove the benefits of one method over the other. The debate is over whether to intervene if there is a simpler, more humane, and less traumatic way to help the newborn. According to Santiago, "In a natural birth, babies cry minimally. The baby is born and is moved by the environmental surprise and cries, but if you respect the cord, then the child cries two, three, four times and then looks around a bit, gets sleepy, closes his eyes and keeps breathing calmly." At this point of his narrative, Santiago is stressing the importance of offering comfort and helping babies transition to their new life outside the womb. "One needs to try not to make babies cry. I insist to them [the students] that you cannot examine a child if he/she is wailing." In a case when a baby was crying, he instinctively and gently caressed the baby's face between the forehead and the nose with downward pressure from his thumb, and the baby stopped crying. Now he teaches it, half-serious/half-jokingly, as a "calming maneuver." Someone told him that it made sense because there is a chakra in that area.

Both interventions and noninterventions are meant to help babies according to their needs; both require careful attention and attunement to the baby and respect for nature. If things do not go as expected in a natural way, according to Santiago, it does not mean that you abandon nature and initiate invasive procedures. "Even in caesarean sections, you don't need to clamp immediately. You keep the cord, then you apply what we call thoracic massage (the compression of the thorax so that it expands, getting air inside the lungs on the one hand and blood on the other) so that the child slowly gains vitality." Vitality, another "ancient" medical term used by indigenous medicine and in the West at the time of "naturalistic" understandings of medicine, is highly relevant for rethinking medicine's goals and methods in a time when the assemblage of market/science/technology is becoming more and more oppressive.[42] KMC, "fuente nariz," respecting the cord, and trusting breast milk to provide enough iron are all about the vitality of love transmission to the newborn in fluids, air, and warmth. In reducing invasions and assuming that the role of the health care team is to facilitate and to give back to babies the possibility of gaining that necessary vitality in the first critical moments of life, Santiago replicates KMC's idea that mothers and children have the most powerful tools for caring and healing. Such an epistemology of care offers a critical reversal to hegemonic ideas that understand medicine as the social institution that saves the lives of passive patients through modern technology.

"Nowadays," Santiago explained, "there is a growing consensus about the advantages of delaying clamping the cord, but there is none yet about reanimation with an intact cord. But we do marvelous things [while reanimating with an intact cord]." He is referring to the very intense moments after the birth of a severely deprived newborn, in which the medical tendency is to perform several maneuvers as quickly as possible to get the baby to react. In those moments, the cord is cut and babies lose the chance for contact with their mother as they are rushed either to one side of the delivery room or to a separate room. In general, with a great deal of intervention through catheters, suction, and medications (such as adrenaline) babies perfuse their lungs and breathe. "What we do [in terms of reanimation of an unresponsive newborn with an intact cord]," Santiago continued, "is absolutely exciting, moving, marvelous, surprising, fantastic." These words capture the experiences of people who get to see him in action and then incorporate his teachings.

"In this birth," Santiago says, referring to a video he uses for teaching purposes, "the baby is unresponsive. His cord is intact and we give him a thoracic massage. Notice how he expands after the compression. He winked a bit so I know he is coming. He opened his other eye a bit. I reinforce the cardiac massage. The child is not looking good. I am going to start the 'fuente nariz' that I mentioned before." At this stage of the video, about two minutes have passed, and tension is growing in the delivery room. Nurses and residents look at each other suspiciously. Although his voice remains calm, he acknowledges being stressed when one piece of equipment for the "fuente nariz" was too thick and was impeding his speed. At some point, the mom asks how the baby is doing. "As oxygen is flowing," he continues in the video once the "fuente nariz" is working, "one can see how it returns from the stomach; because of the noise [that is coming from the stomach] I know he is starting to breathe." Even though he is now confident of the baby's reaction, the crowd's anxiety shows in a mix of furrowed brows and nervous smiles. Four minutes postdelivery, the baby "is starting to gain color, but the lower part [of the body hasn't] yet," explains Santiago. "Then I tell the students and the gynecologists that I am going to do a quick bit of psychotherapy with the mom. I tell her that she did an excellent job, that the baby needs a bit of help from us, but that she did great, so that she won't start blaming herself for what is going on." A minute later, the baby starts gaining more color and giving slow kicks. He finally produces a low cry. The crowd is shocked; the head nurse grabs her head with both hands and turns around, looking back and forth between the wall and the baby, while students and residents give nervous laughs of relief. The gynecologist says "No, no, no . . ." Santiago now turns everybody's attention to the cord. It has remained intact and pulsating, giving the blood to the baby. Once the pulsation stops, the cord is clamped. Santiago Currea shows the baby to the mother, tells her again that she did excellently, encourages her to give the baby a kiss, and tells her that they are going to help him a little bit more so that he can breathe more strongly. As he talks to her, Santiago has grabbed a blanket and starts drying the baby profusely "so that he doesn't lose heat."

"You have to see it to believe it," or "it is a life-changing experience," people say about the experience of seeing an unresponsive newborn gain vitality with the help of an intact cord. "Once you have seen those kiddos that are born half-dead and how they get activated without invading them," Santiago concludes, "nobody can convince you [to do] otherwise." The graduates from La Nacional/El Materno Escuela carry that conviction with them and "fight for the cord tooth and nail" when doctors trained in other escuelas want to rush and clamp the cord immediately.

The power that results from combining careful observation with tuning in to nature as an emotional and analytic exercise means that "one has not invented [anything, whether a specific innovation like KMC or a solution like clamping the cord]. It is the child who offers you the answers. So, this is just about your disposition to pick up what the child is showing you, just that, plus the refusal to abandon the child after two minutes." Children, he insisted, are the ones who teach, and observation demands patience even during emergencies. "Over time, one sees how they [the international community of neonatologists] are arriving at our conclusions [of delaying clamping the cord] and it is not because they have read us or because we have convinced them, it is because the patients teach you."

That babies teach you the right moment to clamp a cord eludes "evidence," Luis Carlos concludes. Besides, Santiago comments, "since we are convinced of its benefits, how are we to do a study clamping a group and not clamping another? That would be an [ethical] absurdity." Nonetheless and in spite of the ethical and technical difficulties of producing "strong" evidence for KMC, respecting the umbilical cord, the Velasco spatulas, progress in the use of nasal positive air pressure devices that avoid ventilators, improvements in toxemia care, breastfeeding, and so forth, now appear in meta-analyses, scientific studies, and guidelines that support their use.

A combination of critical thinking, knowledge, philosophy, ethics, and language has resulted in many simple alternative solutions to complex problems with powerful clinical and emotional implications. While many of these might fail to be statistically significant, they are clearly "nonstatistically fundamental."[43] Some, like KMC and respecting the umbilical cord, have been experienced and described as having "miraculous" results. Fortunately, the power of love among humans still escapes scientific efforts to explain how and why it works. However, other health-related miracles that happened at El Materno show that, like love and committed care, religious forces can play a powerful role in healing mothers and babies. In these cases, doctors do not claim that all "subaltern health innovations"[44] result in miraculous results but that clear-cut "medical miracles" demand alternative explanatory frameworks, as we will see in chapter 3.

CHAPTER 3. Religion and Caring in a Medical Setting

In chapter 2, caring and love were described as fundamental socioemotional principles necessary for KMC babies to thrive. This chapter underlines the emotional trope of "being a family" and the importance of religious figures in promoting an epistemology of care in which devotion and faith play a fundamental role in the healing process.[1] While the importance of faith in Western medicine remains marginally understood,[2] this chapter further shows how the religious presence at the hospital—the nuns and the priest—united the hospital staff and infused the building, its workers, and its patients with faith. In this chapter we will narrate a medical miracle that might symbolize the need for alter-rational approaches to understanding the boundaries and connections between humans, the building and its objects, and spiritual forces.[3] At El Materno, caring, love, and faith from families, workers, and religious figures, including the Virgin Mary, influence bodily improvements and successes.

Care and caring offer profound analytical interpretations of the interconnected acts of caregiving and receiving care.[4] Chapters 2 and 3 show how *caring* at El Materno is largely driven by a commitment to another's well-being and happiness. At El Materno, such politics of "caring for" means that caring extends beyond the individual patient to include family and health care workers. It also means the efforts to satisfy immediate and practical needs, such as food, shelter, or clothing, as well as emotional needs. We will read about humanization work and pastoral duties, which complement traditional areas of

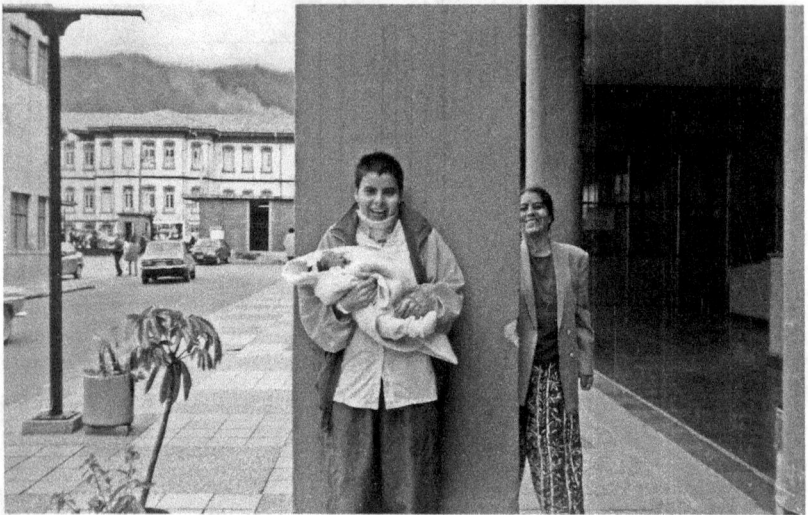

FIGURE 3.1. Photo courtesy of Gina M. Rodríguez.

care in medical settings, bringing a full ethos of caring beyond biomedical techniques. In chapter 2, the social, economic, and political aspects that surround the patients' lives were discussed as the main aspects incorporated into medical practice as a kind of "clinical social medicine." In chapter 3, the emotional aspects of patients and health care workers' experiences are incorporated into the institutional culture with the help of the religious presence and its ethos of devotion and humanization. By strengthening the spiritual connections among people and between people and God, Jesus, and the Virgin Mary, the religious presence at the hospital helped build an "emotional community"[5] symbolized, in people's minds, as "El Materno family." Indeed, one could argue that hospitals without this religious presence do not have such decisive politics of caring, emotional communities, or miraculous outcomes.

Of Family Miracles and Health Miracles

At El Materno, "care" was not simply medical or patient care. Patients, as we saw in chapter 2, needed emotional support, education, encouragement, and confidence. Love was understood to be a powerful force for healing babies and helping them thrive, but in order for parents to transmit love to their babies (as in KMC), El Materno had to take care of people's lives—not just their diseases. The blurred distinction between hospital and household meant that many clinical activities (such as weighing babies, taking temperature, or giving oxygen and medications) happened at home. Similarly, particularly for patients who stayed at the hospital for long periods, everyday activities that usually happened inside the household or in neighborhoods far from El Materno were common at the hospital. Patients and relatives would sleep, bathe, and eat at the hospital. They would also share stories and solve everyday problems. At times, hospital staff would give patients clothes, extra food, or money to take home. They would also give patients advice on personal and family matters and follow up with them at the hospital or through phone calls, mixing medically relevant information with other questions about their lives. Often patients would return to the hospital just to pay a visit.

This blurring of boundaries happened for health care workers too. Their commitments to patients and the intensity of the clinical work, both in quantity and quality, frequently resulted in countless extra hours. Everyone from physicians, head nurses, and high-level administrative staff to clinical and paramedical staff would frequently turn their six- or eight-hour shifts into twelve-hour or even longer shifts. Like their patients, workers brought to the hospital many activities that usually happened inside their household or communities. Staff ate, showered, and slept at the hospital. They developed close friendships with colleagues, sometimes finding life-long friendships or spouses among the people with whom they spent most of their days and nights, weekdays, and weekends. Many workers found solutions to household problems and family needs, like loans, child care, and relationship advice, at the hospital. In people's minds and hearts, the "El Materno family" epitomized this logic of caring,[6] which included not only clinically relevant matters but also a larger conception of care for one another that extended to both patients and hospital workers. Key to build-ing this *family* and making it thrive was the hospital's religious presence.

Nuns at the hospital were formally trained in nursing and, as with other nurses, their experience translated to prestige and reputation, which made them highly valued as part of the health care team. Nuns' vows of service aided in the perception that they fulfilled an indispensable and irreplace-able role in the hospital's everyday functioning. They were important not merely for the medical care they provided; in fulfilling their spiritual duties as sisters from the Augustine Missionary congregation, they also carried out nonmedical activities that were equally relevant and respected. Hence, nuns came to embody a dual role inside the hospital: medical care and nonmedical care. Mother Teresa Vecino, who traveled from Spain when the congregation assigned her the mission of serving at El Materno, be-came one of the hospital's most important and legendary figures. Accord-ing to Head Nurse Rosalba Bernal, Mother Teresa "would arrive at five in the morning, she would offer coffee, she would distribute the clothes for the poor, she would receive [visitors and donations] from the rich."

Mother Teresa was the soul of the hospital until she retired in 1990. Not only did she coordinate all the social service activities for the hospital's poor patients and families, but she was also chief of the nursing department: the largest unit at the hospital, which oversaw nurses, nurse assistants, and porters, with a total complex payroll of five hundred employees. Nursing spanned all the different gynecology and neonatology units, including surgery, inpatient, and outpatient clinics. It was clear that, along with the hospital director, the chief of nursing had the most important administra-tive and political tasks and run of the hospital. Mother Teresa remained in her role as directors came and went. The new directors, all men, would rely on her as they learned the many intricacies of their new role and coor-dinated new initiatives. Mother Teresa would instruct them on the many administrative and political issues crucial for managing relationships inside the hospital and between the hospital and other institutions.

Mother Teresa's compassion, love, and devotion were not given solely to patients. "She filed whenever the secretary wouldn't file," Rosalba added, meaning that Mother Teresa filled in or finished up any pending assignment that a given hospital worker had not completed. According to Rosalba, Mother Teresa empathized so much with the workers' everyday difficulties—whether someone was a single mother, had two jobs and was overextended, had problems at home, and so on—that people would take advantage of her. Mother Teresa was the first person Rosalba met at El Materno. Rosalba was finishing her professional nursing degree at a different university/hospital escuela, and in her last semester, she was assigned a one-week "hospital management" rotation at El Materno. "I had to learn about everything the hospital did from the management perspective. So, I arrived and Mother Teresa welcomed me. She offered me her book [as the head of the nursing department she had the nursing function's manual and administrative logs] and I got to access all areas of the hospital. That was a magical thing."

The religious presence was very important for Rosalba, who had always been a devoted Catholic. She remembered the hospital environment as "beautiful, very familiar, very welcoming." Even though it was just a one-week project, she felt very connected. As she was finishing her professional nursing degree, El Materno announced the hiring of two very-low-paying "rurales" positions. "We are talking about June 1985. My workmates would earn COP$200,000 as rurales [in other parts of the country], which was tons of money and at El Materno they offered me COP$19,600, can you imagine? But I said, there is something there, something magic, I am not sure why." As had happened to many others, the hospital had a force that drew her in.

For her work as a rural, twenty-three-year-old Rosalba received fifteen days of training for a position as the head night nurse in pediatrics. "I was going to start the next Monday but then Mother Teresa called me and told me: 'Daughter, the head nurse of surgery has a medical leave so you have to come tomorrow to surgery. . . .' 'But Madrecita [little mother, an affectionate way to address Mother Teresa] what am I going to do there?' 'Don't worry,' she told me.'" The newly graduated and very timid Rosalba arrived the next day to surgery and asked for the nurse assistant, who welcomed her and showed her around. The chief of surgery, Dr. Germán Sandoval, also welcomed her warmly. That same day, after a caesarean delivery, she got to see one of the magical practices of care at the hospital: Santiago Currea performed a neonatal reanimation "with such wisdom and tenderness, such skilled hands. I was looking at the nurse assistant and then he [Santiago Currea turned to her and] said, 'Jefe [head nurse], please take care of the liquids' [which was the next step in the care of the newborn]. I said that I was shocked, that I had never seen something like that. I talked to him later and I apologized and told him that I was just starting and that I had received training in pediatrics but not in neonatology, that I had had a bad experience in my neonatology rotation [during her studies]. All that happened in my first day at El Materno, which had started at 6 a.m. On top of that, there was humanization course from 7 to 10 p.m., which was a requirement. So, I entered at 6 a.m. and finished at 11 p.m."

The humanization course, which was intended to bring up a humane side to clinical care, was offered by Father Adriano, from the Order of Saint Camillus.[7] Known as the ministers of the sick, the Order was in charge of El San Juan's church, El Materno's chapel, and other chapels in neighboring hospitals. Rosalba's first day was a very intense work experience filled with religious, clinical, and interpersonal emotions. Yet she felt supported and respected. The humanization course "was beautiful. It went on a whole week. So, since that time and for the next twenty years [she worked at El Materno] I got used to entering at 6 a.m. and not knowing what time I would leave." Because of the religious presence, however, dedication for Rosalba and other workers was part work ethic and part spiritual devotion.

"Camillian priests had been the chaplains of Colombian hospitals for over fifty years," Rosalba continued, "and they taught us humanization in three domains: patients, patients and their families, and health care workers and institution. Since then, I was hooked on humanization." Nurses from all the hospitals of the area participated in the one-week humanization training and then in monthly meetings that also included Mother Teresa. As Rosalba's year as a rural went by, it combined humanization and "surgery, deliveries, neonatal adaptation, sterilizing, laundry and so on." The mix of work ethics and spiritual devotion became part of who Rosalba was and the way she saw her role as part of a team. "At times, the afternoon head nurse would not arrive and you didn't even have time to call the Department [the nursing department], so I would just bring the keys at 6 p.m. [after doubling her shift], and Mother Teresa would ask, 'But why you?' [meaning that her shift was up at noon], so I would say 'Madrecita, the head nurse of the afternoon didn't arrive.'" Neither overtime nor oversight was the motivating force behind this doubling and covering of shifts; rather, it was about the cultural ethos of caring. In such circumstances, workmates would be concerned about the worker who had not arrived for her shift and concerned about the worker who had stayed late. So, Mother Teresa would tell Rosalba, "Oh daughter, go eat. So I learned to eat at El Materno." For Rosalba, "learning to eat" meant learning to care for oneself and learning to let others take care of you. Caring for patients, caring for oneself, and caring for all members of the community inside the hospital, as the humanization course taught, contributed to the sense of El Materno as a big family—or, as some people referred to it, as "their second home."

SISTER EMITA (SOR MARÍA EMMA MUÑOZ) felt a religious calling since she was very young and decided to join the Augustinian Missionaries congregation after finishing high school at nineteen. As a nun, she was working at a school with people who were so poor that they did not have money "even to pay for a shot [for medications.]" She wanted to study something that would allow her to help. The congregation supported her desire to further her studies and paid for her two-year training course in nursing at El Materno's nursing school, which Sister Emita chose because of its very good reputation. At that time, the presence of the Augustinian Missionaries at the hospitals was such that the congregation had two assigned areas in which to sleep, rest, and eat, one in El San Juan and one in El Materno. She worked shifts for some years until the hospital hired her in 1985 as "nurse assistant, responsible for the ward." In this position, she performed clinical nursing duties with adult patients in one of the hospitalization wards and supervised the other nurse assistants in her ward. She started to work in the toxemia section and then in the curettage section, following up on voluntary abortions. But in practice, her work activities included her assigned clinical and supervising duties with the job of solving any problem that came up at the hospital, especially on weekends when the director or chief of services was not available. "If the boiler broke then they would call us [the nuns] and we would figure out who to bring to fix it. If a woman could not pay, then we would go [back to the hospital] and say it was ok."

Like Head Nurse Rosalba Bernal, Sister Emita often stayed until late in the afternoon, well beyond the six-hour shifts stipulated in her contract, "because there was always something to do; a patient whose relatives hadn't been found, people coming from other regions of the country that needed help." If her official shift was from 7 a.m. until 1 p.m., she thought of the afternoons and weekends as part of her pastoral responsibilities. In the afternoons "we would visit the sick; we would talk with the nurses, we would ask them if they were happy, if they would like anything to work differently. We would go floor by floor, checking on the children, keeping an eye out just in case someone was being rude to patients or families." Thus, the nuns' pastoral responsibilities included interactions with different groups of people with the goal, in her words, of helping. Helping could entail a specific clinical activity, as with Sister Liduvina, who developed such a clinical gaze (see chapter 1) that she was able to identify babies who needed the RhoGAM vaccine[8] just by looking at them. But it could also entail finding someone to repair equipment, instructing health care personnel in humanization, or helping mothers, babies, and families with nonmedical needs. "There were many things that moms needed. Many didn't have any money, didn't have clothes for their children. We would receive donations and we would organize [the donated clothes] and distribute them [among the patients in need]. We would even dress their husbands [out of the men's clothes that were also donated]. Then we had mass every day at 6 p.m., including weekends. We would go and would help those [patients] who couldn't get there on their own; that is, if they wanted [to come.] [W]e would not force anybody." Sister Emita was emphatic in explaining that their role was not about converting anybody to Catholicism but about helping and counseling.

Father Adriano would also visit the sick in the afternoons, hear confessions, and talk to the hospital personnel. Sister Emita recalled, "We [Father Adriano and the nuns] offered trust [to both patients and workers alike]. If a person was sad, we would ask, 'Why are you sad? What happened? If you want to tell me, just think that I am a friend who can listen to you and you can feel relieved [from whatever the person was experiencing].'" And in those interactions, just as they had been instructed in their pastoral work, they learned to be humble, to learn from others' problems, and to discover the other person's needs. Sister Emita remembered,

I remember a nurse assistant who arrived late. I was coming down the stairs and asked her, "Why are you coming so late?" And she responded, very rudely, "You should first ask what happened and then why you are late." I told her, "You are right, what happened?" "I didn't have money for bus fare, I had to come on foot. I didn't have anything for breakfast either and I had to walk." I told her that I was very sorry [for not asking her first what happened,] that I didn't want to offend or bother her. So she calmed down. And then I asked myself, "God, what do I do?

Sister Emita gave her some of the saved money that they collected from the donations, money that was meant to be recirculated back to the hospital. "We would [use that money] when people needed money to buy medications, when they didn't have money for the bus. If there was a woman from a different city who didn't have money for the intermunicipal bus, we would give it to her, if a husband hadn't eaten and there was nothing left in the kitchen, we would go out and buy him something to eat.

Sometimes, peoples' challenges could not be solved with money. "Let's say someone would arrive from Tolima [province] at 7 p.m. [after a six- to eight-hour bus ride], and it could be a while before the woman would get hospitalized," Sr. Emita remembered. While the woman was hospitalized, "Where was the man going to stay? So, you set something up for him so that he could rest and gave him food because he could be starving. Then the next day, we would give him breakfast early, find a place for him to shower and only then did he have to leave." Of course, to be able to help people (patients and relatives) with nonmedical needs, Sister Emita clarified, "you would ask the physician for permission," which was always granted. Given the hospital's long tradition of charity for the poor, the act of sheltering someone without a place to sleep constituted a historical continuity. In fact, shelters for the homeless and the elderly existed at El San Juan. The fact that the person was asked to leave early the next morning, however, meant that it was clear to both workers and patients that this help was offered as a temporary and emergency solution. There were, however, exceptions, such as an unhoused teenager who was raped, had an abortion, and ended up living in the hospital for several weeks. Another more institutionalized exception was a special ward/shelter/play area that was set up for abandoned babies who could end up living at the hospital for several months when child protection services were not up to date on bringing children to orphanages or finding them places for adoption. In any case, since the children were officially the hospital's patients, the health care personnel had more autonomy in deciding when a child was medically "cleared," and, in cases in which children had won the health care team members' hearts, they could stay "a bit" longer than medically necessary. According to Sister Emita, "Those were elementary things one would do." Humanization, listening to people, and thinking about their needs as an "elementary thing" changed staff practices and habits, including blaming patients for not following the doctor's orders perfectly or arriving late.

Workers developed this kind of devotion to patients not just because of the examples set by the sisters, Father Adriano, or other workers, but because they had also benefited from the special kind of care the hospital provided. Many workers took courses offered at the hospital that helped them advance their careers. The hospital administration—mostly because of Mother Teresa—was accommodating to workers who wanted to study for a new position at a higher level and higher pay grade. In many stories, workers who had not completed primary or secondary education were encouraged to finish schooling. People remember proudly that before the hospital was closed down, all workers had at least completed high school. Many would even continue with technical courses, often in nursing, and then be promoted.

In addition to formal education, many people, including physicians, head nurses, and paramedical staff, received humanization training in Father Adriano's courses. Through those courses, Sister Emita remembered, "People would awaken the feelings of love, of charity, and we came to be a beautiful family." Members of the El Materno family developed close relationships and moved on with an ethos of work ethics and devotion. Over the years and using humanization, El Materno worked to shift from the colonial perspective, which saw the dispossessed as deserving pity and charity, to understanding their difficulties and helping them improve their lives. The discourse of rights had not made its way into the institution, but the importance of social conditions to health and well-being was clearly articulated. Thus, a legacy of charity was being reordered by a more political take on people's needs and the hospital's mission.

Echoing what Santiago Currea said in chapter 2, Sister Emita said, "Patients teach you." While Santiago Currea was thinking about clinical attentiveness to following the patients' needs during treatment, Sister Emita was arguing for social and emotional attentiveness to understanding the patients' needs and offering relevant help. Sisters were known to have a better set of skills when it came to talking—or, rather, to listening—to patients. Frequently, doctors would call on the sisters and tell them, "Sister, this woman is very sick or very agitated or doesn't want to accept [a particularly difficult diagnosis or prognosis]. Come and help us. Try to see if you can calm her down." In the physicians' minds, calming people down was important because being upset could interfere with patients' treatment plans and the general environment of the hospital. In the nuns' minds, calming people down was about finding out what the women needed. Talking to patients did not mean that nuns would interfere with social work, social services, or psychology, all of which were available at the hospital—quite the contrary. By listening to patients' needs, they would be able to refer patients to certain services or direct specific services to certain patients. "So, we would go [to the psychology professor] and tell him, 'Profe, there is a woman that I think needs your help.'"

Because they worked closely with patients, physicians, and the priest in charge, nuns were in a privileged position to understand each group's expectations. The special trust that people developed with nuns, aided by strict confidentiality, allowed them to advise patients so that they would get help or benefit more from interactions with physicians or priests. Sister Emita remembered how "they [the mothers] would tell you whatever was going on [in their lives], and one would advise them to go and tell the doctor. We would even prepare the moms for that [interaction with the doctor]. 'I am embarrassed.' 'Don't be. Don't you see that doctors study precisely to understand everything that goes on in the body? Go with confidence and tell him and you will see that he can help you.'" Mothers articulated shame and embarrassment as reasons for delaying or doubting the benefits of interactions with doctors or priests—both male figures that embodied many social hierarchies.[9] Therefore, we can see how nuns helped empower mothers to get past the social hierarchy. When the issue was not medical but spiritual, or when the issue had a medical and a spiritual component, nuns would encourage patients to talk to the priest.

Sister Emita mixed personal rapport with information about the expectations of the medical and Catholic institutions and, in that interaction, she gained the mother's trust of both her and the institutions. She also redirected the ways in which mothers should speak to the people who could offer them help and support. She further explained the importance of rapport and teaching expected behavior: "You have to learn how to take the stress off people, so they [the mothers who were the ones who frequently sought the nun's advice] start laughing and start telling you. You don't have to come and tell me your sins," she continues, explaining to the mothers how her role works, "I am here only to help you understand how [to tell the priest or the physician their problems.]" Understanding "how to talk" to physicians and priests is very important, "so that they know [why you came to them] and can orient you, otherwise it is hard." Besides caring directly for patients' medical needs, listening to them, and helping them with nonmedical needs, the nuns played a crucial intermediary role in training the mothers in the social conventions of interactions between patients and doctors and between the faithful and priests—conventions that included important language norms of respect, trust, and a focus on important relevant information.

The religious "not-judgmental" approach was central to patients' trust; it was God alone who could judge the ways in which people repented or continued their sins. This was very important, given Catholicism's dominance as the main religion in the country. Although the nuns' counseling was meant to provide nonjudgmental help, it was not neutral when it came to preventing actions that contradicted Catholic principles. In cases of women who wanted to terminate unwanted pregnancies, which was illegal at the time,[10] or who expressed desires to abandon their babies, religious figures would try to convince the mothers to do otherwise. Sister Emita remembered how she interacted with women who wanted to end their pregnancies: "Please forgive me. Do not think I am here to pry into your personal life. I am just here to ask you, 'Why did you become pregnant in the first place?' 'I didn't know [that this act would make me pregnant],' she would say. And I would say, 'You know that a pregnancy is about defending a life, and you are thinking about killing your child who was conceived with love and so on and so forth.' At those moments God illuminates you [as to what to say,] and then the women would say, 'I will think about it.'" According to Sister Emita, many ended up deciding to keep their unborn babies or not to abandon them, although she is cautious in claiming that all interactions were "successful" because many women might have felt pressured to offer the answers the nun was expecting. "One wonders if the woman really kept her baby, who knows, but you have to talk to them with love, with affection. It is really hard but you end up satisfied that you did something for them."

Difficulties, challenges, and moments in which people were very upset were perhaps as common as satisfaction. But satisfaction could happen anywhere. "People sometimes tell me you were the sister at El Materno, you provided clothes for my son, you were very caring. Once I was in a bus and a man came in and started to sell candy [as a street vendor] and he told me, 'Sister, please accept this candy and do not pay for it because it is the only thing I have to pay you for what you did for my son at the hospital.' [There were] many cases like that one."

THE HOSPITAL ALSO HAD rituals with both religious and nonreligious elements that brought people together and contributed to their experience of the hospital as a family. Many workers' marriages were celebrated at El Materno's chapel. Almost all employees, including Head Nurses Rosalba and Patricia Farías, whose history we will get to in later chapters, gave birth to their own children at El Materno. The esteemed gynecology professors "received" their babies and the equally respected pediatricians became their children's doctors. In these cases, work space and family space were further conflated as people shared the most important and vulnerable moments of their lives. Such medical, familial, and emotional bonds were strengthened when the priest baptized the children and, in later years, celebrated their first communions and confirmations. Workers' children would grow up in and out of the hospital, where they were born, came when they were sick, hung out while their parents finished their shifts, and took part in religious celebrations.

These religious celebrations "were also part of our [pastoral] job," Sister Emita commented. El Materno's chapel was not legally authorized to conduct all of these rituals, so they would prepare at the church in El San Juan but offer the mass at El Materno, which was in the same priest's jurisdiction. After the mass, "We had to take all the paperwork back to the El San Juan church." Religious activities were not limited to mass or special religious celebrations inside the chapel. Often doctors would ask nuns to visit a child and apply holy oil whenever they felt the child was about to die. If mothers wanted, they would do an "immediate baptism" to protect the baby's soul. When a child died, nuns would be called to console the grieving mother, "using all the tools that God gives you [at those difficult times]," Sister Emita said. Nuns offered grief support not only for patients but also for workers or relatives of workers. "Everybody would support the person and pay their respects. If a nurse's mother died, we would go there and pray the rosary and be with her for a while [for the wake and burial.]" When a physician got very sick, he received constant visits from his colleagues, and when he died his family was "accompanied" by hospital workers at the wake.[11] The sisters would accompany the sick or the family, sometimes by themselves, sometimes with other workers or with Father Adriano.

"Every year, once or twice a year," Sister Emita added, "we celebrated *la familia hospitalaria* [the hospital family activity, which became an internal holiday celebration]." The initial humanization training by Father Adriano that turned into the humanization interhospital committee, which had evolved into humanization groups at each hospital. El Materno's humanization group was led by Head Nurse Rosalba Bernal, Sister Emita, and another nurse assistant. For the hospital family celebration, they would go to each hospital section and ask the workers to join in the planning. According to Sister Emita, they would arrive to a unit and tell the workers, "We are going to celebrate the 'hospital family,' but we cannot do it by ourselves, it has to be everybody. So, we would come up with the program [which included activities for the workers' families, food, music, performances, presents, prizes] and ask for their opinion." Usually for special occasions such as Christmas, Halloween, or the Colombian day in which love and friendship is celebrated, the humanization committee would go around the hospital to get people involved. Some people were reluctant, but, according to Sister Emita, one way or another people from every department, from every floor participated. At some celebrations, "there was mass and then music and people would dance a bit," Sister Emita remembered. "What I think was the most important aspect was the fraternity that we sowed at the hospital. The kind of work we did makes you realize that it is not us, it is God who makes these things happen."

VERÓNICA AND NATALIA WERE identical twins and the oldest of four siblings. As in many small towns, religious life was very important, and the children participated in all the church activities, including becoming acolytes for the mandatory Sunday mass. At seventeen, when they were finishing high school, they took the admission test for La Nacional. They both graduated with honors and were the first students from their town to pass the university test, a feat that made their father proud. Their high marks in the countrywide high school exit test made them eligible for the government scholarships offered to high-achieving students from poor municipalities, which covered tuition costs and included a small stipend.[12] The family of six decided to move to Bogotá, which Verónica called "a monster of a city." Two and a half years later, in 1997, when they were in their fifth semester, Natalia started to feel very sick, "horrible, and I would ask myself, 'God, what is happening to me?'" A friend of hers suggested that she might be pregnant; Natalia said that it was impossible. Then, since twins have special sensorial connections, including bodily manifestations, Natalia and her friend concluded that it had to be Verónica who was pregnant.

They were correct. Verónica had met Miguel on her first day of orientation at the university and since that day, they had a special connection. Verónica knew that her father was very strict, "very *machista*." She was afraid to tell her parents about her pregnancy and told Miguel that they should postpone telling them until the end of that fifth semester. Her pregnancy had started to show. In Bogotá she had managed to hide it with loose sweaters and jackets, but that strategy was not going to work in the warmer climate of their hometown. The next day, after arriving at the town, her father told her mother, "Something is wrong with that girl. Let's take her to the doctor." Verónica had to speak up, "I don't need a doctor. I am pregnant."

"That was so terrible for our dad," Natalia commented. "We had never seen him cry and that day he cried like a small child." For a man with traditional values who had always insisted on the importance of religion and education and had always told his daughters that they made him so proud, Verónica's unplanned pregnancy was a blow to his manhood.[13] In his mind, the only solution was "to find the person responsible and have them marry." Following gender norms of the machista culture, Verónica's mother called Miguel's mother, whose son had already told her about the pregnancy, and they arranged for Miguel's family to visit the small town to "sort things out." The meeting, which took place on December 24, was "horrible," filled with insults and accusations by Verónica's father, who accused Miguel of shirking responsibility for what he had done to Verónica, and sharp replies from Miguel's mother, who defended her son's integrity. Miguel's mother also argued that it was up to the young couple to make their own decisions about the future. In the end, Miguel agreed to marry Verónica. Verónica wanted to leave with Miguel's family immediately, but she remained in her hometown, hesitant to leave her mother.

January 18 was the agreed-upon day for the wedding. On January 8, Verónica decided to leave for Bogotá so that she could start organizing the paperwork for the wedding. Natalia offered to go with her. "No," their father said. "You stay here and let her [Verónica] leave and fix her life." Natalia stood up to their father and told him, "I am going with my sister." An uncle was traveling to Bogotá in his pickup truck, and they decided to ride with him and enjoy the open air of the cargo space. Verónica was trying to forget the horrible vacation and focus on everything that needed to happen in Bogotá.

At some point during the ride, at around 1 p.m., the uncle saw a tractor-trailer coming at them and lost control of the vehicle. The pickup truck flipped three times before stopping on the side of the road. Natalia was the only one who flew from the car; she landed on the hot pavement. When Verónica felt that their uncle was losing control of the car, she thought, "We are going to be crushed." Sitting on the makeshift bench, she managed to bend down and protect her belly with her hands. When the truck finally came to a stop, she felt something hit her at the base of her skull. "I never lost consciousness and I was aware of everything. Half of my body was inside the truck and half outside. I tried to fix my glasses, but my hand wasn't working. It just hit me in the face. Then I realized things were bad. I started to call for Natalia and somehow I looked over towards the road and saw that she had been hurt very badly." Natalia was unconscious and people thought she was dead. She had a very bad head injury, her skin was badly burned by the pavement and there was blood everywhere. The traffic jam that followed the accident brought people out of their cars. "Thank God, there was a doctor [among the crowd] and he started first aid, took my vitals and said, 'She is alive.'" People put Natalia on a wooden board and transported her to the closest hospital.

As people worked to rescue Verónica, she cried, "My baby, my baby." Assuming she had an infant with her, people looked inside the car for a baby until she clarified that she was pregnant. Two men took her out of the truck and carried her back to the road where a taxi driver offered to take her to the hospital. Someone laid her down in the back seat, but she wouldn't fit. "[Each time] they tried to close the door they hit my head. And so I told the guy, pull me from my feet. Take my feet out through the window and pull so that I fit and you can close the door." At the hospital, they rushed to do a sonogram to check on the baby. They also took X-rays and saw that Verónica had a severe spine injury. Verónica's parents were called; a physician told them, "She has a very high medullar section on the spine. She will never walk again."

Verónica and Natalia were transferred to a private clinic in Bogotá, where an uncle worked and where their mother's work-related insurance could cover some of the costs. Verónica remained in the intensive care unit for eight days. New exams confirmed a full medullar section in the cervical region, from C_3 to C_7. She would never walk again. "I couldn't even sit. They had to hold me from both sides otherwise I would fall. It was depressing and I knew it was going to be a hard ride." After a week of cephalic traction, Dr. Fonseca, a neurosurgeon, told Verónica that he would perform a surgery to stabilize her neck area, "so that I could at least sit in a wheelchair." The surgery, with local anesthesia, was very long, from 8 a.m. until 5 p.m. "They took out a rib and put it in here [neck area]," and fixed it with wires to the vertebrae.

Natalia suffered severe amnesia; everything from forty minutes before the accident to three months later, when she got a call from Verónica, who was still in the hospital, was a blank. The day her sister called and her memory returned, Verónica told her, "You have to help me because I had an injury. I broke my vertebrae and I am quadriplegic but you, Natalia, have to help me. You have to help me stand up from this wheelchair." Natalia was studying occupational therapy at La Nacional and was about to start her clinical years. She started to do massage therapy on Verónica's legs, which she remembered "were already hypotonic," and to straighten her fingers, "which [had] started to show contractures."

Whenever the neurosurgeon came to check on Verónica, she insisted that she was going to walk again. "I am going to be fine in a couple of months, doctor," she would say, asking him for a referral for physical therapy. Instead, the neurosurgeon asked a psychiatrist to help Verónica deal with her denial.

Every day the goddamned psychiatrist would arrive at 10 a.m. and start telling me, "You have to restart your life from a wheelchair." And I would tell him, "No, I am going to finish my career [in biology] and my career requires me to be in the field." And he would say, "Perhaps you can do a lab-based career [rather than a field-based one.]" Finally, I got so sick of him that I told him, "Look, I promise you that I am going to walk. Next time I come to this clinic I am going to look for you, and I am going to have my daughter in my arms and I am going to show her to you. Look at me, doctor, I am a scientist, just like you. You did your part but you know what? Let God do His." Then, he said, "So you believe in God?" And I said, "Yes. I am a scientist, just like you, but I believe in God." And he said, "You better keep on believing because that is the only thing that will lift you up from that bed." And I said, "I know you have to do your job and fill out a form that says that you did therapy. But please do me a favor—next time you come, just sit quietly. If you want, I will sign agreeing that you did the therapy, but it is better if you keep quiet." "Yes, ma'am, we will do that then," he said. And it went like that. He would come and sit in the chair by the corner, he would write some things and bring a book and read. After one hour he would say, "Goodbye, have a good day."

The psychiatrist would talk to Verónica's mom for help, showing his concern that Verónica should put her feet on the ground [a metaphor which means to confront reality]. But Verónica's mom would add to his frustration by building on the metaphor: "My daughter is indeed going to put her feet on the ground when she walks again."

One day, the woman in charge of cleaning the hospital room asked Verónica's guests—Miguel, both of their mothers, and Natalia—to wait outside. Then, they heard Verónica yell. They rushed in and asked her what was going on and Verónica said, "I can move my right foot." She asked Miguel's mom to lift the sheet and they all saw that the foot was moving a little bit. They hugged and cried. When they told the doctor, he said that it was just an involuntary reflex and nothing else. Despite his skepticism, he ordered electrode therapy. Mónica, the therapist, came every day. Verónica said, "I just moved and moved and moved my foot because I thought, oh God, if I stop moving it, it might not move again."

Even though they all appreciated the care Verónica received at this hospital, they did not think it was the best medical care available. And then their money ran out. Miguel's mom started to inquire about the kind of services Verónica was entitled to as a student at La Nacional. The answer was care at El San Juan and El Materno. Going from the individual rooms of the clinic, equipped with TV and private bathrooms, to the large communal wards and poorly painted walls of El San Juan was "really terrible." She was first transferred to the rehabilitation clinic, the San Lucas Pavilion, which had a women's ward and a men's ward. "People [there] were in really terrible conditions. The day I arrived at El San Juan was the only day I really felt defeated." At San Lucas, therapies were central, but they were not the sort of individual, intimate care offered at the private clinics. The therapist, who moved in a kind of assembly line from one bed to the next, "was brutal" in his handling of his patients' bodies. Suddenly, "I had a threatened miscarriage. I was only twenty-five weeks pregnant." They found that Verónica's skull wound, which had been caused by one of the pickup truck rods, was badly infected. She also had a urinary tract infection caused by her lack of sphincter control.

Verónica was transferred to the septic unit at El Materno, where they shaved her hair to treat her wound. At El Materno, everything was different. "It was cool. I remember that the sister and the priest would come every morning and pray. Every morning they would come, talk to me, pray and leave. The social worker would say, 'Whatever you need we will accommodate, because dedicated families like yours deserve everything.'" After the septic unit controlled her infections, she was transferred to the high-risk unit, where she was to complete her pregnancy. She continued with therapy and slowly regained some movement in her arms. At the high-risk unit, pregnant women usually ended up having caesarean sections. Verónica would see these women afterward in pain and think, "Oh God, I don't want that. I want to have a natural birth for my daughter." Verónica would also talk to her daughter and say, "Please baby, have a natural birth because your mommy doesn't have the strength [for a caesarean]." But another urinary tract infection set in and proved very hard to control. No matter what "pregnancy-friendly" antibiotics they gave her, her fever continued to rise. She was thirty-seven weeks pregnant. The doctors decided to schedule a caesarean section for the next day so that they could start her on stronger antibiotics. When they took Verónica for a presurgery bath at noon the next day, she fainted. The doctors, worried, ordered extra tests and delayed the surgery. The next day, as usual, the priest and the nun visited her at 7 a.m. and at 8 a.m., a resident named Cristian "came and asked me how I was doing. I said that I felt fine but that I felt that my belly was kind of hard, very hard. They checked on me and, surprise, my water had broken and I was already 7 centimeters dilated. So, he said, we have to start labor."

At 9 a.m. everybody arrived, including both mothers, Miguel, and a crowd of friends from La Nacional. At around 11 a.m., they gave Verónica Pitocin and her contractions grew stronger. Miguel reminded her to breathe, and when she said it hurt, a doctor checked and said, "You are already delivering." They transferred her very quickly to a stretcher and rolled her down the hallway but they weren't sure where to go: natural deliveries were on the third floor and caesarean sections on the fourth. Around the hospital, word spread that Verónica was in labor. People who finished the morning shift stayed to see what was happening. It seemed impossible that Verónica would have a natural delivery. Besides, everybody knew that she was just eight months into her pregnancy. Sister Emita, who had arrived to check on Verónica, followed the crowd. Once in the delivery room, no doctor wanted to help with the unexpected complications of a quadriplegic and infected woman's natural birth. Finally, two female gynecologists stepped up. Verónica remembered a big crowd inside the delivery room. When the doctor told her to push, she replied, "What do you mean push?" "Strongly," the doctor said. "'With what sort of strength?' I replied." One of the nurses pushed on her belly "and I tried as much as I could and my daughter was born."

The moment the baby was born, at 1:14 p.m. after that last push, Verónica found herself in a sitting position on the delivery bed. "It might have been all the strength. I am not sure. I felt something like electricity running through my body. My legs moved, everything moved. They [the doctors and nurses] had the baby in their arms and they looked at me and asked me, 'Are you sitting?' I said, 'Yes, I am!' That was absolutely crazy, we all cried." After the doctor received the baby, she gave her to Sister Emita, "who sat with her in a chair. I am guessing she prayed for her. She would look at her and pray." At 2450 grams and 48 centimeters, "María," the name they finally chose, "was very pretty, with a head full of hair," Verónica remembered.

Given the many complications during the pregnancy, María was put in an incubator for observation. Seven days later, a worker from the clinical lab was washing a white sterilization tray and saw an image in the tray that resembled a face. When Sister Emita returned from buying flowers for the upcoming mass to celebrate the annunciation,[14] someone told her that the administrator was looking for her. She asked me "Sister, what do you see there?" And I say, "Yes, I can see a face." Sister Emita was recognizing the Virgin Mary's face but, following the instruction of prudence that the church conveys in those moments,[15] she wanted to avoid fanatic interpretations; "You have to respect and follow what people see, not what you see." Sister Emita called Father Adriano and he, as well, said he saw a face. He also said that if people believed it was Virgin Mary, then it was.

The next day, Sister Emita and Father Adriano paid a morning visit to Verónica. Father Adriano told her "the Virgin appeared [in a tray and She is] at the chapel, ask her with faith to help you stand up from that bed." Verónica wanted to go and see her, but Father Adriano suggested that she should just pray with faith. However, Sister Emita, who according to Verónica was more of a "partner in crime," told her to ask her relatives to help her to the chapel, where she could see the tray. When Natalia and Miguel arrived, they wheeled Verónica to the chapel. Verónica grabbed the tray and started to cry inconsolably. According to Miguel's mother, the Holy Spirit touched her.[16] "Sister Emita told me to ask her with faith and that is what I did. I asked the 'virgencita' to stand me up, so that I could raise my daughter."

The following day, María was discharged to the care of Verónica's parents. Verónica started to feel a stronger and stronger desire to walk, to leave the hospital and be with her daughter. Natalia remembered one day when she arrived and found Cristian, the resident, trying to console Verónica as she wept, "I don't want to be in this chair, in this bed, I am tired of being here, I want to stand up because I have to see my daughter grow, I want to carry her, I want to educate her." "So," Cristian told her, "why don't you stand up?" And Verónica said, "And if I fall?" "Then we help you back up," Natalia interjected. From that moment, they were committed to getting Verónica back on her feet. One day, Miguel said, "Let's make you stand." At first Verónica refused, but slowly Miguel convinced her to try. They decided to wait for both their mothers and for Natalia. Once everybody was there, they inclined the bed to a sitting position, held Verónica, and moved her to the side of the bed. When they pushed her up to her feet, she remained still and stiff. Everybody was helping, even the security guard, who held the wheelchair behind Verónica in case she needed it. Miguel dropped to the floor and started to bend her knees and move her legs little by little. "I did three little steps that first day," Verónica remembered. Everybody at the hospital soon knew that Verónica "had walked."

Verónica was transferred back to the rehabilitation ward at El San Juan, the San Lucas Pavilion where she slowly continued improving. She was soon able to feed herself without making a big mess, and then, with a great deal of effort, she managed to move herself from the bed to the wheelchair. Therapies at San Lucas were intense, which was good, according to Verónica. The downside was that they were very strict about visiting times and had no considerations for privacy or dignity: showering consisted of being naked in front of everybody while "a man hosed you down with cold water." They allowed María to visit only twice a week, "which was good and bad," according to Verónica. "Bad because I didn't get to see her and good because from that moment on I just got down to business" so that she could leave the hospital as soon as possible. She spent most of the time at the physical therapy studio, even meeting Miguel there at night to do extra exercises. For Mother's Day, Verónica received a special permit to go home for the weekend to celebrate. Three weeks later, she was transferred to the outpatient rehabilitation program, where she had thrice-weekly appointments. With forearm crutches and a very slow, unstable gait, Verónica walked out of the hospital.

One of the first things Verónica did at home was ask Miguel to help her to the university to apply for readmission. Once readmitted, she traveled there by bus; it took her forty minutes to walk from the campus entrance to her department's building. In the beginning, she would fall dramatically along the way. She would bring María in the stroller, which served well as walking therapy. Six months later was the time that the neurosurgeon had mentioned for the wires that secured the rib bone to the vertebrae of her neck to be removed. She scheduled the appointment with Dr. Fonseca, the neurosurgeon who performed the operation at the private clinic. Dr. Fonseca said he had put those wires there to help her be in a wheelchair and not to help her walk, which was scientifically and medically impossible. He said he would not operate on her again because he was afraid of what could happen. Disappointed, Verónica then told Miguel, "Let's find the psychiatrist." María was already six months old and she was "very chubby, very pretty. I was carrying her in my arms and I knocked [at the psychiatrist's door]. He opened the door and turned white. The only thing he managed to say was, 'I'm sorry, I don't have time to see you.' Then he closed the door."

WHAT WAS THE MIRACLE? Was it that Verónica, Natalia, and María survived the accident? Was it that Verónica was able to walk after a medullar section, the fact that even with that injury and further pregnancy complications she was able to deliver a full-term and healthy baby vaginally? Was it that Verónica never lost faith or strength? Was it the apparition of the Virgin Mary?

Medical miracles and Marian apparitions are most often described in different terms. Religious readings of medical miracles concentrate on the blessings bestowed upon one individual life and on the remarkable powers of that healing act. In such faith-based miracles, like charismatic healing, the person's life changes dramatically from one moment to the next.[17] Verónica's body doesn't fit the image of a faith-based miracle, in which all wounds are healed and the body shows no marks of the past; Verónica's body shows permanent signs of her long journey. Verónica loved dancing and playing guitar and sports, and she regrets not being able to do any of those activities anymore. She still has some minor finger contractures, lack of feeling in one of her fingers, a slow and somewhat unstable gait, and occasional urinary incontinence, all of which make her, at times, feel down. Her body proves that this medical miracle, or rather, this miracle that defeated medicine, was not a full change from injury to health, from bodily manifestations of physical injury to full normality, from living with pain to being pain free. And yet, miraculously, she is able to walk, have a job she is passionate about, to care for her daughter and watch her grow and depart for college.

Verónica's medical miracle at El Materno joined individual strength, determination, and faith with a larger community of loving family members, friends, and care professionals who also showed strength, determination, and faith. Verónica and her family think humbly of faith and perseverance as forces that everybody has, and they think that the many prayers from many people from different religious affiliations helped in achieving their final and desired outcome. When Verónica was at the hospital, she would ask everybody, from all kinds of religious affiliations, to "pray," "preach," or "meditate" for her. In her hometown, they offered a mass for the two sisters after the accident and, afterward, everybody was praying for her, like a chain of prayers. Since her first days at the private clinic, her uncle's wife would go daily to sit by her and pray for her health for several hours. Miguel's mom, a very spiritual person, would also invite people to her home to meditate and pray. So, was the Virgin responding only to Verónica's strength and faith or to the many people from different religions who got involved in praying for her health and recovery?

In Marian apparitions, academic efforts concentrate on understanding the role of the person who "sees" the vision and the role of the "community" in interpreting and validating the apparition.[18] Decoding the message the Virgin wants to convey is an important part of understanding why she decides to appear in particular times and places, and to particular groups of people. The miracle, for Verónica, was not that the Virgin Mary appeared but that she appeared precisely at the time and place María was born. In addition, Verónica thinks that the apparition was not itself the miracle but a testament to everything they had gone through, including their faith and their strength. As in other apparitions, by taking an earthly presence, the Virgin Mary furthers people's faith.[19] However, for Verónica, the miracle made sense in the context of their lives, in which she and her family were always surrounded by many people willing to help and to pray. In a sense, the Virgin Mary did not appear to bring the miracle about but, as Miguel's mother argued, to testify to the miracles that spiritual strength can accomplish. The miracle is, in a sense, a tale of persistence and faith that defied a medical absolute. The Virgin Mary did not appear to show a path but, it seems, to help in a longer history that made the impossible possible. Perhaps, just like the nuns at El Materno, she listened and came to help.

The Virgin, according to many of the workers, came to show them that it was possible to fight for the hospital and to keep it open. The Virgin appeared in 1998, five years after the market-based health care reform was signed and a year after the end of what was called "the transitioning period," in which the government still transferred some resources to public hospitals like El Materno—and after which, hospitals had to compete in "equal" economic terms with all the other health care institutions. In the minds of the professors, Sister Emita, and other workers, the hospital's painful end reflects a failure of faith. Religious forces operate only when people have faith and thus, so it seems, in the absence of faith, spiritual forces could do little to stop the advances of neoliberalism. Nonetheless, according to some workers' interpretations, neoliberalism came with other religious beliefs: particularly the Protestant Christianity competing for the Catholic faithful across Latin America. While people still tried many strategies to keep El Materno afloat and remain truthful to its epistemology of care, not even the appearance of the Virgin Mary was able to contain what was about to happen.

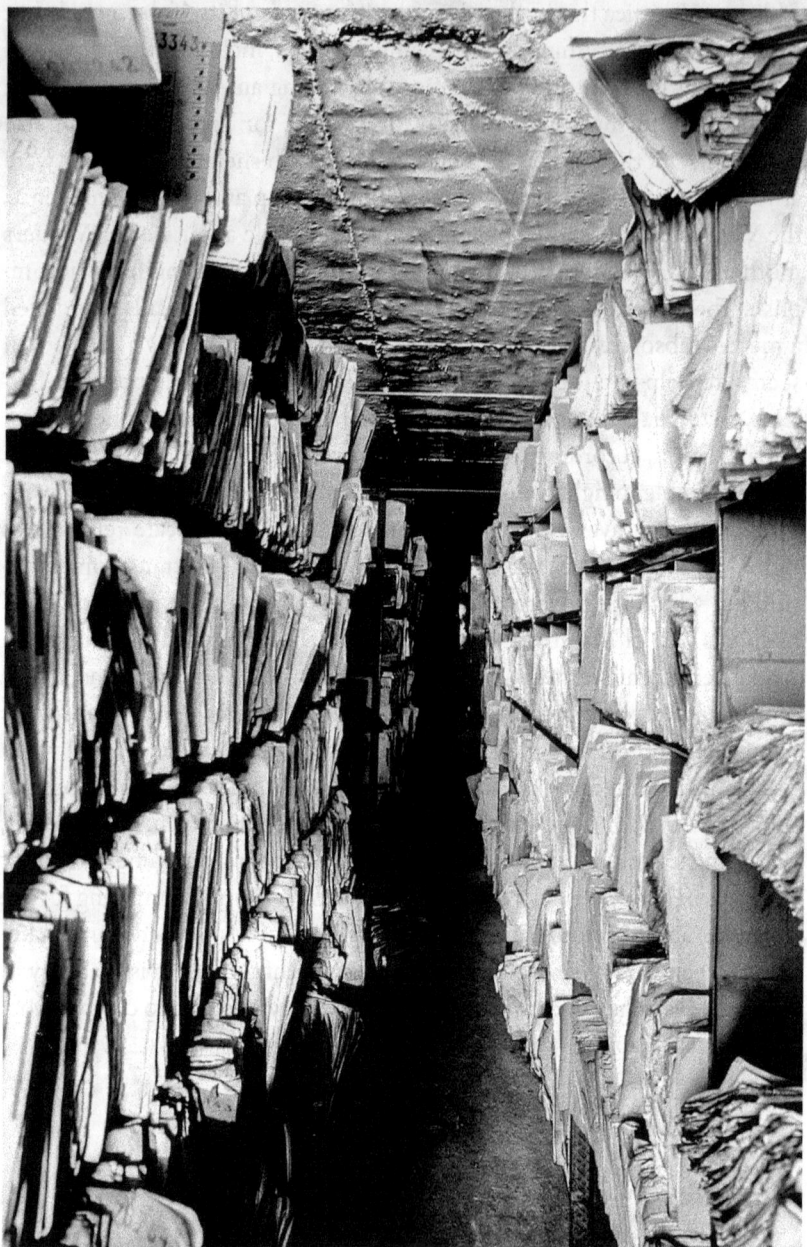

FIGURE 4.1. Photo "Archivo muerto" [Dead archive] from Series Postcards. (Courtesy of the artist: María Elvira Escallón. Technique: color photography.)

CHAPTER 4. Hospital Budgets before and
after Neoliberalism

This chapter offers a narrative of hospital administration before and after the market-based health care reform. It shows how health care administration depends on the conditions set up by corporate governance in health care (i.e., how health care market forces shape the state),[1] by the historical legacies of the institutions, and by health care workers' efforts to manage the tensions between their epistemology of care and market logics. It is clear that hospital budgets were dramatically transformed by neoliberalism. Hospitals moved from a welfare-like system, in which money was transferred directly from the state, to a market-competition model. This chapter argues that more important than an economic discussion of administrators and administrative strategies is an understanding of how the state-hospitals-health triad is transformed. If before neoliberalism, people's health was considered an important expense that ensured a mass of healthy workers who benefited the economy, laissez-faire ideology acknowledged that health was a special kind of commodity that needed some sort of a "regulated market."[2] As a commodity, ideas of social insurance or publicly financed health care institutions had to be abolished. Rather, health as an individual commodity had to be understood as an individual responsibility to be purchased in a "regulated" insurance market.[3] "To individuals according to their insurance policy": meant to individuals according to their purchasing capacity.

This new moral formula of neoliberalism has translated into inequalities, "stupid deaths," and denied and delayed care.[4] In contrast, neoliberal government officials and international sectors used to applaud Colombia for increasing the rate of people "insured" by individual insurance. According to a highly criticized WHO analysis driven by the neoliberal ideologues of health care reform, Colombia's market-based health care systems ranked among the best in the world. More recently, insurance companies' corruption scandals and the catastrophic situation of health care in the country have led government officials and international organizations to stop presenting Colombian health care reform as a global standard.

This chapter illustrates how, for hospital administrators, the reform meant extraneous efforts to transform their structure and administration to match for-profit logics, as well as confronting the medical auditors' attempts to deny hospital bills. Many administrators were unable to do so—not because they lacked administrative knowledge, but because of the transformation of health from a social service seen as part of the post–World War II social pact between government, industry, and workers to an individual commodity. Such transformation of health ideology instigated transformations in medical care and in the institutional culture of health care institutions. The winners, measured not in terms of health standards but in terms of financial profit, were the insurance companies. For insurance companies' administrators, the goal was to reduce payments through denials or price negotiations in order to increase profit margins.[5] Health care institutions that are surviving and "prospering" are those that were established under, or could be transformed for, the new for-profit logics of neoliberalism. These institutions see health care primarily as a business and increase their income through the new forms of labor exploitation that neoliberalism introduced.[6] Hence, the questions we are asking should not be about techniques of administration. Hospitals like El Materno—with its particular epistemology of care, its respect for workers' contracts, and its lack of political relationships with insurance companies—were destined to be outcompeted. This chapter shows how El Materno did not surrender to a for-profit mentality that disregarded quality of care and employee well-being and how workers and administrators tried their hardest to remain economically viable.

Catholic missions were crucial for the colonial expansion of the Spanish crown in Latin America and elsewhere. In addition to their evangelical work, Catholic priests and nuns ran schools, asylums, and hospitals, including the Colombian San Juan de Dios Hospital complex. This complex is dated alternatively to 1564, when the first private religious hospital was built, and 1635, when the San Juan monastic order took over the hospital's administration and made it public. The secularization and modernization of medicine in Europe during the seventeenth and eighteenth centuries also brought transformations to colonial hospitals, where religious figures progressively took on more administrative and social roles while physicians led clinical and scientific activities. Colombian independence (in 1810) reinforced the idea of building a secular republic with secular hospitals, even though Catholicism remained entrenched in the country's everyday social, political, and economic life.

The republic's first president and liberator, Simón Bolívar, signed a decree in 1828 regulating El San Juan's budget reports and administerial functions in order to help the hospital gain more independence from the church.[7] With the creation of La Universidad Nacional's Medical School in 1867 and the signing of decrees that named the school as the hospital's academic regent, the powerful health care delivery/education relationship between El San Juan and La Nacional emerged.[8] The Beneficencia de Cundinamarca (Beneficence of the Cundinamarca Province), created in 1869, became the hospital's third wheel as the new administrative unit that promised to further the separation between the state and the church in dealing with disadvantaged and vulnerable groups. Despite the efforts to move the hospital from a charity model, in which the poor and the destitute were seen as deservers of religious pity, to a beneficence model in which they, as citizens, were part of the state's responsibility, charity and religion remained ingrained in the hospital's institutional culture until El San Juan's final collapse in 2000.[9]

The idea of having a hospital with three "wheels" (health/education/administration) proved to be very complicated. El San Juan and its maternity unit, El Materno,[10] served simultaneously as the city's, province's, and nation's major public hospitals for the poor; as a teaching facility for La Nacional's physicians in training; and as a "welfare" unit administered by the Beneficence of the province.[11] The lack of clear hospital policies and financial plans, the pervasiveness of a charity-oriented institutional culture, and the lack of clarity about the roles of the city and province Health Care Secretariats, the Ministry of Health, the National University, and the Beneficence—all this contributed to a juridical ambiguity and an amalgam of administrative problems that never found adequate resolution. Historically, all of these groups have claimed the hospital complex's successes; no one accepts responsibility for its failures.[12]

From 1950 to 1975 Bogotá grew from 600,000 to 3.5 million inhabitants. In that twenty-five-year period, the only new clinic built was San Pedro Claver, a part of the Institute of Social Security (ISS) health care network.[13] Other city hospitals administered by the Beneficence suffered from severe organizational and budgetary difficulties, verging on bankruptcy. But while most public city hospitals were able to generate income by running some hospital sections as private services (called *pensionados*), more than 90 percent of the care at El San Juan and El Materno continued to be charity based.[14] To make things worse, a 1974 tax reform eliminating important incentives for donations reduced the hospitals' resources.[15] Even after efforts in the 1970s to organize city hospitals according to geographic areas, El San Juan was responsible for the largest coverage area of the city; on top of that responsibility, a large majority of its patients (around 60 percent) came from different city areas and from other regions of the country.[16] El San Juan was the only health center in the city that offered free twenty-four-hour emergency care; El Materno was the only free-of-charge maternity hospital in the city. Their budgets were never adequate, and the hospitals started to be perceived by the government as a problem with no solution. Spatial and budgetary crises became increasingly frequent.

In light of the difficult working conditions at the hospitals and influenced by events throughout Latin American and the world, overworked and underpaid workers at the hospitals, clinics, and sanatoriums of Bogotá and Cundinamarca unionized. On International Workers' Day (May 1) 1972, SINTRAHOSCLISAS (clinics and hospitals workers' union) was created and affiliated with the country's main union, CUT (Central Unitaria de Trabajadores, or Unified Workers Central). If the hospitals' operating budgets—with contributions from the Beneficence, the Ministry of Health, the city, alcohol taxes, and income out of direct provision of services—was already insufficient, the union made things worse. After SINTRAHOSCLISAS started to protect workers' benefits and demand respect for their condition as workers, the politics around the allocation and flow of resources became even tenser.

The Beneficence shifted from a nineteenth-century administrative solution to, in the later twentieth century, one of the hospital's main obstacles to confronting its consecutive and overlapping crises. The Beneficence remained as "intermediary" in the highly politicized management of the hospitals' resources. Throughout the 1970s the budget deficit was such that hospitals were not able to pay providers and personnel, and many services started to reduce their operating capacity, delaying nonurgent clinical activities and ending certain treatments altogether. By 1975 El San Juan was described as having "insufficient capacity to treat the sick, with obsolete infrastructure, undefined organizational structure and constant budgetary crisis."[17] The hospital also lacked "autonomy to manage resources, [and] suffered from administrative intermediation from the Beneficence whose workings depended on political relationships."[18] As personnel grew demoralized, the quality of care and research was compromised. As a result, the hospital's public image began to suffer.[19]

The year 1975 was particularly important. The reorganization of the country's health care around a national health system[20] resulted in further discussions about the hospital's ambiguous legal, economic, and religious character. On July 21, 1976, the Assembly of the Cundinamarca Province signed an agreement turning the administration of the hospital over to the National University, while a commission established by the office of the university president studied the wisdom of this restructuring. The findings indicated that the hospital lacked clear accounting and budgeting. Even basic information such as hospitalization periods, costs incurred per activity, or income generated was lacking. Purchase and supplies were handled without clear time frames or via petty cash. Providers were not paid on time, financial obligations were not being met, purchase estimates were inflated, and there was an irrational use of supplies because the hospitals lacked any mechanisms for distributing medications. Personnel and technical equipment were lagging; existing equipment was not maintained. The commission concluded that the university had the human and technical competency to run the hospital but that the administrative and financial chaos was likely to result in service failures that could harm the university's prestige. The commission advised against the university assuming administrative responsibility for the hospital and suggested it be returned to the directorship body of La Beneficencia.[21]

But the Beneficence refused to take the hospital back. The Ministry of Health was forced to intervene and establish administrative control in the figure of the "director/auditor"—a position intended as temporary, but which became permanent. Under this administration, the hospital was incorporated into the new National Health System as a public tertiary care hospital. Although the Beneficence had surrendered administrative control over the hospital administration, it continued to own hospital land and buildings, and created a foundation to oversee and take care of these assets. At the same time, La Nacional wanted to keep its presence as the hospital's academic and scientific regent and to find legal mechanisms to enforce and extend original hospital/university agreements.

A final "resolution" came during 1978 and 1979, when the central government signed decrees that linked the origins of the hospital to the 1564 private hospital.[22] These decrees considered that the sixteenth-century institution was in effect a private foundation, regulated by civil law. Under new statutes, the Foundation San Juan de Dios could be administered by the Foundation's directorial body. In this process, La Nacional was excluded from the hospital's directorship body for the first time. The Foundation's body was composed of representatives from the Ministry of Health, the province governor's office, the mayor's office, Bogotá's archbishop, the Beneficence, and the president's office.[23] Legally, the shared directorship granted the hospital autonomy from the Beneficence's political handling. However, the charitable orientation and the chaotic possession by a multiplicity of government and religious actors continued to cause problems. Given that no agreement concerning the new hospital director was reached, the Ministry kept the "director/auditor" position until 1991. Even though the Foundation structure and the intervention by the Ministry helped the hospital survive one of its major institutional crises, administrative confusion, juridical ambiguity, workers' protests, and economic deficits—primarily due to the practice of cutting promised budgets—continued to be the norm throughout the eighties and early nineties.

Even though its funding responsibilities continued throughout the Foundation/Ministry's intervention, the Beneficence stopped making its promised contributions. The central government and the city government resentfully covered parts of the gap when doing so was politically expedient. It became the norm for hospitals to receive only a portion—sometimes half, but often less—of the operating budget approved at the beginning of the year. Both budget allocations and budget flows throughout the year were variable, irregular, and arbitrary, dependent as they were on the political and interpersonal skills of each hospital auditor/director. In addition, as part of the Foundation, the hospitals lacked a clear legal status; all their functions were concentrated in the director/auditor, who quickly become a figure with too much power and too little regulation.[24]

Since the 1980s the figure of a private foundation administering public hospitals had been disputed as, at best, inconvenient, and at worst, illegal. For example, workers who signed contracts after 1979 were considered public employees in terms of salaries, but private Foundation employees in terms of benefits.[25] In 2005, after El San Juan had closed, El San Juan workers prepared a legal document demanding the nullification of the 1978 and 1979 presidential decrees that had created the Foundation. Using extensive archival and juridical research, the workers argued that El San Juan was a public hospital and that the national government had bought and/or received the lands where the hospital was located as donations under a mandate to provide public health care services.[26] The Colombian Council of State agreed with their petition. The supporting documents that El San Juan workers had carefully compiled clarified that, since the El San Juan hospital complex was public in character and belonged to the province, the national government did not have the legal standing to alter its juridical nature. The nullification of such decrees meant that the hospital complex was run from 1979 to 2005 under an illegal figure, the Foundation.

IN 1975 CARLOS PACHECO was an intern. He remembers that after the university's failed attempt to gain full control of the hospital, El San Juan remained open under the Ministry of Health's director/auditor figure. Many of La Nacional's clinical residency programs, however, remained closed for several years. When Carlos returned to Bogotá a couple of years later after finishing his rural and working as the director of a small provincial hospital, new cohorts for plastic surgery had not been announced. He was forced either to postpone his residency training in plastic surgery or to choose between the gynecology and pediatrics residency programs offered at El Materno, which remained open throughout the crisis. He decided on the National University's residency program in gynecology offered at El Materno and passed the admission test. Unfortunately, the Ministry of Health signed a decree ending interns' and residents' traditional status as hospital employees. This meant that, even though he had received a small salary during his internship year from 1975 to 1976, he was not going to receive any payment during his 1979–1982 residency years.

The decades-long lack of investment in El Materno showed itself not just in the hospital's infrastructure and equipment (see also chapters 1 and 2); the building itself was also collapsing. Carlos remembered that when he started his residency in 1979, the state of the hospital was such that "there were rats and you would go with the stretcher and, suddenly, a wheel would get stuck in one of the holes of the wooden floors." He remembered that the conflict between workers and the administration was intense. Rumors started to circulate, saying that El Materno might close. In 1981 the university mobilized in response, arguing that the hospital needed resources rather than threats. Other sectors started to echo this call.

At such critical moments, hospital directors and the dean of the medical school usually started moving their political alliances to get help. When Carlos was finishing his residency in 1982, he remembered how some personal connections between then-director of El Materno, Luis Eduardo Santamaría, and the country's president, Belisario Betancur (both from the conservative party), flipped the threats of closure into funds for remodeling El Materno. El Materno returned for one year to the seventh and eighth floors of the main general hospital at El San Juan, where Carlos finished his residency. "I am not sure how they managed to do it," Carlos said, "but they got to avoid going through the city and the province [for funding], and they got the central state to transfer resources directly to the hospital out of tax collection." With those resources, they did what they could to transform the building into a modern facility. "They knocked down the wood floors and put cement plates [and tiles]." Metal and plastic panels served to create semiprivate rooms in which six to eight patients shared a bathroom.

Despite being guests in El San Juan's main building, professors and employees kept their institutional identity as El Materno and considered strategies to help the hospital move forward. KMC "inventors" Edgar Rey and Héctor Martínez, along with Santiago Currea and other highly respected La Nacional professors, created the nonprofit Fundación Vivir, which was tasked with the effort to raise funds to improve human and technical services in neonatology. Fundación Vivir also promoted academic, social, and cultural events, including bringing renowned speakers to continuing education courses attended by national and international health care workers.[27] Workers and professors worried that despite everybody's efforts, El Materno's reopening could be thwarted by politics. When the remodeling surpassed estimated costs, workers agreed to use resources from their pension fund to cover the gap.[28] Happily, in February 1984 El Materno returned to its remodeled building on the east side of 10th Avenue and 1st South Street.

ROSALBA BERNAL ENDED UP staying on as the head nurse chief of surgery after that first day in 1985 filled with religious, clinical, and interpersonal emotions (described in chapter 3). As head nurse in charge of the surgery department, part of her role was to organize personnel activities and make sure that materials and equipment were always ready. She was immediately dissatisfied.

> There were some glass cabinets in the surgery storage area in which you could find everything you needed, which was worth a fortune. You'd take out three dozen catgut [sterile suture] sizes 1, 2, 3, and you'd leave the extras [accessible so that people could use them]. But people would just grab them! I thought, "What is going on?" For example, I would take out the sutures [from storage], and there were fifteen deliveries and I would leave out three dozen chromic catgut 3-0, and they would be all gone. "How come? Where is the rest?" So, I figured we had to start counting and, like any good nurse, I started keeping track. I have always liked statistics, so I would say "for fifteen deliveries you spend at most two dozen chromic catgut, then for so many caesarean sections you need about such and such amount." So, I started to leave just the right amount out for the surgical assistants and I would ask them to help control the flow of equipment.

To facilitate control, Rosalba came up with a log system.

This kind of proper administration translated into many changes that benefited everybody. Dr. Sandoval, the physician in charge of surgery, became a close ally and friend in Rosalba's effort to straighten things up. She asked him to help her calculate the necessary amount of medications and materials per shift, and he grew interested in what seemed like the unit's overuse of materials. "So I started to do my statistics and I would be able to say, here [in this shift, looking at her logbook] this much went missing. And I started to send reports to the hospital administration with a copy to the director. I figured they needed to know because that storage area accounted for so much money."

But this reliance on Rosalba's personal initiative meant that there was still no institutional culture of hospital administration. The hospital still lacked function manuals, and inventories were separate from purchasing needs.[29] Hoping to improve the surgical unit's organization, Rosalba became friends with the surgical assistants [in charge of handling the surgical tools to the surgeon]. She learned about conflicts between surgical assistants and nurses, and about corrupt practices that led to mismanagement and uneven distribution of residents' work duties. "Imagine, if at one point we had run out of sutures or if I had no sutures in storage for a caesarean, then you had to tell the mothers, 'If you want a caesarean, here is the list [of needed materials], and they [mothers/family members] had to find the suture. And a group of residents [there were three groups corresponding to three shifts] would come and say, we can do the surgery because we have sutures." Rosalba connected the dots. When she took out sutures from the storage and they all disappeared, it was not that people were stealing them; it was that the residents "saved them." "That was how things worked. So you had some groups that operated because they had sutures, and other groups that didn't." Rosalba felt that no action was being taken, whether from waste, disorganization, corruption, or a combination. But nurses' professional skills include hospital administration; her hard work slowly paid off and surgery developed from a poorly managed unit into a well-oiled administrative machine.

Rosalba was about to complete one year as head nurse chief of surgery when the hospital director's secretary asked her to meet with the director. The nurse assistant who had been acting as the chief of pharmacy was going to retire, and the hospital was looking for a professional nurse to take over that role. The director wanted Rosalba to be the new chief of pharmacy. Apparently, Rosalba was already on his radar because of her success in the surgery department and the high esteem in which Dr. Sandoval held her. In the director's mind, Rosalba was the one to handle pharmacy—the unit, strictly supervised by the National Audit Office, that managed the largest sum of the hospital's operating budget. "For me, pharmacy opened the doors to all [clinical] services [of the hospital]. Since we [pharmacy] would fill purchasing orders, I could go and exert control." Again, she started to ask questions about the unit's disorganization; for example, "How come the hospital ran out of Pitocin and the services still have some reserves?" Using the same strategies that were successful during her time as chief of surgery, she managed, little by little, to create an organizational system for purchases and demands and to change the institutional culture of scarcity that led to staff hoarding medications and supplies.

BY TRADITION, DIRECTORS OF El San Juan and El Materno were proposed by La Nacional's School of Medicine and ratified without objections. Being the director of either hospital certainly conferred intellectual and clinical prestige, but it also meant having to deal with the many administrative and political tensions between the hospital and other institutions, between the hospital and the medical school, and inside the hospital. In 1987 Santamaría, the former director of El Materno who successfully oversaw the remodeling of El Materno, was acting as vice-dean of the medical school. He called Carlos Pacheco, who by that time had been an attending gynecologist at El Materno and a professor at La Nacional for five years, and told him that the school administration needed to make him director of El Materno. "I told him, 'No profe, I don't want that job, and tons of people here do want that job. I don't want problems and there are other people with more tradition and prestige.'" After careful consideration and after receiving advice from a close friend, Carlos decided to accept the directorship role. Among his reasons for accepting was the fact that not doing so could cause him personal and institutional difficulties. "I stayed for four years. I had to deal with everything before Law 100 [the 1993 market-based reform.] I was the director from 1988 until 1992."

Being director of El Materno at that time was not an easy task. A small percentage of the hospital budget came from beer taxes, but over 90 percent came from national taxes transferred to the province and the city, which worsened the hospital's political dependency. Internally, El Materno's organizational and administrative chaos was all-encompassing. The institution didn't have an official organization chart, instruction manuals, internal regulations, or any comprehensive disciplinary regime. Hiring was disorderly; some employees were hired through public processes and others just with interviews. A single worker could simultaneously have permanent and temporary contracts, a separate hiring resolution, and an appointment as a public employee from an entity without legal autonomy.[30]

Despite Carlos's seriousness, Rosalba said that "Dr. Pacheco was an incredibly visionary man, an excellent administrator, and very organized." One of the first things that shocked Carlos was when he saw how very expensive supplies were left unused and allowed to expire. About a year and a half before he became the director, he witnessed how a senior professor requested a certain number of supplies, and given his seniority and prestige other purchases were stopped to please him. "There was not even a purchasing body," he commented. While Carlos started to bring new administrative ideas to the hospital, Rosalba was starting to systematize the pharmacy. Using large graph notebooks, she filled in by hand a column of medications, then entered in rows the amounts used by each department, and the purchases per day, week, and month. "It was rudimentary because it was pre-computer," she said, but working with clinical services and the pharmacy team (a female secretary and a man who handled the storage), the hospital started, under Rosalba, to count how many medications came into the hospital and how many were being used. Rosalba also remembered that despite having its own director/auditor, El Materno's pharmacy and other purchasing departments depended on El San Juan's pharmacy and purchasing departments. This was a problem for El Materno: "If we run out of something, it could turn into a tragedy. So, we started to develop relationships with people from [El San Juan]." The goal was to head off emergencies by establishing an interdepartmental barter system based on personal connections. If they knew that a given department at El San Juan had a medication El Materno needed, then Rosalba or Carlos would ask, "'Who is friends with so and so?,' and the barter would begin. 'If you give me a Ketalar I can give you a Fentanyl,' and things like that," Rosalba remembered.

Carlos commented that part of the inconvenience of having to run things through El San Juan's administrative structure was that it made El Materno vulnerable to the personalities and politics of El San Juan. Petitions, purchases, transfers, and the like could go smoothly, or they might be delayed without explanation. "If we needed something, the director of supplies would say, 'I can give you this part [of the order] but not this part.'" El San Juan's dysfunction, according to Carlos,

became part of our problem. [El Materno's auditor from the National Audit Office] was a young man and we became friends. He was always very cordial and respectful and realized what we were trying to do [straightening things up at the hospital]. I let him participate in many messy [meetings and negotiations] so that he would see how things were. In exchange he would say, "Whatever you need, Doctor, you just need to ask me." One day I said to him, "I am so fed up with this situation. Isn't there a way to get us out of San Juan [in terms of separating the administration]? You know they could take us down with them [given that their economic crisis was much bigger than El Materno's]. Without the autonomy to manage our own budget, there was no way [to get out of the crisis]." "I have the solution," he told me. "There is a resolution [signed in 1980] that separates the administration [between San Juan and El Materno] and hasn't been made effective." "No kidding," I said. "Please help me." And he did. The administration of El Materno became effectively independent of El San Juan.

Carlos turned to Rosalba with a clear goal: "Let's finish cleaning up this mess." Rosalba remembered how "he had an Apple [computer] in his office [the hospital's first computer] and he would call me in. I would bring my graph notebooks and he would tell me, 'Jefe [head nurse], let's systematize.'" Early in the morning and every afternoon, Rosalba entered her data:

"I was able to tell him how much of X, Y, and Z [medications] the hospital was using per month." Little by little, planning and managing budgets began to make sense to Rosalba and Carlos. The approved hospital budget for the year had to cover all activities; by counting, they could assess how they were doing in terms of spending, identify where savings could be made, and predict what supplies might run out. And systematization did not just allow for improvements in purchasing and budgetary decision-making; clinical events were detected, such as the higher budgetary demands in "harvesting months." Harvesting months included September, when babies conceived during end-of-year holidays were born, and April, when women who had undergone clandestine abortions of holiday pregnancies arrived at the hospital with infections and were hospitalized in the septic ward. The new systematization allowed Carlos and Rosalba to see those peaks in terms of budgetary demands and to establish a purchasing plan so that the hospital had enough supplies for the increased need for deliveries and caesareans in September and antibiotics in April.

Other unpredictable but important data were also uncovered. Rosalba says, "I would find two prescriptions for Rhesuman [the brand-name vaccine offered to the mother in case of mother-child Rh incompatibility] six months apart in the same patient's chart." This meant that young women with spontaneous abortions had not gotten the vaccine because they couldn't afford to purchase it at their local pharmacies; the practice was to treat the abortion and its complications then send the women home with the Rhesuman prescription rather than administering the vaccine at the hospital. Rosalba showed Carlos that finding and from that moment on, Rhesuman, cost notwithstanding, became a medication that "we had to have at El Materno."

Usually, toward the end of the year, around September or October, the hospital budgets ran out or began to see delays caused by the government's deprioritizing of health and social spending. Carlos and Rosalba's new administrative organization allowed them to plan better and offer stronger arguments for extemporary allocations or specific petitions. Nonetheless, approved resources often failed to materialize in full, and even the promised annual budgets often corresponded to only 70 percent of projected expenses. When budgets ran out or were delayed, the politicking began. The director had to persuade the Beneficence, the Ministry of Health, or the health care secretariat of the city to give the hospital extra resources. Carlos remembered that around the time the budget ran out—usually in September or October—the hospital found itself in a race against time as supplies dwindled. Carlos remembered "fights [with the authorities] so that additions to the budget [would] materialize." Rosalba remembered that Carlos, despite being a very good manager, did not have strong political connections. He would work his way up the chain, calling the city's health care secretariat and saying, "Dr. So-and-so, we have gloves for barely a month, maybe for fifteen days." If the health care secretariat would not provide the funds, Carlos would call the Minister. If the Minister would not respond to Carlos's phone calls, he would tell the Minister's secretary, "Could you please tell the Minister that I am going to call all the media and tell them that he won't speak to me, and that I will be forced to close the biggest maternity hospital in Bogotá." That usually worked.

IN 1990 MOTHER TERESA VECINO announced that she was retiring from her duties as chief of nursing of El Materno and returning to Spain. Discussions began about her potential replacement. As in other nursing departments previously run by nuns, professional nurses were taking over, appointed according to their seniority and experience. Carlos Pacheco had to find Mother Teresa's replacement. He knew that the sisters and Mother Teresa in particular managed the very complicated interpersonal relationships of the nursing department. He respected Mother Teresa "because of her history, because of everything she meant for the hospital. I had met her as a student." So he asked her, "Mother, who should we name as your replacement? There were several [professional nurse] candidates, some with very strong personalities [who could handle conflicts]." But Mother Teresa had her own perception of what being a good chief of nursing was about. For example, there was a head nurse in pediatrics who was very organized and an excellent worker, but she was very harsh, and Mother Teresa told Carlos, "No, that head nurse cannot be chief of nursing because she is inflexible. She will just create a big mess for you. So I said, 'You know her better, Mother.' And she said, 'We need someone more flexible, someone who understands, who listens, who talks to people.' I asked her, 'Tell me, Mother—who?' And she said, 'Rosalba Bernal.'"

Rosalba remembered that Mother Teresa left everything very well organized: upcoming personnel shifts, vacations, extra shifts and *compensatorios*, extra paid days that the union negotiated for workers who worked nights, weekends, or holidays. "Daughter," Mother Teresa told Rosalba, "you already know how things work." Besides, Carlos said, "Rosalba already knew all the people from all services [through her role as chief of pharmacy] and people liked her and respected her." Moreover, Carlos trusted in one of Rosalba's strongest skills: "She was good at talking to people."

As chief of nursing, Rosalba continued her administrative duties but was able to return to working with patients and to implement what she had learned in the humanization courses. Her initiatives included organizing sensitivity trainings, screening films, and encouraging better patient interactions, all to build a stronger El Materno family (see chapter 3). But she had to fight to break out of Mother Teresa's image, given that some people expected her to continue Mother Teresa's many pastoral activities with patients, families, and workers. For example, people started to expect that, just like Mother Teresa had, Rosalba would distribute the morning coffee. A staff member from the nutrition department left her twenty pounds of coffee each morning to distribute to all services. She refused. "I don't have to distribute coffee just because Mother Teresa did. I took over her job duties, but I did not put on [a nun's] habit, so stop bugging me." Just like the hospital director, the chief of nursing had to handle many interpersonal conflicts stemming from the colonial legacy of seeing the nurse's role as a religious one.

The chief of nursing was also at the center of many political tensions with the union, dealing with workers who were corrupt or who did not fulfill their duties. Because Mother Teresa's empathy had resulted in people taking advantage of her, Rosalba found herself working to separate professional responsibilities from personal problems. Rosalba started to change the way workers saw their responsibility to El Materno through subtle and difficult negotiations. Workers were protected by the union; their contracts and agreements had to be respected. Negotiation was the limit of what the hospital could do without embarking on a direct confrontation with the union. The understanding was that workers who were not working all their contracted hours could work their pending hours at other times. Negotiations were tough, but "If you had things straight and organized, you just showed them [how things worked and how they were supposed to work]," Rosalba concluded. As Mother Teresa predicted, Rosalba did not come in with a hostile attitude; her goal was to make things work. Rosalba's managerial approach, in her own words, was, "I can give you a break but not a pass." Negotiating meant ensuring that all workers worked all their contracted hours, even if that meant adjusting schedules when people arrived late.

Rosalba Bernal joked that she retained the 6 a.m. to 11 p.m. schedule of her first rural day. As chief of nursing, she would arrive very early and, depending on the needs of the department and of the different units, participate in the morning, noon, afternoon, and night shift-change meetings. By staying at the hospital for so long, she got to know all the workers very well and developed friendships with employees in all departments on all shifts. She often brought her work home, programming and planning in her off hours. In her mind, and in all the workers' minds, it was clear that Rosalba was available 24/7. "I would receive a call at 3 a.m., saying, 'Jefe, the union is going to take over the hospital. They are planning to come and close the hospital at 5 a.m.'" Everybody knew that the union carried a lot of power inside the hospital. The phone calls came from "close allies," appreciative workers who were crucial to Rosalba's supervisory success, particularly when it came to interceding with union members so that their planned activities would not interfere with the provision of clinical services. At other times, she would be alerted to ongoing corruption. Dealing with corruption was challenging. There were threats, and some workers took advantage of union protections to cover their poor performance; expelling a unionized employee was virtually impossible.

But "there were some really beautiful people," Rosalba remembered, "people who would call me and say, 'Jefe, someone is planning to steal the transductor [a very expensive piece of ultrasound equipment] tonight.' Because things like that were true. People knew who the mafias were and my workers [those under her supervision]," were sometimes involved. She would show up at the beginning of the shift when the theft was planned and announce as loudly as she could, "I am coming to tell everybody that tonight someone is going to steal the transductor. So watch out. If you need to go to the bathroom, you take it with you or tell someone to keep an eye on it. Keep your eyes open, because it was announced that it was going to happen tonight."

IN 1992 CONGRESS WAS debating social security reforms. Initially, pensions and health care were treated separately, but the government ordered Congress to present a unified reform.[31] Even though it had not yet passed, it was clear that the social security reform was going to promote a market-based scenario in which direct government funding of public hospitals was going to end; all health care institutions would have to sell their services. The way the health care market would operate was up for debate, but the logic of self-financing public institutions had already begun with a 1990 decentralization law that ended direct financial transfers from the central state. It was also clear that insurance companies would act as intermediaries in the administration of health care resources, as had been already proposed for pension reforms. Questions remained as to the system's technical specifics, but it was clear that the reform was intended to end the understanding of social security and public hospitals as resources for, respectively, "workers" and "poor people." In the new scheme, every person was to be treated as a customer[32] with a health plan based on individual insurance. Health care professionals, La Nacional professors, and the hospitals workers started to discuss the implications of the reform. Health care services, whether public, from the social security sector, or private (whether small medical offices or larger health care centers), would have to offer their services via insurance companies. Thus, direct payments from patients would stop and the insurance companies would become the center of the system: they would receive all the system's resources, sell individual insurance to the country's population, and sign contract services with providers.[33]

Inside El Materno, Carlos and Rosalba's administrative and organizational efforts had paid off; the usual deficit was now replaced by financial equilibrium. In Carlos's mind, however, it was very hard for the hospital to get past that barrier—to make a profit. The "financial equilibrium," Carlos corrected, had to be put into quotes, because often the money was just enough to pay providers and salaries, but not to cover employee benefits. For Rosalba, "it was not as if we could start charging poor mothers for their care either." The scenario after the market reform seemed tense but manageable. According to Rosalba, if the expected contracts with the insurance companies were followed and they paid their bills on time, the hospital could be self-sustainable and survive the transition from administering resources transferred from the government to administering resources from contracts with insurance companies.

ALTHOUGH IT IS VERY hard to prove, directors of El Materno and people in other directorship roles think that the costs associated with union benefits, which had grown, constituted a real threat to confronting the new market-based scenario. Rosalba Bernal remembered, "Working at El Materno was just like working in heaven." Rosalba explained the case of nurse assistants, particularly those who worked night shifts, which brought them extra benefits such as each hour being paid at a higher rate than their regular day time (usually at a 1.5 rate) and having "*compensatorios*," meaning paid days after a certain amount of night shifts in which workers were entitled to a paid "rest" day. Being able to claim several compensatorios a month and pay for shifts to coworkers allowed workers to have multiple jobs, which made up for the fact that, benefits aside, salaries were not very high.

However, some people took advantage of the hospital's flexibility, the administrative chaos, and the lack of supervision. During night shifts, Rosalba explained, "people would take turns with one group sleeping from 12 to 3 a.m. and the other from 3 to 6 a.m." One particular night she had to go to the hospital in the middle of the night, at 1 a.m., and she discovered what the hospital was like during those hours. Rosalba found workers in pajamas and with hair rollers. "In a shift at a service where there were supposed to be seven workers, [I would find only three] because the other four were sleeping. Mothers would be without blankets while nurse assistants lay on three or four blankets on the floor, with pillows and everything. They kept everything [for sleeping at night] in the fake ceiling. You could lift up the ceiling panels and find everything there." She connected the dots once more: "The majority of the accidents that patients suffered happened between 1 and 3 a.m., why? [Since nurses were not doing their jobs,] a mother would fall down, another would bleed out. In pediatrics where there were supposed to be five nurses for twenty babies, there were just one or two [in the ward], so that's why babies would be hypoglycemic [given that they were not being fed as regularly as they should in wards with adequate nurse to child ratio]." Rosalba's descriptions show how the pervasiveness of a charity-based care (in which the poor are seen as deservers of pity and expected to be grateful for any care they receive) mixed problematically with tensions around health care labor, corruption, and lack of motivation, resulting in very low quality of care both in clinical and human terms.

"I called the union and said, 'For the love of God, don't do that [meaning compromising the quality of care of the patients by doing a poor job], our mothers are dying.'" After Rosalba addressed the situation, "some people hated me but some others loved me. I don't think I was unfair, I was fair in many respects. I also made mistakes; [you improve] as you grow up too [meaning that she was young and over the years learned better ways to handle many aspects of her role]. There were also people who allowed me to say I am sorry. All of that amounted to a beautiful experience. But," Rosalba continued as if analyzing how that part of the history of the hospital is relevant for future developments and the eventual closure, "we were not generous with the hospital. And you pay in life for your wrongdoings."

WHEN SANTIAGO CURREA BECAME the director/auditor of El Materno at the end of 1995, the public image of the hospital was as ambivalent as it had ever been. El Materno was going through very difficult years but was still considered an amazing institution. On the one hand, the flow of resources worsened and workers' demands for improvements in their working conditions and salaries frequently turned into strikes. On the other hand, El Materno celebrated its fiftieth anniversary, the government recognized El San Juan and El Materno as the "most important hospital complex in the country," and more of their subaltern health innovations were receiving national and international recognition.[34] Multiple social mobilizations fought for the hospital, asserting its importance and demanded that the government support it.

Santiago had served in administrative roles as director of academics and director of the pediatrics department at the medical school. Directing the hospital was particularly challenging given the new market-based scenario imposed by the 1993 health care reform. About those years, he remembered that "it was a progressive discovery of how things worked. I had never studied administration. And besides, it was not as if you could study how the model worked anywhere [in the world] because it was a novel health care regime. So, you had to discover it along the way."[35] While newly created health care institutions with a clear for-profit mission could more easily learn how the system worked and figure out how to make it work for their own interests, older hospitals had to work with older infrastructural, legal, and cultural structures. Profound transformations meant massive layoffs, exploitation of workers by changing their working conditions, and hiring new personnel, who were more easily overexploited. Adapting older hospitals to the new scenario could also mean compromising quality of care by offering only profitable services, establishing mechanisms to be able to charge even poor patients for services, or incurring significant debts to transform equipment and infrastructure in order to be as competitive as newer facilities. Depending on the particular hospital, the administration was able to enforce a combination of drastic changes and minor adaptations; if that was impossible, they had to find creative ways to become competitive. The system, it was clear, had been created with the interests of insurance companies in mind, and the companies rapidly began to see exponential profits.[36] Hospitals and other health care providers were forced to adjust or left to fail. Just a few years after the new system began, many hospitals around the country had already gone bankrupt.

While Carlos and Rosalba created and improved the hospital's administrative logics before the new law, Santiago worked to transform several aspects of the institution's everyday dynamics. Nonetheless, it was clear that the hospital was not going to compromise its quality of care or trample on workers' labor rights, as was becoming the norm at other institutions. The newly created system had stratified the population into two sectors: those with "enough" income from formal or informal jobs, who were required to purchase insurance, and those classified by the state as "very poor," who were entitled to receive subsidized insurance. Subsidies, however, had to be factored into the state budgetary plans for future years; not all of those classified as "very poor" would be able to receive insurance immediately. Thus, in practice, a third sector of the very poor and as-yet-unclassified uninsured would continue to receive care directly at public health care institutions, entities that would charge the health care secretariats for all the services provided. El Materno could, in theory, either sign contracts with insurance companies providing either contributory or subsidiary plans or bill the health care secretariat for treating the uninsured.

While the previous system was organized around private, social security, and public sectors, the new system formalized class-based inequalities in health; the "contributory regime" (i.e., the health care plan of those who were forced to purchase insurance because their income was above the poverty line) covered much more care than did the "subsidiary regime" (i.e., the health care plan of those who received subsidized insurance).[37] Expense-related health inequalities increased as poor people with unstable or informal jobs who had previously resorted to "free of charge" care in public health care networks were now forced to purchase insurance out of meager, irregular incomes. An important additional change was that all groups (contributory, subsidiary, and uninsured) were required to pay out-of-pocket expenses in the form of recovery cost quotas such as copays.[38] Furthermore, the different plans managed different tariffs for each specific service provided and each material used[39]; each health care institution negotiated different prices with the insurance companies. This created a poorly regulated and unsupervised market; eventually, the allowed insurance companies were implicated in one of the most scandalous embezzlement cases known in Colombian history.

Despite the worrying financial uncertainties, Santiago described the two years he served as director/auditor of El Materno, from late 1995 until the beginning of 1998, as "a very beautiful experience." In institutions with so much history, such as El Materno, directors had to face the new challenges imposed by the market-based system while still addressing the many old and unresolved challenges. The first task that greeted him as director was a formal complaint from all El Materno's chiefs of administrative services against the hospital. "They were right," Santiago said. "For a series of juridical reasons, their salaries were undervalued in comparison with their [same-level] peers from El San Juan; their complaint was justified. We solved that through a dialogue process, a conversation in which they resigned retroactivity in their aspirations and the hospital agreed to level off their salaries. It ended up as a dual contribution: both on their part and on the part of the hospital."

Besides this formal complaint, he got to negotiate with the union and sign a new *convención colectiva* (collective agreement). "When people ask me how I did that," Santiago said, "I always say that it was with respect." Being a leftist militant himself—even since medical school when his politics got him expelled but the students' social movement got him readmitted—Santiago sympathized with many of the issues raised by the union. He had served as representative of medical school professors and participated in the country's medical union but now, as director, he had to change sides and represent the institutional interests. His political history, however, made him popular with the workers, which facilitated the compromise. The dialogue, nonetheless, "was very, very tough," he remembered. Still, unlike previous attempts to sit down and negotiate with the workers' union, which usually resulted in strikes and back-and-forth insults, this time "was very rewarding."

The language and communication used in the negotiations were crucial "because it shared that we were in a process based on respect. The new collective agreement was signed in 1996 [and] meant that workers were resigning very important [labor] rights." But part of the negotiation also entailed recognizing something that was very important for workers' struggles: temporary contracts. So as part of the negotiations, workers agreed to give up pensions and retroactive *cesantías*[40] in exchange for contracts for all temporary workers, even those who were not tenured. It was a good deal for both sides. Temporary workers had never imagined formalizing their status as hospital employees, because the hospital's financial situation made hiring more personnel impossible. "So, the final outcome," Santiago concluded, "was really gratifying." The idea was that as older workers retired, a process projected to conclude around 2015, all hospital workers would eventually be operating under the new agreement, which was closer to the stipulations included in new labor reforms and meant important reductions in the budget through savings on benefits.

Nonetheless, Santiago indicated that this negotiation process and final agreement were dramatically different from the norm at other institutions undergoing promarket transformations. At El Materno "there was not wiping out, there was not massive firing, nothing was taken away from anybody." Quite the contrary, he said. "We reached an equilibrium [between what the workers conceded and what the institution agreed to] so that people could work in dignified conditions." Temporary work—a key part of labor flexibility—sometimes meant meager payment, job instability, and a lack of benefits—all indignities of a sort that pushes people to reconfigure their lives in conditions of precarity.[41] But along with the acknowledgment of how difficult it was to work under temporary contracts and renouncing to large benefits of the past came "a significant increase in workers' salaries; otherwise the union would not have agreed." Salary increases were a central part of the negotiations. Both the unions and the government knew that employee salaries at El San Juan and El Materno were lower than the standard at other health care institutions. "We had the worst salary level in . . . the country," Santiago said. The salary increase was seen as irresponsible in certain circles, but "we were not exceeding the accepted wages for other health care workers in the country at similar levels. [And the salary increase] allowed workers to regain some purchasing power." Santiago concluded that new employee agreements meant that the hospital could move ahead knowing its financial situation would progressively improve as workers protected under the old agreement retired; too, the improved conditions for new workers would allow the hospital to "face the market competition."

In terms of competition, however, the hospital began to see fewer patients as referrals, equipment, and care capacity dwindled. A solution came in the form of a financial plan based on investment of a US$3.6 million financial sector loan. In two years, "neonatology went from having 75 hospital beds to 135. We became the largest neonatology center in the country—I would venture to say, on the whole continent." Over a single weekend, the influx of money resulted in massive investments in "infrastructure and technology," Santiago remembered. "The biggest chunk was allocated to technology. Just as an example, we went from having four refurbished ventilators—artificial respirators for little ones with serious respiratory problems—to thirty-two, none older than two years. We also obtained some new ones but the majority, so as to make the most out of the [loan] money, were not the newest models. We bought equipment for mammograms, we renewed the very old X-ray system. We obtained several sonogram machines, portable X-ray machines. We got to open pediatric endoscopy with some very fine German equipment." The purchasing plan was carefully constructed, with savings in some areas (such as incubators) leaving money for necessary purchases (such as the equipment needed for pediatric endoscopy or mammograms). In conclusion, Santiago said, "We brought the hospital into the twentieth century, [leveling the field so that we could] play on equal footing."

In the new system, securing contracts required offering adequate technology, different procedures, and updated equipment. The most important part of this financial project was a new agreement with the ISS (Institute of Social Security), which had been legally transformed into an insurance company and was allowed to keep its former insured population and expand its "customer base."[42] The ISS agreed to send all neonatal care to El Materno. Thanks to that agreement and the newly completed remodel of El Materno, daily life at the hospital felt like old times: intensely busy, with many patients. "Productivity increased 239 percent," Santiago remembered. "In 1997 the hospital received and paid $1.2 million [out of the loan agreement] with estimated budget projections of close to $100 thousand per month. All of this was important to certify the financial projections; otherwise we would not have received the loan."

For Santiago and the staff, the new agreement, the contract with the ISS, and the signing of formal contracts to temporary workers were steps in the right direction. Rosalba, still acting as chief of nursing, remembered, however, that those decisions generated tensions between Currea and several people, including the hospital administrator, who disagreed with the plan. Some resigned in protest. With so many patients, remembered Rosalba, "We went back to the old Materno [with more patients than beds]. So we started to put pressure on [the patients and employees]; it was really bad. 'Please help lift up that mom and sit her in that chair so that we can accommodate another one.'" Rosalba indicated that the high volume required speedy turnovers—faster than they were used to or comfortable with. "You had to say, 'I am so sorry, but you have been discharged. Look, you can sit in that chair and hold the baby [while the paperwork was finalized]. We were almost kicking them out of beds, stretchers, delivery rooms. It was that horrible, that inhumane, because the ISS overextended us. On top of that, the ISS did not pay us for any of that."

ISS'S LACK OF PAYMENT was part of a larger problem; a culture had developed throughout the health care system of refusing to pay hospital bills. This was a symptom not only of the complex and bureaucratic insurance administration introduced by the reform but of the corruption through which insurance companies ensured their own exponential profits. After that first year of contract with the ISS, which was "successful" in that the flow of patients and bills was high, but a bitter failure in quality of care and the payment of those bills, the contract was cut in half.

About this time, head nurse Sonia Parra remembered how "we fought the biggest fight to keep the hospital functioning." She remembered that Dr. Ariel Ruíz was appointed as the new director. He "called the most senior head nurses—there were five of us—and he sent us to the Universidad Nacional and he asked us to learn [about the intricacies of hospital administration under the new system]. What an extremely bright man. He sent us to learn for free and then, after that, he handed each of us a service and told us: 'Now you are the owner of such area and you are the owner of such area,' as functional units were called. I was in charge of admissions, which meant that I had to verify everybody's rights." The "rights verifier" was a new figure imposed by the insurance-based administrative structure of the new system. The rights verifier assessed all patient documentation regarding insurance payments, insurance coverage, and institutional contracts. Once individuals had the right kind of insurance (meaning that their insurance company had an active contract with the hospital), were up to date on their monthly payments, had a copy of their ID, and paid the required "recovery cost quota," then they could "get in" to the hospital.[43]

Talking about Ariel Ruíz's strategy to have them trained and then run the different functional units, Sonia recalled him saying, "This is it. We have to do it and we have to play by the rules. I am delegating the responsibility for making this work [in terms of improving the administration of services], because we need to get out of this [financial crisis]." Playing by the rules meant doing things "as the health care secretariat wanted us to," Sonia remembered. The health care secretariat, the main contractor with the hospital, served the poor population, primarily the uninsured. As the ISS contract dwindled, more and more patients from the health care secretariat had to fill the hospital, and those bills had to be paid. Nonetheless, further negotiations were required to make sure that bills were in fact paid, since refusals were common from state institutions. Sonia remembered that contracts and payments between hospitals and insurers were hammered out, and how prices were subject to negotiations within the range of government-authorized tariffs.[44]

Shifting from directing clinical services to managing functional units felt like "a big responsibility," Sonia Parra said. "[Dr. Ruíz] sold us the idea very well. Now that I think about it, he got to do what nobody had been able to do in my whole life, which was to make me think all the time about El Materno. For instance, I would be on a trip or running errands and I had my cell phone on and received calls: 'Jefe [head nurse], can we do this [admit a patient or conduct a given procedure that will be covered and paid without problems]?' Yes, no, do it this way, do it that way. I was living just to make this work." Unlike other health institutions in which administration and bills represented a form of "savage capitalism" characterized by refusals to see patients,[45] El Materno tried to remain faithful to its history by refusing to deny high-quality and comprehensive care to anyone, particularly the poor. Besides, Sonia explained that the country's legislation grants special protection to minors and pregnant woman, which El Materno workers became very skilled at using both to protect patients from being refused care and to justify bills and prevent payment refusals by insurers. This was a difference that she saw clearly between the way she and head nurse Elsa Myriam Pedraza, in charge of hospitalizations, handled administrative problems. Sonia explained, "She had to deal with billing for hospitalized patients, while I had to deal with billing for patients who were just coming in [admissions]." Each area had different challenges. But in admissions, an initial approval almost always warranted the full payment of the bill since all treatment resulted from the initial admitting diagnosis, while for outpatient and hospitalizations, new procedures and treatment plans were generally considered additions that needed to be authorized, or else the bill would be unpaid.

BY THE TIME CARLOS PACHECO was asked to serve as director/auditor of El Materno for a second term in 1998, after Ariel Ruíz's short term, he had finished a master's degree in administration. "I always liked administration," he said, and with his newly acquired management tools, he had a better understanding of the hospital's catastrophic situation. The biggest problem in Carlos's mind was that the hospital had increased its personnel from 750 to 1300 workers, which generated additional costs in terms of benefits and nonfiscal mandatory payments that the hospital, after the significant reduction in the ISS contract, was unable to pay. Carlos remembered that in 1998 the hospital debt was "around $4 million.[46] I had to renegotiate with the laboratories; there were accounts receivable that amounted to around US$1 million. Ninety percent of our bills were glossed (*glosadas*)," returned to the hospital by insurance companies for "technical" problems; these bills needed to be fixed and resubmitted before the payment could be authorized. Ninety percent of those glossed bills came from the ISS—still the hospital's main contract. The scenario was very bleak. Carlos remembered, "Accounts receivable of around 1 million, unpaid bills with providers of around 4 million and non-fiscal payments of around 4 million. When I came back [as director/auditor for the second time], salaries were delayed by three months already."

"One of the first things I did" in his second term "was to meet with the team and start to analyze what had happened, why the financial hole grew so big." The ISS had fallen into its own financial crisis after Law 100 and continued to reduce the number of patients sent to El Materno. "So we started to fight with the health care secretariat to compensate for the difference [in projected number of patients,] but the secretariat also had to attend to other hospitals. . . . Finally, we got the secretariat to approve a minimum quota of $250 thousand, [which gave the hospital] some chance at profitability."

Each service was trying its best to "produce" as much income as possible. Internal competition strategies were created to encourage employees to work to solve the crisis. Head nurse Sonia remembered when Dr. Pacheco and Dr. Mercado (working now as subdirector) sat down with the five head nurses who had received training in administration during Ariel Ruíz's term as director and who were now in charge of the different functional units. Sonia recalled how Carlos would start comparing numbers: "At the unit where Consuelo Forero worked, which was exclusive hospitalization, he would say, so many patients and produced this much. Then, Elsa would say in my unit we had this many and produced this much, and then the other one, and then it was my turn and I would ask, 'And how much did I produce? I am not even there because I am admissions, so I am not part of this. So, what does this mean that I only produce glosses?'" Sonia's comments were meant to be humorous given that people knew that her unit, admissions, was the one that funneled into the other services; the final bills from other units also reflected her efforts. These meetings allowed for a managerial assessment of the hospital. Indeed, as Sonia said,

> In these meetings we could see how much we were producing and what our improvements in production were. It was a time in which the idea was to give as much as we could to the hospital. It generated great satisfaction, because we got to do things we never thought we could. We also trained a lot of people. We brought the knowledge we gained at the university and people got encouraged and started to further their studies. Jaqueline, for instance, she was a nurse assistant and she studied and became the chief of the billing department. We

all started to have a different vision and we started to sell the idea [of the hospital as part of a health market] to others; we emphasized that we needed to work around that [idea] and that we had to work hard. So, Jaqueline was the chief of billing and we all worked around her. That was a really wonderful time.

After experiencing many crises and many defeats, being able to "play the game" on the system's own terms and make progress did feel like a step toward a promising future. Whether working directly with patients or assuming administrative tasks, people started to see progress and morale lifted. "Even without [extra profits], if we saw that this was starting to work, it was worth the effort. We started to get the money, we got to start receiving payments monthly and that was very gratifying," Sonia remembered. Still, their goal was to combine a new managerial mentality in which the hospital generated enough income to operate, and, ideally, some profits, while maintaining an ethos of comprehensive and high-quality care in which nobody was refused treatment. "For us, it was impossible to refuse care, we could not conceive of such idea in our minds," remembered Sonia. To solve this paradoxical situation between market impositions and their impossibility of refusing care, they implemented new strategies. "You always tried to find a way. In the meantime, bring her in and lay her down. Then, call the insurance and ask them what they are going to do." They learned strategies to deal with the new systemic "fight over patients" that happened as insurance companies tried to balance their contracts with different institutions while preferentially funneling insured clients to more profitable contracts at health institutions with cheaper rates or those vertically integrated into their systems. Sonia remembered, "We learned that the best thing was to call the insurer and inform them that a patient had arrived here [at El Materno]. For example, if the woman was supposed to go to San Rafael [another hospital] but she ended up here. They [the other hospital] would be furious and say, 'But we told her [the woman] that she should come here.' El Materno workers would say, 'Yes, but we cannot send her there, if you want you can come and pick her up,'" which they knew implied incurring extra costs in ambulance transport. Too, usually because of the patients' medical characteristics, whether a high-risk pregnancy or a woman already in labor, it was not clear that they would be able to transfer her on time or without creating additional risks to her health. Sonia remembered,

We learned that things were handled like that, by fighting over patients. But then, the problem became the medical auditors. They would be sent [by the insurer] to check the medical record and they would write down "paid under medical auditing"—a threat that we had done some extra things and they were not going to pay. But they always ended up paying because it is very hard to fight a woman's bills, especially a pregnant woman with a newborn. They ended up paying for everything even if they initially refused. For instance, they would say you ended up using five extra syringes. Then, ok, [we would say,] don't pay that but the rest you must. You negotiate and you end up with your bill paid, which does not happen in general medicine.

Another management tool Carlos implemented was revisiting purchasing to cut down expenses. Also since there were so many workers with so few patients, it became the norm that workers would go to the hospital to "knit or sell stuff around." He remembered, Toxemia had twenty-five beds and only half of those were occupied. When a patient arrived, only one [nurse out of two] would work. High-risk pregnancies had twenty-five beds and only twelve patients, so what did I do? Since this [toxemia] is high risk and this [another high-risk ward] is too, we will just keep one open full speed and close the other one. That meant that people who had to work were working 100 percent or 90 percent." And "whenever a worker finished his/her contract, that was it, [we didn't renew any contracts] until we went back to having around seven hundred workers."

Rosalba also remembered how "we started to 'fix' problems." Fixing problems meant turning monetary hospital debts into "paid" time. Given that vacations, compensatory days, and *primas* (1.5 salaries per year paid as extra benefits according to collective agreements) could be calculated as a percentage of salary, "We started to fix it. If they [the administration] owed us primas, vacations, compensatory days, then we turned all that into days [meaning "paid" leaves]." This did not mean that workers received any money, but they were free to use that time searching for work or working shifts somewhere else, while keeping their job at El Materno. Hence, some of the hospital monetary debt with its workers was "paid" with time. This strategy also meant that fewer workers showed up for hospital shifts, which helped to manage the chaos of too many workers and too few patients.

About six months after Carlos came back as director/auditor, "we were able, once again, to pay salaries on time," he remembered. Besides improving billing and building a collegial competition among services, Carlos remembered that another important aspect of balancing the budget was when "I asked Manuel Mercado, the hospital subdirector, to gather all the nurses who were just wandering around and get them to begin working in one room [by the director's office] going through each of the hospital bills, one by one." Checking bills meant going through every glossed bill that the insurance companies or the health care secretariat had returned for alleged technical problems and fixing the problems. "It was a group of around fifteen nurses and they were all very happy doing that because the [economic] problem affected them," Carlos remembered.

Dealing with glossed bills meant, according to Rosalba, jumping through many "stupid" hoops imposed by the new system's medical auditing culture. "Imagine, the contract [with a given insurance, the health care secretariat, or the ISS] said that the needle was [caliber] 21 and you used [caliber] 20." She remembered how the "[external auditors] would come and say, "How come this [procedure] was done horizontal rather than oblique?" I would say, 'Dear God, what is this?' And then, they would say, 'Because of that we are not going to pay you.'" This meant that the bill could be deemed unpayable and glossed; such clinically and medically irrelevant mismatches (which, in addition, both needles cost the same for both hospital and insurance) were used as administratively insurmountable obstacles. "Law 100 made us do that [enforcing an auditing culture]. We had to put pressure on the nurses, please write down everything, because you had to bill for everything, for everything." This meant not only "accounting" for everything used in the clinical records and other paperwork required for billing but also managing resources incredibly carefully to avoid waste.

Fixing the billing problems meant identifying minute issues in bills or supporting documents flagged by the auditors: a missing signature, a missing procedure code, a medical order in the clinical record without a corresponding annotation in the nurse's log proving that the medication had been given or the procedure performed. People from the billing department were terrific in that effort, Rosalba remembered. When the team of "bill-fixing" nurses found problems, they would work to solve them, which might be as simple as entering a missing code but could also involve searching for a given physician to sign the form, or finding the misplaced form and refiling it in order to resubmit the bill for another round of auditing. The hospital started to embrace a "medical auditing culture"[47] in which they not only fixed the problems but also learned which problems were likely. As such, new conversations and training happened at the hospital, educating everybody on the administrative demands, like double-checking that all the forms complied with the expected auditing.

Thus, part of the new auditing culture meant being careful with the amount and type of material and the specific techniques used, since for any given procedure the hospital could bill only the precise amount of materials and medications under the correct code and for the specific technique named in the contract. Medical costs had been broken into an array of minuscule components of bills. While given procedures had a billing code and an agreed-upon cost, every aspect of the operation also had separate billed codes: a caesarean would include billing for the anesthesiologist's time, the anesthetic, the breathing tube, the gauze, the sutures, and so on. A failure to document and match everything to the contracts' administrative lists could jeopardize particular aspects or even the entirety of the bills.

Through the efforts of the bill-fixing nurses, thousands of glossed bills were fixed and new bills started to be approved. Approved bills, however, were not paid immediately. The system created a convoluted flow of resources, and the insurance companies systematically refused to pay their bills. They also engaged in other illegal practices, such as establishing vertical integration with their own clinics, which harmed the logics of market competition, and denying covered care to their insured population. The result was that hospitals faced a set of challenges: glossed bills and fixed bills that insurance companies still refused to pay. The insurance companies equivocated, arguing that the government owed them money and, cynically, that the business of health insurance was not becoming as lucrative for them as they had anticipated when they started.

The largest bill that was fixed but not paid was that of the ISS. Carlos remembered that after fixing all the ISS's glossed bills, they had an approved but unpaid bill of around US$1.5 million. So, Carlos set up a meeting with the person responsible for payments and walked out of the meeting with the payment authorization for half of the bill. When the money finally entered into the hospital's bank account, it was a huge relief. "I paid providers, I paid pharmaceuticals."

While El Materno was slowly stabilizing its finances, El San Juan's situation began to seem irresolvable. The hegemonic neoliberal mentality in administration led to many proposals that did not make sense to Carlos. "El San Juan's pharmacy department," for example, "was handed over to a third party," he said. And Carlos was asked to do the same with El Materno's pharmacy department. "But why?" Carlos asked. "All insurance companies are doing that and other hospitals are doing that," was the answer. "And so I told them 'no' because I already had the numbers." He explained to them "the only good income at El Materno comes from pharmacy. I get

30 percent out of every single drug because I can bill it for one price, but I can get it for less, plus it allows us to establish control inside the hospital [to make the medications supplies last]. If I give up pharmacy, then that's it [for our financial situation]."

Carlos remembered the first discussions about closing El San Juan and how he voiced his disagreement. At the meetings, there were even discussions about bringing police tanks to evacuate the buildings, as was happening in other newly privatized institutions. El San Juan received its biggest blow in 1999, when the Ministry of Health signed a letter addressed to all health care institutions in the system; the letter prohibited everyone from referring patients to or receiving them from El San Juan. Institutions that failed to comply were threatened with fines.[48] El San Juan had been blockaded. The last remaining patients were transferred to other city hospitals and, soon after, the electric and water companies cut off service. Their workers, however, were not officially fired. After many months of unpaid salaries, many lost their houses. Homeless, some decided to move into El San Juan.[49] At El Materno, the "closing" of El San Juan in 2000 felt apocalyptic.[50]

Despite El San Juan's closure, El Materno continued reorganizing the everyday activities of the new auditing culture, getting bills paid and paying their bills. Their success was significant, bringing in enough resources to pay salaries and reduce debts. At the end of Carlos's second term, in 2001, the hospital was once more in a "stable situation. However, what were we unable to pay? I reduced the providers by about US$1.8 million, but there was still a US$750,000 debt. What couldn't we pay? Nonfiscal contributions [like health insurance and employee pensions]. Money was scarce; everything was scarce. When something ran out, we just had to make purchase and dig ourselves another hole." Carlos created a model to project hospital expenses over time. With this model, he concluded that the existing and accumulating debt in terms of nonfiscal contributions was what made equilibrium impossible under the existing conditions. Nonetheless, there was a path that could lead to future solutions: additional resources, a new employee agreement, and steady contracts would all help deal with the problems imposed by the existing hospital infrastructure, the large staff, and the many malfunctioning parts of the new market-based health care system. Things were not looking good for Manuel Mercado, who became the director when Carlos stepped down. But they were not as bad as they had been. It still seemed that something could be done. Nonetheless, soon after Manuel started his term as director/auditor, the Ministry decided to assign an external auditor in charge of overseeing all the hospital's finances,[51] leaving the hospital director with the mere role of directing the provision of services.

The external auditor, a private firm, was supposed to assess the situation and offer solutions, but it in fact crushed all the preceding efforts to keep the hospital afloat. After charging sizable contracts that were paid out of El Materno's meager resources, the different auditing firms, particularly McGregor, simply concluded that the hospital was in a deep financial crisis. Soon, an additional problem hit El Materno. Not only did ISS stop its contract completely, drastically reducing patients and income, but, spurred on by its own financial crisis, the ISS also went after El Materno for nonpayment of mandatory nonfiscal contributions for employee health. Under Law 100 (1993), all El San Juan and El Materno workers had become "contributors to the system," which meant that they had to end a fund they created to receive care at El San Juan and El Materno. Instead, they were made to pay a portion of their salaries to one of the insurance companies and use that company's health care networks. They had been officially affiliated with the ISS, which had been transformed into a market-based health insurance company. Given El Materno's economic crisis, the hospital had made very irregular and infrequent payments for the workers' health policies, which had two important results. First, when workers and their families were sick, they appeared in the system's computers as in arrears, and the rights verifier would confirm, if they sought care, that they were not "active in the system." Second, the ISS petitioned to seize El Materno's bills to secure the delayed payments.

By 2003, in constant meetings, workers articulated how alarmed they were by the amount of money the different auditing companies were charging and how frustrated they were by useless reports that offered no strategies or alternatives for addressing the obvious conclusion that the hospital had a severe financial problem. It was becoming common for the auditor to refuse to authorize the release of funds for the hospital's minimum operating expenses. It seemed to El Materno staff that McGregor was pushing the hospital in the same direction as El San Juan.

Even though Odilio Méndez had already retired in 2000 after almost thirty years of work as a pathology professor at La Nacional, serving initially at El San Juan and then at El Materno, he started to go back to the hospital to participate in the meetings. According to Odilio, "There was a huge crisis in 2003, and around September, the hospital community [workers and professors] asked me to serve as [the hospital's] representative in mediation with the auditor firm to facilitate the hospital's functioning. Operating expenses were basically frozen. So, we went to talk to McGregor but obviously we [the auditing company and him] had differences."

After this meeting, Odilio Méndez was named as interim director for October and November. In December he was told that he was not going to continue in that role. "But that helped in generating a very interesting movement here [at the hospital]; the El Materno Defense Committee was created, and I was named as its president," he remembered. The committee pushed the Foundation and the Ministry to accept Méndez as director/auditor in 2004 and end the expensive and useless external auditing. He tried a new set of initiatives and strategies to defend the hospital, including a campaign to raise funds and awareness following a symbolic ritual: people stamped a kiss for El Materno in a piece of cloth that would travel through different parts of the city. A certain sense of normalcy was re-established even as the financial situation was worsening and fewer and fewer patients were arriving. Whenever money did come in, bills and delayed salaries were paid.

On March 22, 2005, with Odilio still serving as director/auditor, a legal decision marked a dramatic turn in the hospital's history. When the Colombian Council of State agreed with El San Juan workers and nullified the decrees that had created the Foundation, the hospitals regained their public character, which meant that their administration had to go back to the Beneficence of Cundinamarca, preceded by the governor of the province, Pablo Ardila. The workers' intention was to protect the hospitals and their workers by forcing the government to provide funds. However, Governor Pablo Ardila argued that given El Materno's debt, the lack of resources, and the presence of a health care network adequate to cover the needs of the province in terms of maternity care, if the hospital was returned to his hands, he would liquidate it.[52] His announcement gave rise to a series of political and academic pronouncements in favor of and against his decision. The hospitals, as always in their long history, were at the center of political debates and agendas. Deans of La Nacional's Schools of Medicine, Dentistry, and Nursing produced an open letter signed August 1, 2005, in which they argued that it was criminally ironic that while the governments of Latin America, including Colombia, were creating strategies to improve maternal health and reduce neonatal mortality as a way to comply with the Millennium Development Goals, governmental authorities were threatening the closing of the country's main child and maternity hospital. Both right-wing president Alvaro Uribe, who had introduced Law 100 to Congress when he was a senator, and Bogotá's mayor Luis Eduardo Garzón, elected under a leftist agenda, claimed that they wanted to save the hospital.

Inside the hospital, anxiety about the future and the progressive empty-ing out of the wards felt like a physical and emotional withering that ex-hausted both the building and its people.[53] At that point, they were seven months behind in receiving salaries. Stubbornly, they continued with their commitment to "save the hospital." To stand up to the demoralization and its effects on quality of care, the staff emphasized the importance of hu-manization. To face economic scarcity, they intensified individual sells, collaboration, and donations. They even bought medicines for patients by collecting whatever little they had in their pockets. However, the uncertain future began to be replaced by a sense that the hospital, and with it their life's work, was coming to an end.

CHAPTER 5. Violence and Resistance

There are many accounts of direct political violence exerted against health care workers. Indeed, health care professionals, even though invested in medical neutrality, usually side with social justice fighters, since they understand that health and well-being depend on the social conditions of life. Health care professionals, therefore, might suffer direct attacks or aggressions, primarily in countries undergoing contentious political debates or war.[1] This chapter shows how neoliberalism brings about other kinds of violence to health care professionals. It argues that the labor conditions of the health workforce, the type of health care system, and the overall conditions of society are important political and economic domains. In these domains health care workers play an active role and can be targeted by power structures threatened by their sociopolitical importance.

This chapter helps us understand that in the transformation of the relationship between capitalist interests and health from a welfare structure to a for-profit culture, the destabilization of labor conditions constitutes another form of violence. As a difference from, or a complement to, direct physical attacks, there is a chronicity of violence in which the destruction of workers' labor conditions pairs with the disregard of their rights and contracts, and failed promises. In this chapter we see how violence and time work together to destroy a particular workforce. Workers wither away; their salaries are compromised, their daily work activities are transformed, and their role as health care workers, which represented a comprehensive,

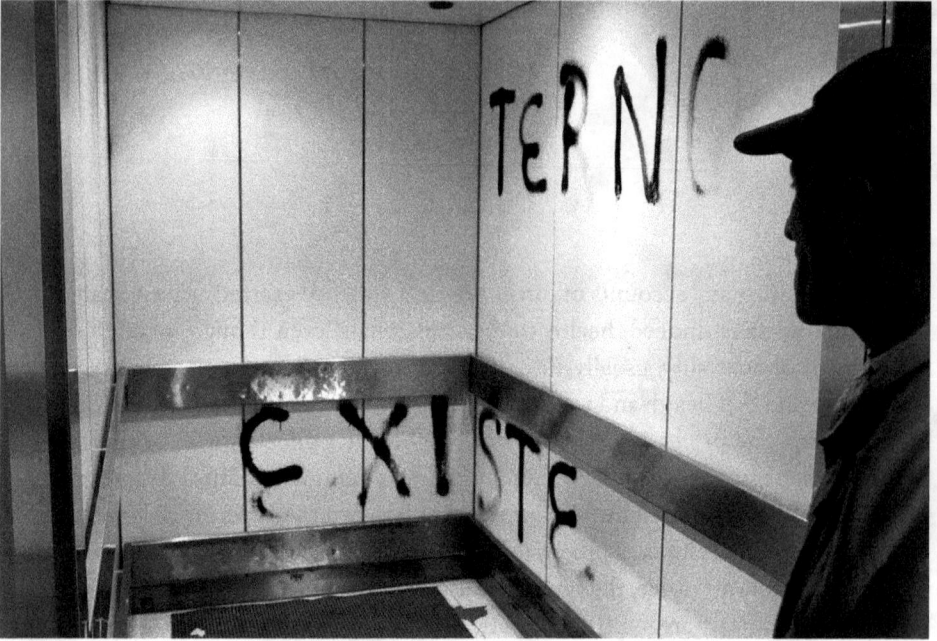

FIGURE 5.1. Photo "Terno Existe." Serie grafitis ["Terno exists." Graffities series]. (Courtesy of Hector Camilo Ruíz Sánchez.)

nonprofit epistemology of care, becomes impossible to maintain. This chronicity of violence acts on the core of human emotions; each individual body, and the collective political body—represented in this case by the El Materno family—is destroyed.

This chapter also shows how throughout such chronic violence and the progressive deterioration of material and emotional conditions, there are moments in which the violence intensifies. In these moments of "acute," "direct," or "visible" violence,[2] the destruction of workers' bodies and emotions accelerates, and their coping skills reach a limit. We will see how all workers, at one time or another, fell apart from the destructive intersection of material violence, emotional violence, and rational incomprehension.[3] Pain and insanity took over the hospital and their lives. Such violence against workers brings us closer to theories of psychosocial trauma, which help us put these workers' experiences of chronic and acute violence in a larger historical, political, and economic context.[4]

Questions, however, remain: Why such violence against these particular workers? and Why did government representatives act so violently, when the workers could have been terminated as they desired, with dignity and with a full recognition of their labor rights? In analyses of violence against political bodies (i.e., groups of people that conform a particular political subjectivity that act within power confrontations), we have to pay attention to what those bodies represent and how the violence directed against them transforms that representation.[5] In this chapter we argue that El Materno workers came to symbolize an epistemology of medical care that threatened the very core ideas of market-based health care systems and the extreme exploitation of the health care workforce that came with neoliberalism. Therefore, their social image was attacked and destroyed by the neoliberal power. To accomplish this, neoliberal power—through legislation, autocratic bureaucrats, and lengthy administrative and political games—attacked the substrate that formed that social image: the workers. True, we will see that there was an instrumental aspect of the destruction that was to force El Materno workers to resign and reduce expenses associated with the severance and with future pensions. But there was also a symbolic aspect to the destruction that came with re-creating the workers as violent and irrational occupiers.

When subverting the order of things is impossible, people resist in creative ways, hoping that the final outcome might shift the balance of power toward their interests. In this chapter, we also see how the workers' resistance actions, like the violent forces against them, addressed their legal standing as workers with rights, their social image as valued members of the country's history of health care, and their material and emotional experiences. Resistance actions can be both individual and collective, but we cannot conceive these as separate domains. Individual actions, like some legal proceedings we will refer to, clearly influenced the collective strategies of the whole group of workers. The opposite is also true.

While some legal actions sought benefits for each individual member of El Materno's workforce, other actions, such as the denunciations of the liquidating agent's actions, were intended to disrupt the whole liquidation process and advance their collective call to be seen as workers whose rights were being violated. The legal battle—what we might call lawfare—included many different strategies and counterstrategies that end up investing the law with the power to put an end to the context of illegality and precarity.[6] Indeed, workers constantly argued that the actions of the liquidator were illegal, that they had contracts that were to be granted by the state. Yet illegal actions continued, and the workers were ostracized for defending their legal rights. Workers illustrated, however, how some additional actions were fundamental to complementing specific legal procedures and advancing their cause. While legal battles continued in the courts, traditional protest strategies such as temporarily blockading 10th Avenue and alerting the media were also important for regaining social understanding, recognition, and support.

This chapter, nonetheless, also unveils how the use of art bridged researchers' activist-oriented approach and the workers' strategies of resistance. Photographs, pamphlets on fabric, video and photodocumentaries, murals and graffiti, and the guided tours illustrate how some artistic resistance strategies work, or fail to work, in the middle of the political battles.[7] Artistic actions can be very effective in articulating the emotional history of the struggle. But they can also be very taxing for those who have to live the story and then retell it to curious and unpredictable audiences. Just like legal struggles, art interventions are subject to political uses by the different sectors involved in the political struggle, and they can be ineffective. More than anything, however, in this chapter workers teach us the importance of being politically aware and informed, being creative, keeping solidarity with one's peers, and, very importantly, persevering. And in order to persevere, the more important strategy is to be physically present. In El Materno's case, this meant remaining in the spaces where the liquidator and the new tenant, a public city hospital called La Cruz, wanted them gone.

"I was so scared the day I arrived here because I was brought in an ambulance and they put me in a wheelchair. I saw this huge hospital and I said, 'Please don't leave me here, I am going to die here.'" Leidy arrived at El Materno one night in October 2005, precisely as the debate about the hospital's future peaked. The office of the attorney general asked the governor of Cundinamarca to revoke his decrees that initiated the liquidation process for the hospital, arguing that the liquidation went against the general interest and threatened Colombians' fundamental right to health care.[8] Even though Leidy did not know the specifics of the debate, her impression of the hospital worsened as a porter helped her to a wheelchair and brought her inside admissions. The lack of even a minimal operating budget and the scarcity of patients made the hospital feel like an abandoned building. "[It] looked like a [haunted] house. Those hallways were all empty and everything looked dark, there was just one light bulb . . . when we arrived there was only one nurse and she said from down the hall, 'Wait a moment,' and you would hear an echo, and I was just thinking, 'Oh God!' I started crying and I told Yerson [her partner], 'Please don't [leave me here], this hospital is horrible, it is a bad hospital, please get me out of here.'"

Even though Leidy's mother delivered all her children at El Materno and spoke fondly of it, the media had given Leidy the impression that "nobody was sent to this hospital anymore. I knew that before the service was good, that's what my mom said, but I was thinking tons of things: that with the problems [the hospital] was now bad, that there were not even doctors. I was scared. I kept on thinking, 'What if they let my baby die?' I thought that maybe, because we have a low [income] level, I had been sent here. I thought that it was because of that that I had been sent here that was now [a] bad [hospital]." Leidy's recollection suggests the idea that the poor deserved worse care. She did not refer to herself as poor, but as "low level," signaling that she had incorporated the new poverty classification schemes of the neoliberal trend in social welfare policies.[9] Leidy had integrated the news about the hospital's economic crisis with the new neoliberal terminology that divided "low income level" deservers of subsidies from those who, at higher income levels, were forced to purchase health insurance. In her mind, the traditional image of El Materno as the hospital that provided the best care for the poor when her mother delivered her children, including her, had been replaced by an image of a hospital that provided bad care and where, as a form of punishment, the poor were sent to die.

Leidy found herself caught between employees who were able to maintain a loving and nurturing idea of patient care (see chapter 3) and employees who seemed burned out by the emotional toll of too few patients, economic scarcity, and debates about whether or not the hospital was going to close.[10] As in other narratives, the traumatic first encounters with the hospital changed once the patient passed through the emergency room or admissions, as pregnant women arrived at wards or their newborns at neonatology. "They took me to the fourth floor and I started to see people, more doctors and nurses. And the fourth floor was full. There were other mothers and the place where they had the babies was pretty and then I thought, 'This is not as ugly as I thought.'" Indeed, it seemed that the hospital had shrunk, half busy with patients and half empty. Patients would stay in the places where medical care was active, but they often saw or had to pass empty, abandoned areas.

WOMEN FROM ALL OVER the country with high-risk pregnancies were still referred to El Materno. They and the staff constantly wondered why the government—the president, the Ministry of Health, Bogotá's mayor—could not inject resources into the hospital. The governor of Cundinamarca province was seen as an absolute enemy. Depending on the news, the staff whipsawed between hope that help was coming and fear of final liquidation. In the midst of that tension, they adamantly emphasized keeping up with *their* commitments to *their* patients.

Despite the governor's threats of liquidation, Rosaura, a secretary, felt that the resolution by the Council of State revoking the decrees that had made the hospital private brought hope "because we now know that we are public employees and someone has to be responsible for us [meaning acknowledging their contracts with their full labor rights]. Whoever it is in the state, they have to take care of us. We know that this [struggle] may continue, but someone will have to respond for us. We are hoping that in about six months things get fixed."

There were different visions of what it would mean to help the hospital; some hoped simply for salaries, and some for budgetary resources and a plan that would allow El Materno to compete in the new system. Economic viability seemed less and less likely; workers recognized that, since their personnel costs were much higher than other institutions', securing a future for the hospital likely meant a drastic restructuring. "If it would secure a future for the hospital, I am willing to resign," Rosaura, like many others, frequently said. On the other hand, it seemed impossible that they would not at least receive their back pay. Again and again, they asked themselves, "They have to pay us what they owe us, don't they?" Rosaura thought that her six-month time frame was realistic: "[I don't want to] imagine that things are going to be solved that rapidly because we have been disenchanted so often. So, if we get entered into the budget [of whatever state institution] then, around March [2006, things should be clear]. If they restructure the hospital, it is not going to be that fast, so it will be a process that takes time. I cannot imagine a very long process, just as a way to keep our hopes up." In Rosaura's mind, a restructuring could mean that some staff would be rehired in better conditions, or that they would be let go with severance, depending on how many people were required for a new competitive structure. "[Any] decision would be better than what we have right now," Rosaura concluded; they could not maintain the current situation of uncertainty and economic precarity much longer.[11]

The hospital's constant economic deficit didn't cause immediate or unheard-of changes; workers were used to receiving their salaries late even before the neoliberal reforms. With the current crisis, however, payment delays became more frequent. Raúl, who started to work in administration and then became a nurse assistant, explained how unpaid salaries built up. "Well, it is not really true that the institution owes us seven months of salaries, that there have been seven months in which we have not received a payment. It is not like that. Let's say it was June, and whoever was the director would say, 'We have enough to pay either the *prima* [additional payment that amounted to a month and a half's worth of salary] or the salary [for that month].' So, we would say, 'Pay us the prima and owe us the salary.'" In their minds, "it will be easier later to demand the payment of a salary than that of the prima," which as an extra benefit out of collective bargaining agreements and former labor laws was considered less of a contractual obligation than salaries. Besides, Raúl explained, "the prima was a bit more [in terms of money] than the salary." Another way in which salary debt accumulated was that, depending on the flow of money, "one month they [the administration] would pay [us on] the fifth and the [next] month they would pay [us on] the twentieth. So you have fifteen days of delayed salary already, and then the next month they pay [us on] the twenty-fifth, and so it happened like that, little by little, until we realized that it was already seven months" of accumulated unpaid salaries.

In his explanation, however, Raúl did not present the situation as a contest between the director at that time, Odilio Méndez, and the workers; rather, these payments corresponded to "whatever the hospital was able to produce in terms of bills and our effort to keep the hospital open.

Obviously, if it had been seven consecutive months without salary, none of us would have been able to *'aguantar'* [endure the fight]."[12] That they were used to receiving delayed salaries since they had first signed their contracts and that the failure to pay salaries was not continuous did not mean that the economic crisis of the hospital had not translated into severe strains on employees' household economies. Raúl remembered that the new collective agreement signed in the late 1990s served to bring their salaries to a more competitive level but, since then, their salaries had not increased. "We had to look for other sources of income," Raúl explained. "Since I am a nurse [assistant], I can cover night shifts at other hospitals. I cover shifts, vacations, and so on." Many workers started to find more jobs, and some even found other six-hour to eight-hour contracts at different hospitals and on different schedules so that they could cover both shifts. In many cases, they were doubling their working hours but receiving only one full salary.

People also began to sell things. "Everybody here is selling something," Raúl commented. "I am selling CDs right now. We come up with all sorts of ideas; we have established a kind of a barter system. Obviously, it is not that they [the administration or chiefs of services] openly say [that sells are allowed], but they do say, "'Just don't neglect your work—sell your stuff but don't neglect your work.'" Workers resorted to having multiple jobs, when available and with important consequences for families' everyday dynamics, since parents had to work all the time and were exhausted, to "sells" and barter inside the hospital, to undesirable loans, and to many other cost-cutting strategies.

The ways in which the domestic economy was affected by delayed and unpaid salaries varied depending on household compositions, social networks, and level of income. In households where El Materno's salary was not the central source of income, families were still forced to make severe adjustments, but the situation was not as dramatic as in families that depended on El Materno's salaries. Just like the health care system, the public education system in Colombia was also characterized by underfunding and inequalities. Public education had a bad reputation, and the differences between public and private education were seen as an expression of class inequalities. Many workers from El Materno made all sorts of sacrifices to enroll their children at private schools. When the economic situation hit the hardest and delayed salaries accumulated, many, like Raúl, were forced to transfer their children from private to public school. This felt like not only a drop in social status but also a painful decision; they felt the quality of their children's education had been compromised by the situation at the hospital.

In the narratives of many other workers, help from relatives, friends, or other institutions was common. Depending on the particular individual and family story, the hospital and household economic crises were more or less manageable. Household economies combined help received from family, friends, and institutions, the occasional payments at the hospital, and, frequently, loans. In Lucía's case, worries grew hand in hand with debts. Lucía reflected on how this process evolved.

> My basic [monthly] salary is around US$233, then if you add all extra benefits like years of service and so on [including education subsidies], it comes up to around $290. Out of those $290, they take $150 from a loan I made to a workers' fund to purchase a house that in the end we could not keep on paying; we lost everything [we had invested on that]. Out of the remaining $140, they take $74 to pay a bank loan I made last year to be able to register my youngest daughter at school, so I am left with around $45 once you take out health and pension. So, every time they pay us here I receive around $40. Then I have to pay around $25 of another loan that we had to ask for . . . I don't even remember when we did that. It was maybe two and a half years ago. So, I am left with $15, can you imagine? Last Friday, for example, the children called me to tell me that the gas company was there and was going to cut our service. I ran to talk to them to tell them that my husband had already paid, but I didn't make it on time and they cut the gas. The children can look after themselves, they can cook, but without gas. . . . So, for the next bill I will also have to pay a reconnection fee, plus the $4 I pay monthly for the gas bill, which seems like nothing, doesn't it?[13]

Lucía's detailed reflection not only makes visible the decreased purchasing power of domestic economies stricken by "systemic violence,"[14] but it also demonstrates how the chronic challenges of living in "survival mode"[15] have been worsened by the economic crisis of the hospital.

Because of the hospital/household economic crisis, many families stopped vacationing. In more severe cases, workers could not pay their rent and had to move in with relatives. Employees who had mortgages started to make late payments or default altogether. Many lost their houses. In some cases, workers and families went hungry. Many attributed divorces to the economic and emotional crises that bled from the hospital into their homes. Even though all the staff lived through the same crises, each experienced these crises differently according to their individual life stories and with their work histories at the hospital. In different cases, the hospital/household crises cut off paths toward independence from abusive or problematic families, destroyed dreams of owning a house, interrupted or ended personal education projects, made caring for elderly parents impossible, and raised the difficult and frightening prospect of aging without a pension. El Materno workers conveyed how the decline of a single hospital resulted in a multiplicity of experiences of loss and precarity.

ODILIO MÉNDEZ, THE LAST director of El Materno, recognized that it was the workers' "understanding [of the situation], their commitment, their sacrifices," that kept the hospital open. He also recognized that Bogotá's health secretariat had been vital during 2005 and 2006—very difficult years in which 70 to 80 percent of hospital income came from bills sent to the health secretariat. Interestingly, this indicated that El Materno was holding up its original mandate to serve the poor, since the health care secretariats paid bills for the uninsured. Odilio also recognized the extreme solidarity "of providers who helped by giving us their products and services as long as we gave our best efforts to make partial payments on those contracts. In addition, [La Nacional] professors and students keep on working with us."

At times, however, supplies ran out. When patients needed specific medications or supplies, the workers would collect whatever little they had in their pockets and buy the necessary items at a local pharmacy. In their minds, the economic situation of the hospital and their own economic situation did not justify failing to provide whatever medical care patients needed. Lida Pinzón, introduced in chapter 2, still had a considerable flow of patients in the Kangaroo Care Program and remembered that she helped purchase antibiotics for the patients at the local pharmacy for a very long time. Once, someone came to her house at 11 p.m. to borrow money for an expensive medication because the workers did not have enough. Similarly, Sister Emita, who worked at the hospital as a nurse assistant and was introduced in chapter 3, remembered another sick child "who needed a medication urgently. So, I called the sister [in charge of her congregation] and I told her, we have this need and we have no money. There is a child who is going to die if we don't give her treatment. And she told me, go buy it and we will reimburse you." In addition, the legacy of charity and donations came in handy. Sister Emita remembered how "we started to go and ask for help from people who knew us. We would go to schools and other places and ask people for help. People would donate medications and we would classify them and bring them to the pharmacy as a way to help ease the situation a bit."

Odilio Méndez explained that, as the situation grew more and more difficult, a final resolution about the hospital future and its workers was in the making. Despite the fact that the Council of State had clarified the public nature of the hospital, "two important obstacles remained," he explained. "First, the transition of the institution from a private to a public character means that the Beneficence has to receive it [but repeatedly claims that it will not], and secondly, someone has to accept responsibility for the hospital's existing liabilities, including pension liabilities. The most equitable scenario is a concurrence—an agreement among government entities to finance those liabilities." As Odilio saw it, the attorney general had been instrumental not only by stopping the governor's attempt at liquidation but also by serving "as a friendly mediator interested in bringing people together to find solutions. He has organized meetings with the three involved governmental entities [the national, province, and city governments] and the workers." It was becoming clear that a financial concurrence among those three governmental sectors was necessary. "The city, according to the mayor, reiterates frequently that it is interested in being in charge of the hospital but that he [the mayor] will receive them [the hospitals, including El San Juan] and keep them running only if the liabilities are all cleared up. That means that the hospital's debts have to be zero."

Head nurse Sonia Parra credited Odilio Méndez with keeping the hospital open. "He is doing all the hospital administration, but he is also reaching out. He is talking with everybody, he goes to every meeting, he talks to the press." In one of those meetings, the Beneficence agreed to receive the hospital's inventory. According to Odilio, this was very important "so that later the inventory could be attested, [meaning that the final assets of the hospital could be estimated] and a definition could be reached about who would administer and protect those inventories and, most importantly, who would be in charge of running El Materno." While Odilio knew that a proper legal resolution was needed to officially delegate responsibility for El Materno to a single authority, some workers started to complain, arguing that he should just give the hospital to the Beneficence once and for all to see what happened. Despite the sustenance the community provided one another, problems became increasingly common among the El Materno family; distrust of Odilio Méndez and other leaders, including the union, started to build. "Now we have fights," recognized nurse assistant Mary. She acknowledged that, for many, the economic crisis was reaching new and unthinkable lows; those who had less social support and a harder time meeting bare minimums "were always tense. If you try to talk to them, they respond very aggressively."

Odilio understood that a final solution could be found only through a conciliation [among key stakeholders of the hospital] or in Congress. However, the hospital was once again caught in a political firestorm. While the Ministry of Finance insisted that the government was eager to support the hospital and a congressional commission worked on a 2006 budgetary proposal for saving the hospitals, the Ministry of Health voiced its disagreement with the congressional plan.[16] In the midst of these tensions, a final agreement, overseen by the attorney general, was reached in June 2006. According to the agreement, the governor of the Cundinamarca province was to designate an agent to liquidate the Foundation San Juan de Dios. The mayor's office agreed to manage the hospital and integrate it into the city's health care network as a unit offering highly specialized neonatal and maternity services. The national government agreed to provide US$30 million, the estimated amount necessary to cover all the pending liabilities of El Materno workers.[17]

Inside the hospital, the news was received with mixed emotions. The hospital was going to be "saved," as they had hoped. Odilio shared that optimism: "All the years we have put in the hospital should serve as a sufficiently strong basis for a better future. I think the hospital will improve significantly." The staff expected, finally, to receive their delayed salaries. However, it was unclear who was going to be in charge of the hospital and whether the employees would keep their jobs, be terminated fairly, or be rehired by the health care secretariat. Maria Teresa, an occupational therapist, commented that "when it was decided that the hospital was going to be closed down, we really started to worry about what to do. It was different from the delayed salaries because you would still have in your mind that those delayed salaries ought to be paid, one day. But the moment you feel that the hospital is not going on, then you ask yourself what am I going to do? Nowadays it is not that easy to find a new job."

The liquidation process was supposed to start on July 1, 2006. The governor had rapidly reappointed Ana Karenina Gauna Palencia as liquidating agent—the same person he had appointed with the first, revoked decrees. However, workers continued to wait for payment while unpaid salaries continued to accumulate. In those months, rumors about the new "owner" abounded, while different institutions (universities and city hospitals) visited to check on the hospital. While the staff was not opposed to having visitors, they felt that payment should be prioritized over surveillance. Workers were losing patience by the time another rumor began—that another city hospital, La Cruz, was going to manage El Materno. "How come," several asked themselves in a meeting, "they [government officials] have hired a liquidating agent, have decided that La Cruz will be the one taking over El Materno, but they are yet to do anything about the obligations to El Materno workers?" For the health care secretariat, the problem was that the new agreement between the liquidating agent Ana Karenina Gauna Palencia and La Cruz Hospital included renting the building for US$50,000 per month, starting August 1. La Cruz's director was complaining he was not going to pay for a building that was not generating any income.

AFTER THE AGREEMENT, WORKERS started to deny entrance to La Cruz officials as a form of protest. They also protested in front of the building. Sometimes, they would stop traffic on 10th Avenue to let the public know "we are El Materno workers and we won't leave until they [the government officials] pay us what they owe us"—payment that had already been officially approved. In response, city officials placed army tanks in front of El Materno and surrounded it with two sets of police: the regular force and the ESMAD (Mobile Anti-Disturbances Squadron), a special police force designed to confront protests. This force received specialized combat training; were equipped with shields, helmets, protective clothing, and batons; and were authorized to use powerful water hoses that connected to the army tanks. Most hospital workers experienced this police presence as "horrible" and "terrifying." The police were not just fulfilling a symbolic role; they were trying to get inside the building and "take control" of the hospital. As the police attempted to come inside the hospital, workers would tell them, "We still work here, don't you know? Go tell them [your bosses] that. You cannot remove the people from the institutions where they work. Tell them [your bosses] that that is illegal."

On August 1, the last day of confrontations, the police made it inside the hospital. This time, La Cruz officials were also part of the crowd forcing itself in. "It was a horrible battle. We were securing the doors. People would rush to the door and [we would] push them out; they'd rush to the door again and be pushed out again," Yolanda, an X-ray technician, remembered. The fight was intense. Many people got hit by the police, and two female workers were badly battered and arrested. Different people have different traumatic memories and experiences of that day. Head nurse Patricia Farías thinks of one haunting image that she wishes she could forget. "The subdirector of La Cruz was kicking and kicking the door. I still see that image and I don't think it is going to go away. It was just too painful, mostly because he was an alumni [he had studied medicine at La Nacional and gynecology at El

Materno]. I ask myself why that image doesn't go away or why don't I want it to go away?"[18] For others, it was the noise of the door being taken down, the image of workmates being injured or harassed, the anger and frustrations mixed with screams, the anxiety of feeling unsafe. Many people ran and searched for places to hide.

From that moment on, the police remained inside the hospital.[19] El Materno workers continued treating the remaining patients, working their shifts, and getting together to discuss their situation. The police had become an annoying presence that reminded them of the days of confrontation, but they started to ignore them and to concentrate on the final resolution of their working conditions. Much to their regret, the liquidating agent now had full access to the hospital. The La Cruz director started to bring people around to plan the reopening of El Materno.

EL MATERNO WORKERS DECIDED to continue their protests in the hospital parking lot, voicing their discontent to the public and denouncing the fact that they had not seen any of the money from the approved liquidation process. On August 28, 2006, they hung a big terracotta tent in the parking lot and set up chairs. They informed an audience of workmates, visitors, and the press that the workers' debt amounted to $22.5 million, out of the $30 million approved, and that while they would continue providing care to the few patients that remained at the hospital, they declared themselves in permanent assembly.

The workers' protest continued in the parking lot. People began to refer to this place as *La Carpa*—the tent. Workers tried to combine their political participation at La Carpa meetings with their regular work activities, even though fewer and fewer patients were transferred. Patients began to be discharged, and as the many workers wandered around mostly empty halls, the energy at the hospital very quickly became surreal. While some staff lavished extra care on the remaining patients, others were burned out. Sister Emita remembered "when they started to transfer patients out of the hospital. [At her service,] there was a woman who had been at the hospital for around three years. She had her baby at El Materno, and I don't recall exactly what happened to her [what kind of medical complications occurred], but she remained unconscious. She was with us for three years, and we all took care of her. Everybody would bring in the things that she needed, for personal hygiene and stuff. We kept her all that time, and she never had so much as a single bedsore." As the ward emptied out, this patient received even more devoted care. Then they "transferred her to another hospital, and it seems she died there. Her transfer hit us all hard because it seemed for sure now [that the hospital was closing down] because they said she was not supposed to remain with us, that it was the city secretariat who needed to take care of her. So, we were left with nothing to do."

Something similar happened in neonatology, where care of a premature baby boy, Juan David, kept the NICU running. Nurse assistant Nancy remembered how she always worked the night shift, and she began to see fewer and fewer babies. "One night we only had one birth, and an ambulance came and took that baby and only Juan David remained." Juan David became an emblem of the hospital's survival; he was mentioned in meetings, he was mentioned by the press. He had been abandoned by his mother and social services got involved. Somehow he resisted as long as he could. At different moments, they tried to transport him to a different hospital, but his vital signs would not allow the transfer. Then, one day, they did transfer him. According to Nancy, "The day they took Juan David away was like killing the hospital."

Odilio Méndez asked administrative and supervisory workers, including Sister Emita, to turn in their keys and inventory. Sister Emita handed in the inventory in front of several witnesses. "All the things we had we turned over. Even the chapel, which was so very painful." All the religious items remained in the chapel, including a piano that belonged to Sister Emita's congregation and the tray where the Virgin Mary had appeared. Some inventories were easier than others. Head nurse Patricia Farías, who led the lactation program at El Materno and was one of the country's experts in implementing Women- and Child-Friendly Institutional Strategies,[20] also had to turn in the keys and inventory of the Teaching and Service Committee, which she led. Her responsibilities included sitting on the hospital's ethics committee, overseeing agreements with a range of educational institutions for internships and hospital rotations, and managing the educational equipment at the hospital. At her office, there were boxes of valuable educational materials produced at El Materno that included, among others, pamphlets, buttons, mugs, pens, emblems, and models with information about breastfeeding, sexuality, and kangaroo care that were impossible to classify.

Even harder than making sense of the educational materials and furniture used in classrooms that could have up to four different identificatory plates was turning in the keys to the La Cruz representatives designated to receive the inventory. Luis Carlos Méndez, whose story and clinical perspectives were shared in chapters 1 and 2, remembered how hard it was for Patricia and other academics to turn in educational materials to a nonacademic institution. The disregard shown by La Cruz representatives, who were mostly physicians from La Nacional and who had done their residency training at El Materno, made the process difficult, even incomprehensible. Luis Carlos remembered, "Jefe [head nurse] Patricia wanted to show them her [educational] material [about breastfeeding].... [They responded,] 'No, we don't care about that. You figure out what you are going to do with that because we are not interested in that. We will throw it out.'" Probably, La Cruz plans addressed only the neonatology and maternity care services. Everything else, including the tradition of La Nacional Escuela, was seen as irrelevant. This was the first sign of the many complications the new relationship with La Cruz would bring for El Materno staff and La Nacional students and professors. "In radiology," Luis Carlos continued, "[we had] Dr. Luis Fernando Novoa Cordero, the best radiologist. He was a professor at La Nacional and he had the most comprehensive collection of radiology for neonatology that I am aware of. It was organized and annotated. I learned radiology because every time I finished my shift, rather than going home, I would go there to learn from his collection, to look at the X-rays, to read his annotated comments. If I had any doubts, I would go the next day and ask him. What a wise man." His collection remained at the radiology department at El Materno, even after he retired. When radiology was turned over to the La Cruz representative, Luis Carlos, pained, remembered them saying, "We don't care about any collections." Given that the radiology films had silver, "They said, 'Let's weigh it instead and sell it by the pound.' *THEY SOLD IT BY THE POUND!*," Luis Carlos continued in disbelief. "They did not recognize [the worth of things that] came before them." Echoing Patricia's pain when the La Cruz subdirector kicked the door to force himself in, Luis Carlos commented, "What hurt us [professors] the most was that they [La Cruz representatives] had been our students."

Besides the disrespect for La Escuela (El Materno/La Nacional's combined history that goes on for generations), turning over places with so much history also meant that from one moment to the next, workers were disoriented, without places to sit, hang their coats, or put down their purses. Chiefs of services turned keys and found themselves in the uncomfortable position of not knowing where to go next. Amparo, a secretary who worked for La Nacional's school of medicine at El Materno's gynecology department, remembered that "first, they asked social work [to turn in their service] and people didn't know anymore where to go. Then, they asked Dr. Clarita.[21] Dr. Clarita did not want to turn in her service at first, but, after an official notification letter, she had to. We [the gynecology department] were kind of the last ones [to turn our keys in]. Even the union left. Then Dr. Odilio Méndez turned over the director's office, and the administrative director turned his keys as well."

Without offices or patients, in a totally "disturbed" environment,[22] El Materno workers started to gather at random corners or at La Carpa. They had not been officially notified about the termination of their contracts and, as had happened to El San Juan staff six years previously, they concluded that they should continue to come to the hospital during their assigned shifts. If they didn't, they could be accused of having abandoned their workplace and be fired without severance payment. Once the last patients were transferred and they had no formal duties or offices, the staff concentrated their efforts on exerting pressure to speed up the liquidation process and attending to the rumors about what the hospital's new administration would look like under La Cruz. Head nurse Patricia commented that, according to the rumors, La Cruz was going to hire back some El Materno workers. However, she was concerned because La Cruz was claiming that out of the eight hundred workers, only two hundred were needed, and those two hundred were only from clinical areas. "They have not said anything about us [the other workers with more administrative, directorship, and supervising responsibilities and contracts]. They haven't said anything about terminating us." She said, "We are just looking to be terminated in a dignified way." Still, the idea of "saving the hospital" remained; two nurse assistants told Patricia that reopening El Materno, even under La Cruz's administration, was a victory: "[Whether or not we remain here], we saved the hospital."

People seemed to be walking randomly throughout the hospital, stopping at specific places such as La Carpa or their previously assigned units, where they wondered about what was going to happen next and how long any resolution was going to take. Corners of some wards and offices that remained open were rearranged; stretchers were pushed to corners or moved to a different space while chairs and couches transformed clinical areas into gathering places. Desks and small tables that used to hold clinical records, medications, and supplies started to hold stoves where workers brewed coffee. Looking out a window, facing the patient-free San Juan, head nurse Patricia sipped a cup of coffee and commented, "What a loss it is for the whole country to have these hospitals closed."

In a different corner, sitting on the windowsills and some benches on which patients used to rest, another group was reminiscing about the hospital's glory days, when toxemic and septic service departments were packed to the brim, when they celebrated the twenty-fifth anniversary of the Kangaroo Care Program, when the last remodeling made the hospital pretty again. "Why did we stay?" this group wondered. "Because we loved our work, our institution, and our patients" was the general conclusion. The conversations went on for hours, days, and weeks, mixing nostalgia, affection, and humor. "What about that story of the mom who came with three husbands and she would be kissing one while the other two were waiting." "Or what about the 'ñero' [a poor and unkempt homeless person, usually addicted to glue or crack] who as soon as someone turned their backs would grab soap and a towel, take a bath, and return the towel back to the same spot until head nurse Elizabeth put aside a towel and liquid isodine [iodine-based antiseptic], and every time he came she would give them to him and allow him to bathe." Toward the end of this gathering, the remembrances turned toward everything the staff did to understand what patients were going through. Amazed and excited about what they had done and accomplished, someone said, "What about all the money we collected so that moms and babies had everything they needed?" "Do you remember that Dr. Lida would travel with the moms in the *transmilenio* [city transportation system] to really understand what it was like for a mom to be discharged with an oxygen tank for her baby?"

One day, as night fell, another group gathered by the stairs and the elevator around Jefferson, an energetic porter, who became a nurse assistant but had to stop his undergraduate studies in psychology because of the economic crisis. Having been a "street child" himself and having received helped from an adoptive family and from the El Materno family, he was grateful for the hospital. He understood clearly that the hospital, like the life he had built for himself, was about helping people. When women who came from distant provinces were discharged but their babies remained hospitalized and the women had nowhere to go to, Jefferson offered his humble household as a temporary shelter. Like his selfless spirit, Jefferson's sense of humor was contagious. While tensions and uncertainties about their future (or lack thereof) with La Cruz were about to explode, Jefferson was a source of relief. He reenacted the funniest times at the hospital or shared a joke, like "when you read lab exams to patients, you sit them down in a line and you start: you are fine, you are fine, you are fine, you can keep on crying, you are fine, you are fine . . ."

THE WEEKS DRAGGED ON. By September 2006 the only results of the June announcement that the government had approved US$30 million to save El Materno had been confrontations with the police and the surrender of the hospital to La Cruz representatives. Workers kept up their protest; the main meeting place remained La Carpa. The health care secretariat acknowledged publicly that the workers' complaints were fair, but he threatened that "if the workers do not stop their takeover of the hospital, the hospital might be definitively closed," because he would terminate the agreement with La Cruz that was keeping the hospital alive. Meanwhile, the liquidating agent, Ana Karenina, explained that the Ministry had not deposited the US$30 million to move forward with the liquidation of workers' contracts; the Ministry of Finance argued that the government needed a promissory note signed by the governor of Cundinamarca to make the money available. Bogotá's mayor was furious because he had moved forward with the agreement with La Cruz and, according to rumors, he was calling the president directly, asking him to put an end to the back-and-forth excuses between the minister and the governor. In a meeting led by a delegate of the office of the attorney general, an agreement was reached: the money was going to be managed through a fiduciary; US$22.5 million out of the $30 million were reserved for paying the hospital's debts to its workers.

As days went by, tensions escalated. The news started to report that El Materno was going to be reopened, but inside the hospital, nothing happened. Rather, rumors that the police were going to force them out escalated. "They cannot expel us from here. First, they have to fire us," concluded a group at La Carpa. At this point, La Carpa started to run like a central office for the collective of El Materno workers. People reported to their workplaces and then came to La Carpa to get updates. In the parking lot, a big pot heated with firewood served to provide food to whomever was around. For many, this was the only food of the day, since La Cruz had not paid anyone since receiving El Materno inventories.

Meantime, Ana Karenina announced that she would be visiting the hospital to talk to the workers. Gloria remembered that first meeting with Ana Karenina. "She got us together on the third floor. She left us speechless. She spoke so nicely and intelligently, she said she was there to help us and to help us establish our legal claims [about their debts and severance payments]. She seemed to have such good intentions. People were in a state of shock, of admiration. I was dazzled, as if I was facing the impossible, like being in front of the president. The union leader did raise some criticisms, but he mostly kept quiet. She said she was the one who was going to save El Materno." The good impression lasted only for that day. The second time, Ana Karenina came to El Materno in a bulletproof car with bodyguards.

"She took all our résumés [which were in the director's office] and told us that we had to leave the hospital. Then she came in a van saying that she had the money to pay us our debts. When people started to bang on the van, she said she was attacked and that she was not coming back."

The workers existed in a constant swirl of confusion, rumors, and misinformation. Ana Karenina would only meet with workforce delegates outside the hospital. The delegates would return to La Carpa and report, "Nothing happened, no news. We have to continue waiting until we receive official letters notifying us that our contracts ended," said head nurse María Esperanza to the crowd at La Carpa. Suddenly, Ana Karenina announced a visit to the hospital to hand in letters explaining the contract terminations, which the staff would be required to sign. Craziness, panic, and terror reigned. According to head nurse Patricia, all of this created divisions inside the hospital. "Some people started to say that that woman [Ana Karenina] was a godsend. . . . At the hospital Catholicism was predominant," but Ana Karenina had announced that she was an evangelical Christian. Many workers had turned to that religion over the years and started to believe that Ana Karenina had indeed been sent by God to save them and to save the hospital. For many, this idea led to devotion; they would support whatever Ana Karenina suggested, even if it meant signing resignation letters in which they renounced their legal entitlements.

Ana Karenina started to announce meetings for people to sign at different places, including the health care secretariat and a university known for conservative values and evangelical religious principles. Groups of workers would go and invite others to go. Many would come back announcing that they themselves had signed their resignation letters or that the majority of their workmates had signed. At another meeting, a workmate said that Ana Karenina had received a phone call from the governor asking her to stop the signing of resignation letters, that the process had no legal basis anymore. "[We were all] so lost. It was just so crazy. I didn't know what to do. I would ask around—should we sign or should we not?" nurse assistant Judith said. The union held meetings explaining to the employees that if they sign they would lose their entitlements. They explained that the workers were entitled to all their collective bargaining agreements, which were still in effect, and that as difficult as the situation was, they had to resist and not sign. Sooner or later, the union representatives said, workers would be able to collect all the money that the hospital owed them and get all their benefits, including early pension.

Finally, Judith decided to face Ana Karenina at one of those meetings. That particular day, the meeting was at El Materno's director's office. People stood in line for two hours. On meeting days, many more police officers came to "protect" Ana Karenina. Police officers were placed on all floors of the hospital and many of them had police dogs. "I did go in," Judith said. They were handing out tickets with numbers to see her. "I asked for a number to get in and she asked me, 'Are you going to sign?,' and I told her, 'I am coming to talk to you.' She said, 'Sign first and then we talk.' I told her, 'No. One talk firsts and then one looks at what one is getting into.'" Using a business metaphor, Judith continued,

> You don't buy first and then look at the product. . . . She stared at me and said, "Well, what do you want?" And I told her, "[I want] to know what you are going to do with my twenty years of service here, because I cannot just leave like it's nothing. . . . I am already entitled to my pension and I cannot just sign [a resignation] and leave." She said, "But you are still young—go work." And I said, "That doesn't matter, I already earned my pension and you cannot just take it away." And so I told her, "I am not signing," and took away my ID from her. And then she said, "Then, I will write down your name here, under the 'special cases,'" which I am not really sure what that meant, if it was based on age or years of service or who knows.

Head nurse Patricia was part of the group of those who had completed or were about to complete their pension requirements. She remembered that day when they met with Ana Karenina at the hospital director's office.

> We didn't know what was going to happen, but we stood in line to talk to her because we were supposed to talk to her. The only ami- cable face I can remember is one policeman. Everybody else had a panicked look on their faces because that woman would have us sit, four or five sitting. . . . She would leave us waiting for even longer because she said she was afraid. . . . But people got upset, and with reason, because she would tell you to sign and tell you you have no rights. How come we have rights to nothing? Then, she would get mad, she would create chaos, she said she was afraid for her own life and ended the meeting.

The general feeling was that those who signed had "succumbed" to Ana Karenina's seduction techniques, to their inability to withstand more days under such emotionally charged environment, or to the promises that those who resigned were going to be the first ones receiving payments and getting new jobs with La Cruz.

Head nurse Sonia remembered how the situation was even more fraught for people who, like her, were caught in what was called a "transition" situation—workers who had signed contracts before the labor and social security reforms of the early 1990s and had completed or were very close to completing twenty years of service and becoming eligible for pensions according to the collective agreement of the time. For this group of workers, "the liquidator had the grandiose idea of saying that she could not liquidate those of us who had been working at the hospital eighteen years or more because we were in the 'transition' phase, and so she did not let us resign. We had to come and sit and do nothing for the whole day. We started to knit, paint, whatever, read magazines, whatever we could do." A transition law was in place to protect workers who had fulfilled or were close to fulfilling pension requirements and meant, according to Sonia, "that they [the liquidating process or the state] had to find you a place to continue working [until you finished your requirements and could file for pension]." Sonia recalled Ana Karenina saying that she did not know "what was going to happen with us, meaning that it was up to the state [and not the liquidator] to decide how to solve their pension petitions."

"We just had to wait," said Sonia. On August 2006, Sonia said, "the liquidator called a meeting at the health care secretariat. She called everybody, all the people who had not resigned. The meeting was in one of the rooms on the first floor and we all went to find out what it was about." Sonia remembers that Patricia stood up and asked the liquidator, "We are part of the transition and we are still here. So, we need to know how you are going to handle our situation, whether you are going to find us a new job." Sonia remembered how Ana Karenina just "looked at us and told Patricia, 'Nooooo, I am not going to do anything. You just have to quit like everybody else.' So we were looking at each other and thinking about all that time [we spent working]." Head nurse Elsa Myriam said, "This is outrageous." "Right there," Sonia remembered, "we stood up, formed a line, and signed." It was dramatically painful, but Sonia remembered that all the head nurses who had been involved in the administration process to keep El Materno afloat during the last years were pushed to the limit and felt defeated. "Still," said Sonia, "there were rumors that six head nurses from El Materno were going to be reappointed to work for La Cruz, that so and so will be rehired, that yes, they are going to pay the liquidation fast. I said, no [meaning she wasn't going to continue in the same situation and preferred to sign], I will leave for Meissen." By this time, Sonia was working at Meissen, another public hospital, in the afternoons. When the economic situation had been critical, she was one of the lucky ones who had been able to land a second position while continuing to fight at El Materno.

THE MEDIA STARTED TO report that the labor situation at El Materno had been fixed. Around five hundred out of the seven hundred workers ended up signing the "voluntary" resignation letters. But they heard nothing about their payments nor about the supposed new contracts with La Cruz. Most of the people who did not sign were in legal limbo. They had fulfilled their twenty years of service, or were about to, and according to the collective agreement, they were entitled to pensions. According to new legal reforms, however, they also had to fulfill an age requirement. A new legal complication arose; Congress had approved the US$30 million for "restructuring" El Materno, but the money had been used for "liquidating" El Materno. This confusion kept the money tied up. The two hundred workers who did not sign started to wonder what else they could do to exert pressure. Another problem was that, without signed resignation letters or official dismissals, they were still considered workers and had to come to their workspace. The La Cruz director and Ana Karenina constantly asked them to leave, but workers would tell them they had to be fired and paid first and that any threats to impede their coming to their workplace was an interference with their labor rights.

On October 23, 2006, after a long process of negotiations overseen, once more, by the office of the attorney general, the city's health care secretariat, the director of La Cruz, and Ana Karenina met with several staff delegates from El Materno and the directors and judicial advisor of two workers' unions to sign an agreement. In the agreement the liquidating agent, Ana Karenina, agreed to use the designated resources, the US$30 million, to pay workers all their entitlements and to notify them of the end of their contracts with El Materno no later than November 20, 2006. The workers were authorized to remain inside the hospital, occupying the areas of admissions, the kitchen, and the fourth floor until the payments had been received in their bank accounts. They agreed to remain peacefully and to allow La Cruz workers to enter the hospital (starting the next day, October 24, 2006), who were to reopen some of the health care services; this made way for the rental agreement for US$50,000 per month between the liquidating agent and La Cruz director. La Cruz agreed to maintain the hospital's name,

"Instituto Materno Infantil," also known as IMI, and to prioritize El Materno workers as new hires. La Cruz also agreed to allow El Materno workers to remain at the hospital, although it reserved the right to restrict access to certain areas in which they would be reopening clinical services.

News reports two days later announced that El Materno had "come back to life" by reopening its outpatient clinic and treating fifteen patients. La Cruz was mentioned as "the unit in charge of El Materno" and its director, Gerardo Cano, said that services would grow slowly, but "we hope to have the intensive care unit and deliveries operating soon, with at least 100 hospital beds and 270 employees, all basically from the old Materno."[23] While some workers had come from La Cruz's own staff, some El Materno workers started to be called on to sign new, renewable three-month contracts without any benefits. The news articles mentioned specific aspects of the agreement, the efforts of all parts involved, and cited the health care secretariat, who said, "What was important was to open el IMI to the service of the people. That is already accomplished."

However, as the agreed-upon deadline for their payments approached, workers announced that they had not received any payments and had decided to continue in permanent assembly.[24] Ana Karenina said she could not pay the workers' debts—by that time, over a year's worth of salaries—because the Beneficence of the Cundinamarca province had not hired the auditing firm to oversee the handling of the US$30 million. Another newspaper column mentioned that in spite of the "coup" or continued occupation by three hundred workers, the Instituto Materno Infantil was open to the public, treating seven mothers and seven hospitalized babies.[25]

Rather than paying the workers, Ana Karenina continued exerting pressure on more and more people to resign. Anger and demoralization peaked as the year drew to a close. Workers saw in disbelief how even an official agreement had been blatantly violated. Head nurse Patricia said, "Chaos increased." On top of the internal divisions, mental illness started to conflate with anger, confusion, and politics. "Josefina started to say that there were unborn children circling around El Materno because they have not been able to be born, because this was the place where they were supposed to be born. Then one could only think that [the workers] were really on the edge. . . . When I did sign [the letter], you looked at that letter, and it said that you were resigning voluntarily. I signed my letter at the very end, the 26th (of December). I signed because I felt I was going mad, and I thought about my sons." Patricia felt too exhausted and felt that she was at the edge of a mental breakdown. "That day, I said I am leaving because I cannot withstand this anymore, physically or emotionally. It felt like I had weights on my shoulders, I could not sleep, I was crying all the time. Everything seemed worthless and everything seemed to say we had lost. Walking around El Materno was so sad. It was a terrible depression." She still had hopes that, even under La Cruz, they could still run El Materno as before, but everything was indicating that the administrative and supervisory roles were being filled by La Cruz; El Materno workers who had been rehired were being mistreated as cheap labor. Resorting to conspiracy theories, she concluded "that we had to leave our own lives [at the hospital] was part of the plan all along."

Death was not just a metaphor. Patricia continued, "Well, I think that the girl [a nurse assistant] who died, she had depression. She got treatment and she handled her problem, but in the end, she locked herself up and died." Some went mad, some had severe medical complications, and some ended up hospitalized or dying. During that fateful 2006, there were six worker deaths—some clearly attributable to the crisis and some more indirectly related to it.

Just two days after Patricia resigned, on December 28, 2006, the remaining workers saw their names in an edict. Several pieces of paper were taped on the windows of the inside corridor facing admissions, where the workers remained. The edict had a long list of their names and IDs, and claimed to be official notification that as of that day they were no longer considered employees of the institution. The document, however, did not mention anything about payments. Whenever a worker searched for his or her name or arrived at La Carpa and was told about the edict, a new round of tears and anger began. At the end of the day, workers concluded that, according to the agreement, they were authorized to remain at the hospital until they received full payments of their contractual obligations, which had not happened.

Six months after the edict informing the workers that they were no longer considered employed at El Materno, the country's most widely circulated newspaper announced that more than fourteen hundred babies had been born at the hospital since La Cruz started its administration.[26] Both the city's health care secretariat and the director of La Cruz hospital declared that on balance, "in spite of the labor conflicts between the workers and the liquidating agent," the situation was good. Cano, the La Cruz director, further stated: "The relationship between investments and bills will soon reach a point of equilibrium since the demand for neonatology and high risk gynecological care is pretty high in Bogotá."[27] He explained, "Nowadays, the institute has 83 hospital beds. Without the takeover of the former workers, the capacity would be 120 beds. Without this obstacle, there would be not only equilibrium but utilities. More than anything, however, we would be able to offer better health care services."

This announcement indicated both that the hospital could generate profits and that the former workers were an "obstacle" to better economic and social results. In the workers' minds, the news generated mixed feelings about whether or not La Cruz had indeed saved El Materno. They argued that the news proved that they had been right in their claim that the hospital could have survived without a third-party administration. Only if political will had been enough to clear the hospital bills, including pension liabilities and debts with other institutions, the hospital could still be running under the workers' supervision. They were enraged to see that the agreement that authorized them to remain at the hospital until they received what they were owed was now being twisted to present them as troublemakers who were "taking over" the hospital. Cano was claiming that they were the reason the hospital was not generating profits and citizens were not benefiting from better neonatology and high-risk gynecology. They had gone from epitomizing strong maternity and child care to being presented as the obstacles to that care. Rather than being recognized as workers whose rights were being threatened, they were being portrayed as people causing harm.

The news omitted the fact that only a fraction of the workers had received their liquidation payments and that those who had received them had been those who signed their "voluntary resignation." The news did not mention either that Ana Karenina, the liquidating agent, had put those who refused to sign on a special list, which over time proved to be a form of punishment that would delay their entitled payments for years. When someone who did not sign did somehow receive a liquidation, it was an unfair and incomplete payment, including only unpaid salaries—far from an adequate liquidation, which would have included severance and all other entitled payments. Often the liquidations came in such ridiculously small amounts that the receipts seemed like sick jokes. In one case, the liquidating agent told a worker that, since El Materno had made no contributions to her social security funds, she was entitled to just 1 peso (about 50 cents in US dollars) of benefits after proper payments. In another case, a person received a check for a ludicrously low amount, only to receive a new letter a couple of days later saying that because of an error, the first amount was wrong and that she would now be receiving even less money. Workers rapidly understood that, while the liquidation process did represent the end of their work relationship with their beloved Materno, it was just the beginning of a new struggle to demand the recognition of their labor rights. The prospect of a speedy resolution turned into years of legal demands and a prolonged "occupation" of El Materno. What they feared the most—becoming like El San Juan workers who were forced to fight for years over their labor rights—was starting to happen.

FOR GUSTAVO, A NURSE assistant who refused to sign a resignation, and whose name was therefore included on the list of "specials," these years of waiting and resisting were particularly difficult. In 2009 he thought that the three years since the 2006 edict had been the most difficult; "the state itself had such confusion [about the legal procedures of the liquidation] that it made us equally confused. We did not know if they [state authorities] were going to liquidate us." Despite the fact that the initial agreement overseen by the office of the attorney general had seemed to clear the path for liquidation, many legal challenges remained that, time and again, seemed to block the process. "At moments," Gustavo continued, "we would ask ourselves, could it be possible that I worked twenty-eight years for the state so that I have to go hungry until I turn sixty?" During those years, one of his most painful moments was when, after years of raising his children on his own, he was forced to ask them if they wanted to stay with him, in spite of the very difficult economic situation, or go to live with their mother. Without salaries or liquidation, he could not make mortgage payments anymore and his house was foreclosed. He rearranged one of the offices in admissions and, like a female workmate who moved into one of the rooms on the fifth floor, Gustavo started to live at El Materno.

Every new legal loss or mockery by the liquidator pushed him to new and unexpected lows. "I have suffered the rejection of the state, the rejection of society because I reached an age at which I am considered worthless, a nuisance. It is hard to accept the reality in which we are now forced to live. The liquidating agent already caused that harm, and now we have to wait for a judge to rule in our favor." Indeed, the majority of workers who received the ridiculous and partial liquidations immediately filed legal claims to challenge the liquidation. Those who the liquidated agent decided to punish by delaying liquidation had no standing to raise challenges. According to Yolanda, an X-ray technician, "I am waiting for her [the liquidating agent] to give me my liquidation so that I can challenge it." Some decided to represent themselves, but the majority worked with lawyers, spending more money that they did not yet have.

Years went by, and the money spent on "justice" began to seem wasted. The legal system proved very slow in responding to their petitions; when it ruled, it almost always came down against them. Flor worked at El Materno in the general services department. Because the hospital liquidation was framed as a problem with health care workers, there was a window of opportunity to protect her labor rights by challenging the liquidation. Flor filed a legal complaint saying that she had been fired unfairly and petitioning the judge to reinstate her. The judge ruled in her favor, much to the La Cruz director's regret. Hired back but despised as a member of La Carpa, she was assigned to clean unused areas, "so that they don't even have to see me," she said. Regardless, she had gotten her job back. Everybody was excited and wondered whether they could use this ruling as a legal precedent to help others from general services be reinstated. However, Ana Karenina, the liquidating agent, challenged the ruling, saying that Flor's petition had come after the stipulated period for challenging the edict had passed. A couple of weeks later, the new judge assigned to review the challenge ruled in favor of the liquidating agent, and Flor lost her job for the second time. Everybody at La Carpa understood that that was the end of that specific legal recourse. In the face of so many legal defeats, Gustavo concluded that "justice [was] completing the process of crushing us down."

Depression, tears, and nightmares were common. Some people could not sleep, and others became paranoid. Even though he had not lost his house yet, Gustavo kept dreaming about the moment when they would come and remove him from his home. He dreamed of being embarrassed in front of the neighbors. In his nightmares, he saw himself as a delinquent who, in the eyes of neighbors, must have done something terribly wrong to be evicted. The dreams were slow and detailed: first, he could not pay the water bill and the water company cut the service. "Then you feel in the nightmare that you cannot do anything, you can't get any money, everything is coming at you, until then, you are not there anymore, you disappear. You feel like [you are] coming very close to dying."

Reflecting on his nightmare, Gustavo thought that his strange feelings of disappearing as he was about to be removed from his house were "part of a mental state. You feel you are a nuisance, then you start thinking about dying. You start talking to people about what dying would be like, wondering about different states of consciousness in which, for example, as some people believe, you can communicate with others who have died." Gustavo suggested that being a nuisance to society meant losing one's social identity (a worker who does not work, a house owner who cannot make mortgage or utility payments, a father who does not provide for his children). Then, "it is," in his words, "as if you cease to exist." Gustavo explicitly linked the losses in his social identity with losses in his sense of self and the alteration of his mental state. Rather than hiding these connections, he and others openly admitted, "We have all been made crazy."

ONE OF THE MOST absurd aspects of the process, according to Gustavo, was that during the liquidation process, the liquidating agent stopped paying for the workers' health care. They were health care workers with many medical physical and mental needs, and they could not get care. In many cases, workers' whole families were left without care. When people raised this concern with Ana Karenina, she suggested registering with SISBEN, the stratification system that classified people based on poverty level; those classified as very poor could be entitled to subsidized health insurance. With this suggestion, she acknowledged both that the liquidation process had made them very poor and that she was not making or planning to make any social security payments for them. Some people thought the liquidation legal documents implied that they should be entitled to medical care, but when they tried to schedule any kind of medical visit, they were reported as debtors. According to the health care system, they were not unemployed, but they were not making any insurance payments. This bureaucratic trap drained more of their energy. According to Gustavo, "Everybody just misinforms you and [then, you think that] all efforts are pointless. You start losing your strength. We have no right to even see a doctor. That is really the limit."

Yolanda was one of the lucky ones who secured a second job at a different hospital. When the El Materno crisis hit bottom in 2006, she worked morning shifts at another hospital and came to El Materno for her afternoon shifts. She fulfilled the other hospital's requirements and started to receive a pension. Even though she was entitled to health care and health insurance payments were discounted judiciously out of her pension check, she too was unable to receive care because of the liquidation process. At one point, she developed a bad pain in her lower back and leg. She asked for an appointment only to be told by the rights verifiers that the system reported that she had two affiliations to the system, one from her pension and one from El Materno. She had to fix the administrative problem first before she could be seen by the doctor. For Yolanda, the aggravation was all-encompassing. Her lawyer told her that "Ana Karenina had taken all of the health care payments out of her partial liquidation," but the "system" reported that Ana Karenina had not made the payments.[28] "So," she concluded cynically, "thanks to Kareninita [little Karenina, a mocking name for the liquidating agent], the only thing I have in terms of medical care is the paper that says that I paid." Even though she had been discounted from two sources toward the health care system, she was still "disentitled."[29]

Health was yet another piece of the legal battle that had no clear timeline for resolution. Many workers were unable to receive any care; some received care for free or in private offices through their social networks. Yolanda had vision problems and needed eye surgery but had to wait even though she was going blind. She followed people's suggestions and managed her problem by putting wet cloths covering her eyes. Only when "Kareninita decided to pay our salaries [the initial liquidation]" could she afford the eye surgery out of pocket. "I was left for the very end [in the list of specials], but as soon as she paid me I went immediately and had my surgery done."

After the surgery and after challenging the liquidation, Yolanda was still wondering about the new timeline for a final resolution. "Every three months [the liquidating agent] promises she is going to pay us. Now they are saying that next month, others say that it is going to be the second week of next semester." Since the official agreed-upon period for finalizing their payments had long since expired, Yolanda insisted, "she is violating all the deadlines, all the agreements. She violates everything. And, [I ask,] who controls her?"

The legal battles continued. There were several congressional sessions during which Ana Karenina was called to report on the liquidation process. Slowly, newer and fuller liquidations started to be paid. Head nurse Patricia remembered, "I was rich for one day." For the majority, receiving their liquidation meant paying off debts. In Patricia's case, she was very close to losing her apartment, and most of the money went to canceling the mortgage. The majority of workers paid off their debts and pending medical care. After waiting so long, they were forced to spend their liquidation in a matter of days and quickly "went back to being poor." Many who had left the hospital and had new jobs resumed their lives with clearer images of El Materno as a dear place where they had their best years. Others continued working with La Cruz and adjusted to the new dynamics. Some La Carpa workers decided to accept the liquidation money, however partial, and not return again; others decided to continue resisting. The new liquidations were definitely better but they did not yet reflect all their entitlements and could still be challenged—and they were.

TO PREVENT THE METAMORPHOSIS of personal and familial difficulty, boredom, and fatigue into mental illness, workers turned to crafts. They began to occupy their time by knitting scarves, bags, and sweaters or embroidering and painting fabric that would become placemats, tablecloths, or paintings. As the years went by, people would bring in new materials and ideas to master new skills. Knitted, embroidered, and painted items would be themed around holidays. Some were kept or given as presents, but arts and crafts also became income-generating merchandise. More than anything, as Yolanda put it, "if we did not have our knitting, we would have gone mad already." For Gustavo, manual activities "help people to be in a different space. One person comes and tells you, 'Look how pretty these flowers [made in crochet] came out.'" Arts and crafts and coffee helped the days pass. Depending on the day and the economic possibilities, communal lunch or dinner would be prepared in what were once the admissions locker rooms and bathrooms.

La Carpa workers felt that no one, other than their colleagues, understood what it was like to go through such a prolonged and absurd situation. Their shared years of precarity, defeat, loss, aggression, and uncertainty brought them together; they developed strategies to understand each other's needs and mechanisms to support one another. One of the most valuable tools was La Carpa itself—a space to keep each other company as the hours, days, weeks, and months dragged on. Gustavo described how, even though everybody knew very well what everyone else was going through, people worked to retain their dignity. "A person comes and tries to hide [their difficulties]—says I will be right back and then disappears. Why? Because you have to go home by foot, or you had to walk two or three hours to get to work [having had only] a cup of coffee. But you are an adult and you are supposed to be working [and earning money], so those things are very painful." Gustavo emphasized the importance of La Carpa: "You look forward to being with your *compañeras* (female workmates), because we are all sharing the same painful mental state."

For Gustavo and the other workers, being surrounded by people in the same situation allowed them to find solace and distraction. Yolanda went home every day, but made sure to return every afternoon: "I get up and I organize, prepare lunch, eat, and come [to La Carpa]," she said. "What am I going to do at home, just stare at the ceiling or the walls? Then you start wanting to cry, you start remembering all the people from your generation who have died and you start feeling lonely. You get such sadness and nostalgia that it becomes unbearable, so you come here and start knitting. I don't have any money, so what else am I going to do? I just knit." The relationship with workmates from La Carpa represented a reconfiguration of the old El

Materno family, even though fights and breakups became more common over the years of the escalating liquidation crises.

AS THE YEARS WENT by, waiting at La Carpa became the new normal. Often, there was no news. Sometimes, someone would announce that another person had received a liquidation or that Ana Karenina was making new promises. La Carpa workers knew that those who had refused to sign their termination letters had done important work; having their names listed in an edict was not the same, legally, as receiving individual letters terminating their contractual obligations. It was clear that a contract could only be terminated with an agreement signed by employer and employee, which had not happened in their cases.[30] As such, workers thought that they could still be considered active workers and had to fulfill the duty to come to their workplaces. Perhaps, all the weeks, months, and years might pay off if that "work" time was included in the future severance package of a final and proper liquidation. According to the lawyers, conciliations were possible. While some workers considered conciliation, which could get them some money and end their fight, many figured that the call for conciliation proved that they were in the right. The majority agreed: "If we have waited for so long, why not wait a little bit more?" Years of accumulated salaries and benefits, plus inflation, could result in a substantial amount of money, which could make the effort over all those years worthwhile.

Workers resorted to constitutional mechanisms to protect their rights; in addition to challenging the liquidation, they filed several petitions explaining their situation. They told the judiciary that their labor rights were still being violated by the liquidation process; they argued too that their rights to health, social security, dignity, education, and so on, had been harmed in the process. Often, the judges' responses acknowledged their situation but concluded that nothing could be done or that nobody was at fault. When one judge started to research Ana Karenina's actions and omissions, she found enough documentation about the legal conundrums to justify delays in specific cases. Ana Karenina would frequently complain that she did not have enough money to attend to the many demands.

Given the complex legal terrain, the country's constitutional court decided to revisit twenty-three liquidation-related petitions made by El San Juan and Materno workers. A constitutional court ruling was important because it could clarify the entitlements for the entire class of affected workers. Importantly, the court's sentence (SU-484, 2008) acknowledged that workers were fully entitled to all their benefits according to their respective collective agreements. A fair payment was important, according to the court, because it promoted the workers' rights to labor, minimum vital, health, and social security. Nonetheless, the court capped the time-span that these contractual obligations covered. San Juan workers were entitled to payments up to October 29, 2001, and El Materno workers until August or December 2006. The court ordered that the necessary resources for the fair liquidations should be distributed among the Ministry of Finance (50 percent), the city (25 percent), and the Department of the Cundinamarca province and the Beneficence (25 percent). The new timeframe for the payments to be made, according to the Court, was one year. While workers celebrated the official recognition of their rights, they quickly argued that the Court had overextended its functions by determining a date for the end of their contractual obligations. "The Court," they intelligently remarked, "is not our employer." Some entered new legal petitions asking to be omitted from the court's mandate because they still considered themselves employees of the institution. Some judges agreed with them; this reopened the possibility of reinterpreting the Court's ruling.[31]

BY AUGUST 2008 AROUND EIGHTEEN workers, sometimes more, sometimes less, were still waiting for their first payments, including Marisol, the new leader of La Carpa. Resistance activities at La Carpa included monitoring new developments with Ana Karenina, maneuvering everyday activities with La Cruz, managing information with the media, and continuing to offer each other support, company, and unofficial therapy.

Over the years, the relationship between La Carpa and the director of La Cruz was tense—at times cordial, at times embattled. El Materno workers started to notice that the agreement allowing them to be in certain spaces at the hospital while La Cruz reopened some clinical wards did not address all areas of the hospital. Many areas were "no man's land," and the workers noticed that things started to go missing. Just like at El San Juan, valuable assets—including colonial paintings, expensive medical equipment, material assets with historical importance—and things that had no value at all began to disappear.

A mix of theft and "rearrangement" seemed suspicious to the workers and incited them to take action. They remembered that El San Juan workers had lobbied a politician to declare the hospitals (San Juan and Materno) national monuments and educational centers, which happened in 2002 with the signing of Law 735. They rapidly concluded that it was up to them to not only take care of their labor rights but also to watch over the hospital's assets. Because the agreement authorized them to remain at the hospital, workers at La Carpa also worried that they might be blamed for things going missing. More than just a sense of moral responsibility, being the hospital's "guardians"[32] gave the workers a new sense of meaning in an absurd situation. It also served a political purpose: they could try to use the legal system to counterbalance the immense power held by La Cruz and Ana Karenina. If the law had failed them with respect to the liquidation, it might still help them protect their hospital—and indirectly, their cause. Quickly, the workers began registering what went missing and when; they sent reports to the Ministry of Culture, in charge of overseeing the national patrimony.

They realized that Ana Karenina was behind the "disappearance" of hospital assets; she felt that, as the liquidating agent, she could dispose of and sell all the hospital's assets. Ana Karenina had hired former El Materno workers to fact-check the 2006 inventories and was selling whatever she could. Nobody was overseeing the sales; nobody knew how much money she was making or what she was doing with it. La Carpa workers started to take photographs of some areas to serve as evidence. Then they put chains, locks, or just glue-paper seals on the doors of certain areas La Cruz had not been authorized to access. Both Ana Karenina and Cano expressly disapproved of these actions and constantly threatened La Carpa workers with the police. Marisol recalled how the calm period of La Carpa and La Cruz co-occupancy of El Materno transitioned into a new period of stress and fear. "At any point, they [can] kick us out. [But] we cannot leave [the hospital] alone because José [a former Materno worker], who is doing the inventory for Anita, changed all the locks. And we just don't have the muscle to counteract that situation anymore. We just remain here for our own dignity. We are pained [by the situation], but we are thinking that at least we did something for the hospital." Because of the constant threat of police, La Carpa emphasized the importance of well-staffed shifts. "Please, don't be alone during your shifts," Marisol warned people. Anyone found alone when the police came may be arrested.

A new director was appointed to La Cruz, but the situation did not change much. Just like his predecessor, he wanted the whole hospital to himself and threatened the workers with the police. "If he wants to annoy us, we will annoy him back," said a crowd of La Carpa workers. They had a variety of practiced methods for denouncing their situation. Since the early days, they had hung banners in front of the hospital façade, reminding the public that they had not been paid. "The Workers of El Materno have not been paid" and "Long life to the fair fight of IMI workers," read two painted slogans that stayed on the hospital wall facing 10th Avenue for over a year. They also denounced larger national political situations, like the government's investing so much money in war rather than in health care. Since then-president Alvaro Uribe had been the proponent of Law 100 when he was a congressman back in 1993, many of the banners were directed at him. At this time, Uribe's links to paramilitary organizations were being constantly brought up in the media. When someone wrote "Uribe Paraco" on one of the hospital's brick walls, La Carpa workers made another banner, which read, "Uribe, you build battalions and close hospitals." The politicized hospital façade frustrated both Ana Karenina and the La Cruz director, but perhaps worse were the inside walls, which were filled with messages directed at them. "Pay us and we leave," one of them said. The stairs that connected the third and fourth floors had a message that remained for years: "Ana, the massacre maker, get out!" Another permanent message was on the fourth floor, just outside the entrance to the neonatal unit, where a big banner hanging from the ceiling read: "Because of the falsehoods of the liquidator, we, the workers, are in critical situations both emotional and economic."

Other slogans contained messages for patients, visitors, and colleagues, decrying the situation, "informing" them about farcical new promises or clearly stating that the hospital patrimony was being stolen. The La Victoria director tried to contain and eliminate these nuisances by painting over the slogans in the highest-trafficked walls with white paint. Workers saw this as an opportunity to retrench their political messages: blank canvases on which to declare, "Free publicity," "Juridical Hallway," "Work is a right," "Materno, pioneer of the Kangaroo Care. The liquidating agent is closing it." When time was short or snitches close by, a mere "Thanks for Painting" would appear, or simple colored lines made with any material at hand—paint, spray paint, graphite, or even lipstick. Some messages clearly stated that La Carpa workers were in for the long haul. "Even if you pay us, we won't go. Even if you want to bury the IMI." Such messages promised that even if they were kicked out, El Materno would continue existing. Perhaps inspired by the many ghosts that inhabited the hospital, they warned, hauntingly, "Dead! [Materno] will continue living x ever."[33]

TENSIONS CONTINUED THROUGH 2009, 2010, and 2011, as La Carpa faced internal fractures and countless external threats of finally, for sure, being kicked out of the hospital. Some relationships were permanently severed and others mended. In particular, whenever workers received a new threat that the police were coming or had a new confrontation with

Ana Karenina or La Cruz, La Carpa seemed to come together again. One of the rumors that grew over the years was that Ana Karenina wanted to sell the southern part of El Materno's parking lot. The La Cruz director also felt threatened by this. He saw that the hospital he was renting could be sold out from under him in pieces or that Ana Karenina could, at any point, decide to rent or sell the whole building. Marisol recognized that the new director's anxiety could work to their advantage. They [La Carpa] negotiated with him, allowing him use of the parking lot to bring in oxygen and park ambulances. In exchange, he did not bother them and promised to be attentive to Ana Karenina's mishandlings. Marisol warned him, "You can also be found at fault if national patrimony under your supervision goes missing."

Very early one morning, on June 5, 2009, Marisol called Camilo and told him to hurry, that the police were coming to oversee the official sale of the parking lot to El Materno's neighbor, the Cancer Institute. "Bring the camera," she ordered him. Camilo was a researcher from the critical medical anthropology research group; he had become a dear friend of Marisol's and had helped her record several of the turbulent moments with his camera. When he arrived, police and bureaucrats were already there. This time, however, city officials were there too, to make sure the sale took place. The bureaucrats told La Carpa workers that they could sign as witnesses if they wanted. All the documents seemed legal. Camilo took tons of pictures of the police, the dogs, the computer used to enter information into the official document, the trucks arriving with bricks, and the workers building a wall that divided the parking lot in half. "How could it be possible," people wondered, "for her to legally sell national patrimony?"

In May 2011 someone brought the news that Ana Karenina had put up a website with a list of items for sale from El San Juan and El Materno.[34] Her efforts during these past years to finalize the inventory finally made sense, and people now knew what she had been up to. "What she is doing is illegal," they were quick to point out. Someone announced that trucks were on their way to El San Juan to pick up the "inventory items for sale." Quickly, people circled the trucks and made photocopies of the authorizations and some items the truck drivers were supposed to pick up. They also took pictures. It was the first time that they obtained proof that Ana Karenina was selling the nation's patrimony. They brought copies of the new pictures, the list of items to be picked up, the website information, and testimonies to the Ministry of Culture, the city's office of patrimony, the general audit office, the attorney general's office, and the people's ombudsman's office, adding them as evidence to previously initiated complaints.

In their denunciations and legal collective action, workers were assisted by a human-rights attorneys association and an NGO where we (the research group) were also members in order to protect the hospital's patrimony and legacy as an educational institution. And their efforts paid off. After presenting the new evidence and the legal material of the collective action, a judge opened an investigation that showed several inconsistencies in Ana Karenina's handling of the liquidation. In June 2011 the judge signed precautionary measurements to protect the hospital's assets and ordered Ana Karenina to "stop any process of liquidation, sale, expropriation or handling of any title and of any material asset that is property of the Centro Hospitalario San Juan de Dios [that is, San Juan and El Materno]." The judge reminded Ana Karenina that she was supposed to liquidate the Fundación San Juan de Dios and handle the workers' liquidations but that at no point was she supposed to consider the hospital assets her own. Ana Karenina tried to counter the precautionary measurements by arguing that they were keeping her from accessing the money she needed to fulfill her role as liquidating agent. Marisol and the other La Carpa workers emphasized that the money came from the Ministry of Finance and was managed by a fiduciary—it did not come from selling off hospital assets.

In addition to the precautionary measurements, another small victory was that Ana Karenina was left without money to run the liquidation as her own business. She was forced to fire seventeen people, including José, the former El Materno worker who had helped her with all the inventories. "She lost power and we are calmer," Marisol said. In April 2012 Bogotá's health care secretariat also denounced Ana Karenina's action in the media.[35] He was part of an administration that was finding Ana Karenina an obstacle to their plan for including El Materno and San Juan in the city's health care infrastructure. He was quoted in the media saying that Ana Karenina had sold the parking lot illegally, according to the 2002 cultural patrimony declaration. Besides, he said, clearly discontented, "She has to report what she is doing with the [fifty thousand dollars] that the health secretariat and the Hospital La Cruz are paying monthly to renting the Instituto Materno Infantil, and she has refused to make those reports."[36] Ana Karenina and her team of lawyers defended the legal character of the sale with a study showing that the specific area sold was not included in the zone declared as patrimony. The study, however, seemed doctored by Ana Karenina herself, and was dated after the sale had been completed.[37]

The final victory against Ana Karenina came in October 2013, when the national audit office found that after seven years as liquidator, Ana Karenina had not fulfilled her duties—that she did not know how much money she had nor how much money the Fundación San Juan de Dios owed.[38] In addition, there were irregular tax findings, amounting to close to US$5.8 million, which raised the specter of disciplinary and penal processes. In particular, the auditor's report mentioned that Ana Karenina self-assigned an exorbitant salary without clear procedures backing her honoraria; her salary amounted to close to US$700,000 during those seven years. Other onerous honoraria for other members of the "liquidation team" were labeled "liquidation expenses," and an auditor's visit to the hospitals showed that assets and equipment were not properly placed, identified, registered, nor accounted for. Besides the dismantling and deterioration of equipment, the auditor's report warned that the buildings were at high risk of becoming ruins.[39] The national auditor asked the attorney general to stop the sale of the hospital complex and suggested that the governor of the Cundinamarca province fire Ana Karenina. Four days after the national audit's report, Ana Karenina resigned, claiming to be a victim of political persecution. A new liquidating agent was appointed.

CAMILO, LIKE MANY MEMBERS of the critical medical anthropology research group, thought that academic writing and helping workers find useful data were not sufficient—that politically and emotionally involved researchers could and should do more at El Materno.[40] An artist himself, he believed that art could help advance some of the workers' political fights, gain them more visibility, and influence the larger political debates around the hospital. In his mind, art could help the workers achieve a speedier resolution of their labor demands. With some other artists and friends from the research group, Camilo created a video documentary, a photo documentary, and other art-based initiatives, now available on YouTube alongside many other materials created by journalists, students, artists, and politicians at the hospital. Some nationally acclaimed fine artists and photographers have even received prestigious awards because of their work depicting the situation of the hospitals and the workers.

Camilo was fond of these artistic expressions and inspired by the workers' use of art-based interventions inside and outside of the hospital. Camilo saw the painting of walls and fabrics with different materials to convey powerful ideas as fitting within the subversive logics of graffiti artists.[41] In 2011 he partnered with other artists to include El Materno on a list of places to which the city's office of patrimony was promoting public visits. The idea was that visitors would come on three different Saturdays and get to know, smell, see, and hear El Materno. Camilo formed an artists' collective called "IMIenEspera" [IMIWaiting]. The group started to visit the hospital frequently, working with La Carpa workers to realize their vision. The effort involved in creating a guided tour inside El Materno would be significant. More political art spaces had to be created, and the workers had to be tour guides, explaining to the public how different areas of the hospital were connected to different moments in the hospital's history and in their labor struggle. Some workers disliked the idea, seeing it as yet another waste of time. Others were apathetic and disinterested, perhaps because, exhausted as they were, whatever little energy they had left was needed for their own legal demands. Marisol, Gustavo, and other workers did like the idea and decided to help the group of young artists.

Over several explanatory and preparatory meetings, workers and artists carefully crafted a guided tour. October 11, 2011, was the first of three Saturdays in which a group of around twenty-five people walked through the hospital, stopping at eleven points of interest. The tour started in the parking lot area, by the broken-down ambulance. Admissions, laundry room, locker room, kitchen, Kangaroo Care, a view of San Juan, a classroom, a view of the wall that divided the parking lot, and the empty hospitalization and neonatal intensive care unit wards completed the different stops. In each area, a worker would tell a part of the story, or the visitors would experience multimodal art installations; videos, audios coming from speakers, acetates, slide projections, and pictures all conveyed different messages. Each tour lasted around three hours and ended with coffee and some conversation, in which visitors shared their reactions of solidarity, outrage, or, sometimes, complete misunderstanding. One of the guests was a military veteran, who made some weird and worrisome comments about war and health; another was a representative from the health care secretariat, who was advertising for his own event. All the work seemed, in the end, to be for nothing.

Six months later, Camilo shared his reflections about the guided tours and the other art-based initiatives with Marisol and César. In general, the work had not been easy, and he was troubled about their lack of effectiveness and limited reach. "How many people have watched the documentaries? How many people went on the tours? What were the results of all that [work]?" he asked. He also realized that working with the other artists, who did not fully understand El Materno history and La Carpa resistance, was difficult. Camilo had experienced what La Carpa knew all along: "visitors" came to El Materno with all sorts of interests, and workers had to be very careful about what information they shared, and with whom.

Visitors were important because they might be political allies who could help them share their perspective with a wider public, especially when the media was involved. Yet, many times, more often than not, their position was misrepresented, edited to convey the opposite of what they wanted or used to discredit the hospital. Efforts to "instruct" visitors were labor intensive and emotionally draining, and they had limited effect; even when their messages were strong and fairly conveyed, nothing concrete seemed to come from newspaper articles or clips aired on national TV. And yet, the individual strategies added up—together, the juridical pursuit of labor rights, everyday negotiations with the La Cruz director, interfering with the liquidating process, and "helping" visitors and the media understand all amounted to something. Marisol told Camilo that patience and intelligence were key in these long-term struggles: "You have to know where you are going and you go step by step, little by little."

"In the end," Camilo told Marisol, addressing the guided tours and the difficulties in handling the other artists, he felt that "one ends up with a big mess and one ends up burned out, like you [the workers] at La Carpa." Marisol agreed with him. Part of the difficulty was that the new group of artists brought in to El Materno did not have a long history with La Carpa. Marisol had trusted them, because they had all worked with us [the group of researchers]. But, Marisol responded to Camilo, "The intention was really good, and I thank you because we had fun doing it, but we did reach a point of total exhaustion." It was too much: planning, setting up all the different stations, reliving the hospital's most painful moments for curious visitors, and "the stress of having to take care of everything. Being attentive so that visitors don't go places where they are not supposed to go." Marisol remembered too that she had to instruct artists on speaking carefully and respectfully to La Cruz workers, not interrupting their everyday activities, not leaving valuable equipment unattended, and making sure everybody stayed together as a group. "It was really stressful," she acknowledged.

Camilo reflected, "I thought that art was going to be more powerful. Now I think that both academia and art are very insular worlds. Who is [the audience for art or academia]? Just a handful of people. And I thought that the visits could change that." Marisol, however, brought in a different perspective on the value of these efforts. "We had fun," she reminded him, sharing good memories from the preparations. She also elaborated on the political praxis that collectivities need to sustain efforts. Her words are so eloquent that we (Marisol and the researchers) decided to share them with this book's audience:

When you have been resisting for six years, you learn that if things don't go as planned immediately, you just need to keep on moving forward. You also have to relax and keep on living . . . the goal you have to create for yourself is to keep on going because if you let setbacks affect you that limits your ability to do more things. If someone opens a window of opportunity, I take it because that might be the game changer in the future. Whatever you decide to do or not to do can be a game changer.

DEBATES ABOUT THE HOSPITAL continued throughout 2013, 2014, and 2015. The health care secretariat and the mayor himself continued to claim that the city administration would maintain the electoral promise to reopen El San Juan and incorporate both San Juan and El Materno into the city's health care infrastructure. The assembly of the Cundinamarca province authorized the sale of El San Juan and El Materno after the superintendent of notaries clarified that the province was the official owner of the buildings and the land. As a public proponent, Bogotá's health care secretariat received priority in the purchase after making an offer for close to US$80 million. The money was to be used to finish paying the workers.[42] The news was flooded with discussions about the expropriation and remodeling of buildings.[43] The Ministry of Culture approved a remodeling plan; El Materno was at the top of the list.[44]

At La Carpa, the general sense was "this is really it. The end is getting closer." This news was received with mockery and tension. Gustavo, who had been living at the hospital for six years now, said defiantly that he had no interest in leaving. "I live perfectly well here," he said. "I have my land, I have my garden, and I don't pay any rent." But things had changed; their actions had affected the narrative. Now, the workers did not have to argue, as they had for many years, that they had rights. Government officials acknowledged the workers' debt. The discussion now was about how much the hospital owed each worker and when the workers would receive their payments. Overall, the news of the sale and remodel got people preparing for an end. But nobody could know that Enrique Peñalosa, the neoliberal and technocrat mayor who took office in 2016, had no intention of finalizing the purchase of the hospitals. Once again, everything came to a halt. No final payments occurred, no buildings were remodeled.

In 2015 journalists had gone back to the narrative that the occupying El Materno workers were the last obstacle to reopening the hospital.[45] Government officials claimed that workers were being offered "houses" through a special subsidy line but that they still refused to leave the hospital. At La Carpa, workers were quick to respond that they were not asking for housing, that they were asking for the fair and full payment of their severance packages. Besides, the promised houses were not even built yet and, according to the plans, they were to be located in the outskirts of the city, in a very undesirable location. Some of the most desperate families were starting to consider the offer, but the majority were against it and made that clear in meetings with government officials.

During the next four years, new moments of hope were celebrated when a particular lawsuit seemed to be prospering. However, more frequently than not, legal resistance strategies started to pile up negative results, and workers progressively realized that they were running out of legal, emotional, physical, media,[46] or artistic options to claim the remaining work-related benefits they thought they were entitled to. Finally, on April 2, 2019, officers from the mayor's office along with members of the ESMAD (the antiriot police) came to make the eviction of the remaining workers of La Carpa official.[47] The same officer that had overseen the selling of the parking lot informed the audience that he had the legal authority to tell the police to detain those who obstructed the procedure, as well as to issue fines if necessary. Another officer from the mayor's office dictated to a secretary who was filling out the official form: "An official document from the Public Ministry confirms that all the work-related entitlements have been satisfied." In the space provided for complaints or disagreements, workers made sure to include that "it was untrue that the workers have received all the severance they were entitled to." Regardless, that was the last day they were authorized to be at El Materno.

CHAPTER 6. Remaining amid Destruction

In the famous prison notebooks, Italian Antonio Gramsci wrote, "[A] crisis cannot give the attacking forces the ability to organize with lightning speed in time and space; still less can it endow them with fighting spirit. Similarly, the defenders are not demoralized, nor do they abandon their positions, even among the ruins, nor do they lose faith in their own strength or their own future."[1] Remaining at a place can have different meanings—nostalgic, practical, economic, and, according to Gramsci, political, if there is a battle between forces aiming to perpetuate and counteract the domination of some groups by others. Importantly, Gramsci speaks of the ideological battles around capitalism. In health, capitalist ideology is expressed as the belief that health can be dealt with as a commodity. Professors and workers remained at El Materno to represent and fight for a set of emotional and historical meanings that surround the provision of care. This chapter argues that remaining became a way to keep El Materno's history alive and came to signify the most important strategy for confronting the system's for-profit orientation. The importance of remaining at El Materno can be seen every time a medical record includes a professor's note and every time a baby receives the special epistemology of care that reflects El Materno/La Nacional Escuela. Remaining is also part of a symbolic battle about the future that is being defined; it allows workers, professors, and students to continue dreaming.

Continuing in this Gramscian trend, remaining could also be understood as a wise political maneuver in a complex and moving warlike landscape

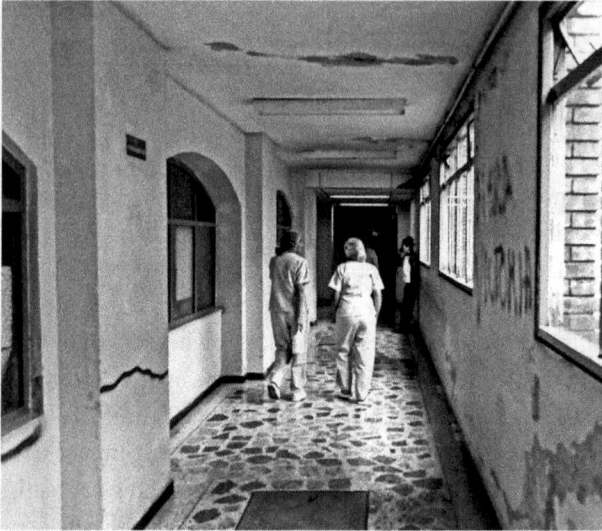

FIGURE 6.1. Photo "Electrocardiograma." Serie grafitis ["Electrocardiogram." Graffities series]. (Courtesy of Hector Camilo Ruíz Sánchez.)

that came to be legally symbolized in Law 100 and became part of the everyday conflicts between El Materno and La Cruz. Indeed, we can think of remaining as a strategy within both the Gramscian war of maneuver and war of position. Interestingly, we can see the coexistence of direct clashes (war of maneuver) and periods of relative calmness (war of position). In this chapter we will see how El Materno and La Cruz, as representatives of the two contradictory ideologies around health care, aimed to gain control over the everyday dynamics in care. While La Cruz imposed its advantageous position as the official administrator of the hospital, El Materno professors and workers remained faithful to their principles and negotiated their presence at the hospital to the best of their abilities.

Importantly, this chapter also allows us to see how history is embodied through particular institutional identities and how people act strategically within such politicized history, even after they leave the institution. Hence, this chapter explains how El Materno does not exist exclusively in those who currently inhabit it. When professors, workers, and alumni leave for different workplaces, they bring with them a piece of El Materno. El Materno remains because it *is* the hospital and what the escuela made of *its people*; hence, El Materno continues to exist in many people and in many places. Without discounting the great destruction of the hospital, its people, and its legacy, this chapter suggests that El Materno has found parallel lives in other settings.

When a worker or a professor leaves the hospital, we might think of this as the loss of a particular battle for El Materno. Nonetheless, if this worker or professor continues to practice and defend the hospital's epistemology of care at other institutions, the confrontation between epistemologies of medical care that are practiced in Colombia, or around the world, remains. Albeit with significant limitations and evident material, symbolic, and emotional destructions, El Materno's epistemology of care continues to be defended inside and outside the hospital, as this chapter demonstrates.

We Are El Materno

"La Cruz's great advantage is that we are Instituto Materno Infantil," laughs head nurse Sonia Parra. She was offered a position at La Cruz two years after finding no other solution than to resign in 2006. Even though the pay was much lower with La Cruz and contracts were "temporary," renewed every three months, she accepted the offer in order to work again at her old institution, asserting "I am El Materno." Indeed, the El Materno workers rehired by La Cruz and La Nacional professors who remained at El Materno in the academic programs in medicine, gynecology, and neonatology constantly battled with La Cruz over recognition, respect, and autonomy. It was always unclear how much of El Materno continued to exist under La Cruz directorship, how much El Materno's existence depended on the workers' and professors' presence, and how much La Cruz wanted to institutionalize a new identity while keeping the hospital's symbolic image as a place of excellence in child and maternal health.

Even though several La Cruz directors openly wanted to eliminate El Materno's history as a way of consolidating their new "ownership," El Materno's legacy brought many benefits, as head nurse Sonia knew. She was reappointed to her earlier post as chief of surgery, and she argued that La Cruz's great advantage was that "the health care secretariat has and wants relationships and contracts with us [El Materno]. We treat [patients] from Salud Capital [the city's health insurance for subsidized populations]. And the majority of the people from Salud Capital are from around the area, so it is very easy [to come to El Materno]. Besides, the mamás [pregnant women and women with sick newborns] already learned that they have Salud Capital, and that we will treat them if they come here even if they have been assigned to a different hospital."

Ironically, La Cruz did not provide any new or specialized administrative knowledge. Sonia said that, on the contrary, all that El Materno workers had learned about the new business intricacies of billing insurance companies and fighting their glosses (chapter 4) was put to La Cruz's advantage. "Another advantage we have," she said, "is that the law protects women, especially during pregnancy. So, they come here [to El Materno site of La Cruz Hospital, as it was renamed] and we call their insurance and we tell them, 'We have a patient of yours here,' and the insurance company says, 'Then, we will come and get her,' [but we know that] is not true." Sonia is referring here to the economic and clinical calculations made in the decision to transfer patients. On the one hand, it was likely, due to vertical integration between insurance companies and their clinics, that the insurance companies had cheaper contracts with other hospitals. On the other hand, transferring pregnant women or a woman with severe clinical complications required the use of a specialized ambulance (called medicalized), which added costs. Besides, Sonia commented, "When a woman is already here at El Materno, it is not that easy to find another hospital bed for her, because they [the patients] come to El Materno because of a special [medical] condition. They have heard that babies survive here, that here babies get such and such treatments. A doctor can even tell a mother, 'Go to El Materno and you will see that they treat you and that babies do very well there.'" El Materno, in spite of the crisis, its period of effective closure, and the new administration by La Cruz, had been able to maintain a collective image of excellence in clinical care, which was known to mothers with high-risk pregnancies and to doctors around the city.

Sonia saw that "many people still don't know [that El Materno changed administration] and still think that this is El Materno." On official stationery and a multitude of administrative and pedagogical signs around the hospital, La Cruz's stamp sat beside El Materno's symbol. Nonetheless, Sonia concluded that people still perceived the building as El Materno. She laughed when she remembered how they would still answer the phone saying, 'Instituto Materno Infantil.' "Now we learned, and we answer, 'Instituto Materno Infantil site of La Cruz Hospital.'" Despite the changes in stationery and administration, Sonia felt that the everyday dynamics at the hospital, both in terms of patient care and collegial relationships, remained about the same as in the former El Materno:

> When La Cruz arrived, we already knew many things [referring to the workings of the new system]. It is not as if they came here to teach, or as if they tried to change us, to change our ideals. After all, there are a lot of us, mostly on the morning shift. We can say that 90 percent of the morning shift is El Materno, everybody, head nurses, nurse assistants, physicians, everybody. I mean, there are still many people from El Materno still at the hospital, [including] professors from La Universidad Nacional. In the afternoon, there are fewer people from [El Materno], but at night the number goes back up. So, it has continued, it is still almost the same.

Indeed, the majority of the people working for La Cruz were former El Materno workers; this allowed, as Sonia said, the idea that things were *almost* the same, in spite of the new administration and the new contracts.

Contracts under La Cruz were renewed every three months, which led to permanent employment insecurity: a contract might not start immediately, and the hospital could decide at any time that an employee's position was no longer necessary.[2] Another uncomfortable change was that temporary contracts had no benefits, so people were forced to pay their own health and pension costs out of their paychecks. Under temporary contracts, vacation time became a euphemism for unpaid unemployment between contracts. "Lucky" workers at other health care institutions who had managed to secure years of uninterrupted contracts would sometimes ask for a gap between contracts so that they could take some unpaid time off and rest.

Head nurse Sonia had begun to work the night shift at Meissen Hospital at the peak of El Materno's economic crisis in 2004. When she was rehired as a La Cruz worker at the El Materno site, she worked afternoons. She continued that double shift (El Materno site of La Cruz in the afternoon and Meissen at night) for almost six years, but she progressively felt more and more tired. Even though Meissen paid her very well, around 40 percent more than her salary at La Cruz, she preferred to stay at the El Materno site of La Cruz Hospital.

> I started to feel that I was very tired. It was just running, running. First of all, Meissen is very far away and the area is tough. So I would arrive early and wait to start my shift [so that she would not be traveling in the dark]. Second, I said to myself, I will remain at El Materno doing what I have always wanted to do, to be with the mothers and babies. I am in the [clinical] area that I like—surgery and delivery. So, I said, I will stay at El Materno even if that means earning much, much less.

Like many others, Sonia still preferred her lower-paying job at El Materno to other, better-paying options. She also, like the other workers, resisted seeing herself as a La Cruz worker and always referred to her workplace as El Materno.

Despite the workers' low-paying contracts, it seemed that La Cruz's finances were doing very well. "They have reached financial equilibrium," Sonia said. Part of their economic advantage over other health care institutions was that "we all now have [temporary] contracts. We don't have rights to vacation time, compensatory, leaves. We don't even have the right to three hours for voting . . . all that is money that goes into their pockets. There are only four regular personnel [meaning with regular/permanent contract], and everybody else is under [temporary] contract. If we cannot be profitable under those circumstances, then there is no institution that can."[3]

Sonia, however, recognized that she was in a privileged situation. She said, "I am in an area that is totally closed off—totally closed off from the public spaces, because it is surgery and deliveries. The only contact with the exterior world is the door, isn't it? That includes administrators, everybody. For me, my clinical area is entirely inside, which means that the environment inside is the same environment I have experienced my whole life. The physicians are the same, the gynecologists are the same, the pediatricians are the same, the assistants are the same. That is, my environment is wonderful, and I cannot complain." Indeed, other workers felt more tension; some people's contracts weren't renewed, and others feared that political quotas could force their replacements. Still others began experiencing harassment at work, particularly when their directors were not former Materno colleagues. Sonia said that people outside her workspace did complain. "You can hear them saying that a doctor is such-and-such [rude or disrespectful], that the other one is like that [even more rude or disrespectful], that they get yelled at, mistreated, threatened, all sorts of things."

THE KANGAROO MOTHER CARE (KMC) program, perhaps the most important subaltern health innovation created at the hospital, as we discussed in chapter 2, also suffered through the economic crisis, closure, and reopening under La Cruz's management. Esperanza, a nurse assistant who worked at Kangaroo for over twenty years, remembered that the 2004–2006 crisis ended with the pediatrician's resignation, "because they were not paying her. She resigned, as did the ophthalmologist." She remembered that "patients would come and there would be no pediatrician. We had to tell them to go to their insurance company and ask to be referred to another Kangaroo program because here it was definitely closed down." However, Lida Pinzón, working as a professor of the National University and serving as director of KMC, tried to keep the program running as long as she could, until the order came to close it down.

Esperanza continued showing up at El Materno but, like many others, found it almost unbearable to see her work unit permanently closed. Like the majority of those who resigned, she presented her curriculum vitae to La Cruz, who called her back in November 2006 and offered her a temporary contract doing night shifts. "I resigned, then they paid me [and then they hired me]." As with head nurse Sonia, her contract was supposed to be renewed every three months, but that rarely happened. The way it was handled was that "every month they give us an 'addition,' meaning a one-month extension of the contract. So, we sign the addition and they pay us every month." With additions, the contract was effectively reduced from three months to one, but workers trusted that the additions would be signed on the first of each month and payments would not be interrupted. Additions were signed at the coordinating office: "You go, sign, make a copy, keep the copy and give the original." Additions were usually signed the day after the official contract ended, but that did not happen every month. "This month [January 2015]," Esperanza commented, "we have not received the addition and it is already January 9th, which means that if they don't want, they don't need to pay us [for those 9 days] because we have not signed anything. Well, La Cruz always delays it a bit, but you always end up signing within the month [and they pay fine]." Esperanza had completed eight years of work with three-month contracts and monthly additions—a new normal that brought with it a sense of dissatisfaction and resignation.

Esperanza said, "The new contract is nothing like the one we had with El Materno. We had everything: social security, vacations, *primas*, *cesantías*, everything entitled by law. Now, we have nothing." Not only did benefits disappear, but the overall salaries were lower; significant extra deductions resulted in a much-reduced monthly check. She explained, "[Salary now] is a bit more than minimum wage, [while before a nurse assistant's salary was between two and four times the minimum wage]." In addition, former salaries from the "welfare era" were recalculated to an hourly rate under neoliberal labor reform, which allowed institutions to eliminate payments for any time workers did not devote to direct labor-related activities included in their job description. It was an administrative strategy to increase workers' productivity and exploitation. "Now," Esperanza explained, "we get paid by the hour. If you work 6 hours, then you get paid 6 hours. Each hour gets paid at around US$3, and I work Monday through Friday from 7 to 1. Every other weekend I work on vaccinations and that is how I complete 40 hours. With this kind of contract, you come, work your hours, leave, and get paid. You have no rights to anything, just to get paid. No prima, no vacations, you just come, work, and leave. On top of that, you pay for your own health [and pension] out of your salary" by way of deductions. "In a month," Esperanza would say, "I make around US$450 to US$500. From that amount I have to pay health and pension, which are around US$100, so my salary comes to around US$350, can you imagine?" In spite of her disappointment with such a low amount as compared to her previous salary, Esperanza knew that in the existing job market for health care professionals, La Cruz's contract was not unusual. She considered herself "lucky" to have a job. Resigned, she asked, "What else can one do? Where else do you find a job? You have to keep what you have."

"On January 3rd, 2007, they [La Cruz directors] told me that they were planning to reopen Kangaroo [and asked] if I was interested. I said yes and we started the process, we started to give appointments." La Cruz pediatricians started to send babies to the program. Of course, the new program was nothing like KMC in its prime. Before La Cruz, Esperanza remembered, the Kangaroo program was very comprehensive, well funded, and well run. "We had two nurse assistants, including myself, and a head nurse exclusively appointed to the program. There was the pediatrician in charge of the program, there were all the therapists, the nutritionist, psychologist, plastic surgery, general surgery, genetics, pediatric orthopedics with Dr. Ramírez. There was also all the laboratory, X-ray diagnosis, everything was here." When El Materno was finally closed down, Esperanza remembered, "The last head nurse left and everything collapsed."

When La Cruz reopened services, it also reopened Kangaroo Care, but not with the same professional team or comprehensive services. Esperanza, who was rehired, noted that, even in 2015, "It's just me and the head nurse, but the head nurse is not just for Kangaroo. She is the head nurse for all the outpatient programs." When Kangaroo reopened, La Cruz appointed a pediatrician who combined her clinical hours with the Kangaroo clinic. Not only were the number of offered services significantly reduced, but the number of patients decreased. Patients now had to face many of the obstacles imposed by the health care reform, which El Materno tried as much as possible to handle. "Now," Esperanza said, "people have to authorize every service. Since Law 100 arrived, people have to go to the insurers and get authorization." She further explained how the system's new administrative "biobureaucracy"[4] was harder for people with meager resources to manage:

People here cannot just say, "OK, I will come back tomorrow," because they don't even have the money for transportation . . . before, you did not need to bill. A baby arrived, you weighed her and the pediatrician saw her, period. Since Law 100 you have to bill for everything. If I take an oxymetry, I have to bill for that. So, that means that the mother has to go [to the insurance] and get authorized. In order to authorize, the doctor gives [the mother] an Annex 3 form. In that form, the doctor writes down all the orders and referrals the patient needs, if he needs to be seen by orthopedics, if she needs a hip X-ray, if he needs to be seen by genetics, by surgery because of a hernia, and so on. Babies with oxygen, we have to do a weekly oxymetry. We give them the order so that they [insurers] authorize a given amount of oxymetries. The mother authorizes them, bills them [goes to the billing department], and then she brings me the receipt. In the receipt it says her name and the kind of [authorized and paid] service and then I can take the oxymetries.[5]

This mandatory authorization process has become, according to Esperanza, "one of the reasons mothers stop coming." Indeed, problems in lack and continuity of care abound in the new system.[6] Even though the program is run *almost* the same as before and by the same La Nacional/El Materno graduates, the quality of care and the progress of Kangaroo babies have been affected. Esperanza said:

> Just as one example, I have noticed that we don't have enough therapy appointments. Many of [our Kangaroo] children need therapy, but they cannot come because there are no appointments. So children start presenting with delays: a baby who is supposed to be sitting and is not, their cognitive development is also affected. For instance, physical, occupational, and speech therapists come daily, but they only come [for their paid shifts] from 10 to 12:30 or 1:00. That's it. So, they get to see only four to five patients per day. So, they cannot see everyone who needs these therapies [and] every day, there is a backlog of unseen babies. The doctor prescribes therapy, and it is not just one therapy, it is five therapies per month. So, lack of appointments has become a huge obstacle to good quality of care and follow-up.[7]

Besides therapies, something similar is happening with other specialties that, at El Materno, were well staffed, since the hospital had all the specialties and subspecialties that La Nacional medical school offered. Esperanza listed subspecialties that have problems with insufficient appointments, many of which don't even have contracted workers: physiatry, neuropsychiatry, orthopedics, neurology. For some of these, there are only appointments when La Nacional professors come in.

On top of all those problems, "there is not enough personnel for adequate follow-up in Kangaroo. For instance, I am alone here and I have to do everything by myself. Another person is in charge of follow-ups [for Kangaroo patients], but that person is also responsible for many other things." "Sadly," Esperanza concluded, "we don't know any longer why patients don't come back."[8]

ESPERANZA BELIEVED THAT ALL the pediatricians who had run the Kangaroo program were excellent. "It is because [El Materno/La Nacional] Escuela is very good. Almost all of the pediatricians have been part of the escuela, and almost all have been trained by Dr. Alcira. She is just so excellent in everything she does: an excellent teacher and an excellent pediatrician." For years, the Kangaroo program was run by La Cruz, but Alcira Muñoz kept seeing patients. The new director of the pediatrics department disliked Alcira's presence and even told her that she had no business with the program. Eventually, thanks to several negotiations, La Cruz offered Alcira two hours a day to work at the Kangaroo clinic. She and Esperanza knew each other very well, worked wonderfully as a team, and decided to rebuild their old Kangaroo program, as much as the limitations of the new hospital structure and health care system administration allowed. Slowly, the Kangaroo clinic started to see many kangaroo babies. Even in 2010, years after it was reopened, the Kangaroo program was far from what Alcira envisioned. In her words, "It is a disaster. What they [La Cruz] called Kangaroo is not Kangaroo." Alcira referred to the challenges she faced in trying to make La Cruz administrators understand what a comprehensive program meant and how to integrate all the services despite the limitations of contracts and the new system's other cost-control mechanisms. Besides the missing therapies, diagnoses, and subspecialists, Alcira was pained to see how the new administration did not help ease patients' experience of the health care system's complex bureaucracies, but in fact added to them, making the interactions between insurers, patients, and hospitals more difficult.

Like other professors, Alcira negotiated with the La Cruz director, who allowed her to handle some aspects of the program as she thought best, but in many respects Alcira still faced a good deal of resistance to rebuilding the old Kangaroo program. In particular, her comprehensive assessment of each kangaroo baby required a longer medical visit and a set of preventive actions that included extraclinical tests, therapies, and social services. She was faced with repeated conflicts with the pediatrics directorship body and La Cruz administration because these extra costs, without a commitment from the administration to find strategies to ensure that all clinical patient needs produced successful bills, would likely result in unpaid bills and glosses (see chapter 4). When they complained about her slower-than-expected pace of clinical interactions, she responded that she was seeing eleven patients in two hours. The directors responded that she was moving slowly because she was also giving clinical instruction to interns and residents, despite the fact that La Cruz was not paying her to be an instructor. She replied that she was also using her hours as professor of La Nacional to extend her time at the hospital, but that even with those extra hours, she still did not have enough time to see all the patients.

While La Cruz administrators increased her paid hours so that she could keep up with the growing demands of Kangaroo patients, they also put a nurse unofficially in charge of "keeping an eye" on her actions. "Since I am, let's say, obsessed with being thorough, I apply the risk-based approach to determine what [each child needs]." The risk-based approach refers to a set of clinical, emotional, and social conditions that help "predict" potential complications and aid clinicians in setting up a management plan that includes preventive interventions addressing the specific needs of children and their caretakers. The risk-based approach and the subsequent management plan ensure that children continue thriving after they are discharged and avoid setbacks and rehospitalizations. So, in any given case, Alcira might order additional tests or keep a baby hospitalized for one more day to make sure that all the risks had been considered in the child's management plan. In these cases, the unofficially assigned nurse would undermine Alcira's authority, telling mothers that Alcira could always find problems with children but that they should not worry because a different doctor would always find the same children well enough to go home.

The everyday conflict between Alcira and La Cruz required diplomatic negotiations and patience with La Cruz directors, given the unknown future of La Cruz and La Nacional at El Materno. But Alcira found herself perhaps too strong-willed, unable to bend her standards of care when it came to doing what was best for the patients. Alcira started to experience the undermining of her medical orders as an exhausting daily routine.

For me it became such an ordeal to hospitalize a baby. In one particular case, there was a child [in the outpatient Kangaroo clinic] who seemed to have a severe urinary tract infection, who was not putting on weight and was not doing well overall. I ordered a blood test and a urine test. The next day [when the child came back to the clinic] I started to notice some respiratory distress, so I thought that we needed to hospitalize him. But since I already knew where things stood [with the administration], I decided to take the urine sample myself with a catheter and order a culture. Well, [the nurse who was keeping an eye on her] reversed my hospitalization order. The next day, I came to check on him and he was not hospitalized. I was told that the child was in perfect condition [and did not need to be hospitalized]. So I go down to the lab and the urine test showed a terrible infection, so I had to call the mom and tell her to come back to the hospital immediately. The mom tried to explain that she was told that it was ok to go home. I said to not worry, to just come in, that I would hospitalize him. The child remained hospitalized for a whole month and the mom sent a letter to the hospital saying, "Thanks to the stubbornness of physicians like Dr. Alcira who insisted [on] hospitalizing my baby, I can now enjoy him at home. I congratulate you for having people like her working at your institution."

In direct confrontations, Alcira was told to stop scaring parents unnecessarily by telling them about other tests that could be done or telling the parents that their children were sicker than they were. "These were daily events," Alcira said. Nursing assistants, head nurses, and physicians were forced to obey La Cruz administration by reporting on whatever steps Alcira took and contradicting her "excessive" orders and "desires" to keep hospitalizing patients, even though she constantly proved herself right.

One day she even had to explain a case in which she had to reassert a hospitalization order that had been turned down by La Cruz's "reference person." The reference person, Alcira explained, "used to be a pediatrician but now is a general physician in charge of coordinating La Cruz's emergency and pediatrics [departments]. This person is supposed to be in administration, but closer to the workings of the department." In reality, this person is a bureaucratic liaison charged with making sure that everyday clinical procedures are aligned with the hospitals' needs in ensuring payments for services. The reference person would also cancel contracts with "problematic personnel" and less profitable specialists. "You better watch out," one patient told Alcira. Indeed, some days later, she found herself sharing her clinical hours at Kangaroo with a new pediatrician and had to find other services in which to fulfill all her contracted hours. However, La Cruz "got rid of [the new pediatrician] . . . it seems she complained about something she thought wasn't right and then [the administration] told her that she could finish her month at the intensive care unit but that her contract was not going to be renewed."

Although Alcira regained all her hours at Kangaroo, the work-related harassment did not stop. One day, "I cried because I just didn't know what else to do." At around the same time, the nurse who had made it a personal project to make Alcira's life at the hospital miserable "accidentally" shoved her in the hallway. "And on Tuesday," Alcira continued, "[one of the babies whose parents she had supposedly worried unnecessarily] was hospitalized with a severe abdominal infection and a perforation. I said, 'Do I have to feel happy that a child got sicker just to prove that I was right?'" The final straw that made her make the very painful decision to quit was when an intern noticed a heart gallop in a baby who was already on oxygen. (Many kangaroo babies go home with oxygen tanks.) "So, I increased the oxygen until he was stable, but we started to discuss possible causes. I sent him to emergency because it was already around 3 p.m. [when the clinic closed for the day]. I stuck around, as I usually do, and the mother and the grandmother came back [crying] after hearing who knows what from the nurse and physicians [at the emergency department]. I was so hurt to see that even other people were crying for me, that someone else had to tell me that it was not just [that they were revoking her medical decisions]." The grandmother told her she was upset by "the way they refer to you, how they mock you, and they laugh at you. And I know you, and I know that the only thing you do here is work and care for our babies. And I was just so shocked that it was the grandmother who was telling me that. It can't be that [a patient's relatives] love me more than I love myself, can it?"[9]

ALCIRA WAS HOPING THAT she could still help the new pediatrician in charge of the Kangaroo program, if not as a hospital worker then through her position as professor at La Nacional. In her mind, the new pediatrician, whom she knew from her residency at El Materno, could see the patients; Alcira could assist her with education and other family activities, while continuing to instruct medical students and residents. But then she was notified that she could not work in the Kangaroo program anymore—not even with students—in part because La Cruz attending physicians' and service directors' lack of affiliation with the university challenged El Materno's hierarchy of knowledge and decision-making. To professors, it seemed nonsensical for their orders to be supervised by nonacademics, who were in some cases their former students. Equally, to attending physicians, it seemed absurd to receive advice or comments from academics about their decision-making. The 2006 agreement approved by the attorney general that formalized the split between workers defending their labor rights and an active hospital had not considered the disagreements about mission that might arise between a city hospital organized around the new for-profit logics of the system and a university hospital with faculty and students.

Depending on their clinical practice, some professors could challenge or circumvent the imposed limitations of La Cruz's administration more easily. In deliveries and neonatal adaptation, for example, clinical decisions are more autonomous, and it is virtually impossible to have different processes approved or supervised. But depending on whether they saw a professor from La Nacional or an attending physician from La Cruz, patients would experience different epistemologies of care. For example, Santiago Currea continued arriving early, and babies were born in the mornings aided by his loving hands and words; their umbilical cords were respected. In the afternoons, La Cruz attending physicians would clamp and cut the cords right away. On other shifts where La Nacional's presence was less evident, Santiago acknowledged, "the situation was kind of half-catastrophic." Stories of complications and infant deaths—things that would not have happened at El Materno—began to circulate.

Like Alcira, other professors were disturbed by the painful changes they witnessed. But some of them opted for other negotiation strategies with La Cruz. Some opted for diplomatic choices. Some avoided La Cruz personnel as much as they could, some tried to collaborate with La Cruz members who were more willing to listen, and some continued negotiating with directors of services or the director of the hospital for elements they considered important to patients' clinical care.

The removal of certain El Materno/La Nacional workers—including professors, like Alcira, who had confronted La Cruz's standards more bluntly—was celebrated in a meeting as an important step toward "purifying" the hospital. But every time a former professor left the institution, it was a big blow. And yet, Santiago acknowledged the cruel paradox: "If it were not because of La Cruz's presence, there would not be any Materno left. It has never been the same as before, has it? We remain in a fragile state, but at least we are still open and can do our things. . . . That is how history works; it tries to get rid of all traces of the past. At least, as long as we are here, that is not going to happen."[10]

In 2015, months after Alcira resigned, Santiago was close to fulfilling his retirement requirements. The situation at the university, however, was tense. He was torn between wanting to retire because sustaining the hospital situation was very difficult for him, and hearing from other professors how important it was for the university that he remained at the hospital. He was a key figure in El Materno's resistance. In 2011 he wrote in the presentation of one of his many public presentations about the hospital that they were "resisting for rebirthing"; some years later, in 2014, he insisted that the most important aspect of this painful history was that "they had remained and remained and remained." Nonetheless, he acknowledged, he was bored with the whole situation because it was "like the invasion of France. But if France had not resisted, it wouldn't have kept its identity. So, La Cruz has that characteristic—it wants to get rid of everything from El Materno, but at least as long as we are here that is not going to happen." He was aware, however, that in the current scenario, it was La Cruz "who calls the shots." Dealing with La Cruz, for him, was like "living in someone else's house." You have to learn "how to handle them. There are many daily conflicts and confrontations, but you have to pick your battles." Nonetheless, the losses had been immense. According to Santiago, "before, services were very integrated; teaching hospital activities were combined with clinical duties.

The teaching approach was parallel or in synchronicity with the clinical activities. Today we have a very different situation: La Cruz has its own professionals and we are just there," in an ambivalent space—not considered instrumental, but still employed. He knew, however, that he had a relatively easy time of it, perhaps because of his area of expertise. The clinical dynamics around neonatal reanimation and adaptation occurred behind doors and in total autonomy, as we saw with head nurse Sonia. Santiago also admitted that "I avoid conflicts, very consciously." In other parts of the hospital, he knows, it is easier to feel annoyed by La Cruz's position. "So there is a certain irritability that grows into conflict. That is unavoidable."

Orders written by professors in the morning could be altered in the afternoon, which made doctors angry and concerned for their patients. Worrisome ruptures of personal ties and old friendships began to appear among the faculty. These interpersonal crises among faculty members were more clearly the result of the situation with La Cruz than had been the case with workers. The faculty tried to keep things civil, although they knew that the department, the relationship among colleagues, and their tradition as "La Escuela" would never be the same. They were aware that they were dealing with La Cruz in order to maintain their presence and some resemblance of a university hospital. The unspoken question was how far they were willing to let the destruction of their academic principles go. The impossible question was whether they might one day be successful in regaining El Materno for La Nacional.

Tensions also grew between faculty members and former El Materno workers, since the workers' resistance strategies disrupted not only La Cruz's activities but also the professors'. While all professors showed immense understanding of the workers' situation, as time went on, some of them started to express bitterness at La Carpa workers for jeopardizing clinical and teaching activities. Workers, on the other hand, had mixed feelings about professors; some had been very supportive of the workers' fight all along, but the workers felt that most faculty had turned their backs on them and were defending the university at the expense of El Materno as a whole—faculty, students, *and* workers. Under the 2006 agreement, the parking lot was also assigned to workers, and in spite of several negotiation efforts, professors were not allowed to park there; they were forced instead to park in one of the public lots and walk a couple of blocks in an area that was not considered particularly safe. La Carpa workers did authorize professors to use one of the classrooms that they had initially secured with a lock.

When the coordinator of La Nacional's pediatric department at El Materno got funds in 2014 for new curtains and paint for the classroom, La Carpa workers initially refused to authorize the painting of the classroom but, a week later, they said that they would let the university paint it if the state's department of patrimony authorized it. The absurdity of having to ask for permission to paint a room demonstrated the precarity of both groups' projects: the workers' resisting through any strategy at hand (chapter 5) and professors' finding ways to keep up with their university mission.[11]

DURING THE MONTHS OF El Materno's closure in 2006, professors searched for alternative hospitals where they could take their students. Santiago remembers that when he accompanied two other neonatologists (Luis Carlos Mendez and Gabriel Longi) to a new, small hospital. It felt like too many professors, but "no babies were being born at El Materno. So, how could we teach anything? We went to the Engativá hospital and made the agreement. They accepted us with kindness, with tolerance. We continued holding classes at El Materno. We maintained a certain academic presence there, but the clinical aspects were impossible [given the lack of patients]. When they finally reopened El Materno, I didn't have any doubts—I came back. I came back to pick up where I had left off. . . . I didn't have problems returning." He did acknowledge that it would have been difficult for Luis Carlos to return to El Materno: "He had built a very valuable presence in Engativá. It is not only the work with the children but with the whole team. You cannot build that [relationship] in two days." Indeed, Luis Carlos Méndez had established wonderful relationships with the team of workers from Engativá, and the students had also found a new place for learning. Luis Carlos stayed, bringing a piece of El Materno to a city hospital twenty kilometers away. For Luis Carlos, the situation with La Cruz was unbearable. He felt they had been "displaced from their own home"—a strong violence metaphor, considering the country's history, but one that he did not use lightly.

Like many others in the El Materno/La Nacional Escuela, Luis Carlos arrived at work early and left late. Luis Carlos remembered that he would arrive at Engativá at "5:30 in the morning and would leave at 3 p.m. absolutely exhausted. But it was so beautiful. How can I put this? I continued being Materno." At Engativá he started at a different pediatric service, which forced him to go back and study more, but he felt that at the new hospital he "could bring all that knowledge from El Materno." The warm welcome at Engativá was so important because, after the painful relationship with La Cruz,

Engativá "allowed us to be recognized as human beings again, to relate to one another. They were offering their space, their house, their institution. They were giving it to us." Unlike La Cruz,

> it was not as if they were imposing on us, quite the contrary, they said it was a pleasure and an honor to have us there. So, when you have been displaced, hearing that is just wonderful. Maybe that is why I am growing roots there. We are also creating a team. For example, the other day, a nurse assistant said to me, "Doctor, yesterday I attended a baby who had meconium, which means that the baby had pooped inside the womb [a condition that can lead to serious complications]. He was born like that and wasn't breathing and so I did as I have seen you do. I started all the maneuvers and said, 'Watch out, do not clamp that cord,' and I waited. It was eight minutes, Doctor, that we were there waiting [for the baby to respond]. And then the baby went home with her mom!" So, what else can you ask in life? And students as well, they say that it is very hard to contradict the attending physician but they are starting to tell them to wait, to see if the cord is still pulsating—they are starting to confront the residents.

These anecdotes point to the resurgence of the escuela, even if on a much smaller scale—an escuela that, like at El Materno, involved not only medical students but the whole health care staff. As at the former El Materno, nurse assistants and other personnel also learned different clinical aspects and became experts in particular aspects of care.

Hence, the feelings of gratitude to Engativá are, according to Luis Carlos, "eternal." In spite of La Nacional's continued presence at El Materno, Luis Carlos agrees with others who conclude that

> it is not El Materno anymore. It is with the deepest sorrow that I say what I am about to say, and it is absurd to say it because I never thought that I was going to say this, but nowadays I prefer staying at Engativá to going back to El Materno. If I had a full time position [as a faculty member at the School of Medicine, where he only has a half-time contract], I would have gone back to El Materno. Besides, both medical students and residents, said to me, "Don't leave here [Engativá], stay with us. We want you here because we can assure you that what we are experiencing here, what this rotation is meaning to us, we are not getting anywhere else."

Nonetheless, Luis Carlos had the same hope as those who remained and those who left. "I hope to return to El Materno, to return to my home, to my escuela. I hope to return and fulfill a dream. It is a dream that the team [of neonatologists] have had [since the economic crisis first began to threaten a bleak institutional future]. We would love it if the Instituto Materno Infantil could become the National Institute of Perinatology and Neonatology." In their minds, an autonomous institute specializing in perinatology and neonatology, like other successful institutes, would ensure both academic autonomy and administrative independence enough to survive within the market-based model. Since the health secretariate of Bogotá was finally authorized to "purchase" the hospitals El Materno and San Juan after the many negotiations and legal and administrative battles between 2014 and 2017, Santiago continues to have the goal of independent administration. If El Materno cannot become a national institute, then, at least, it can become Bogotá's Institute of Perinatology. This dream excites former and current El Materno workers.

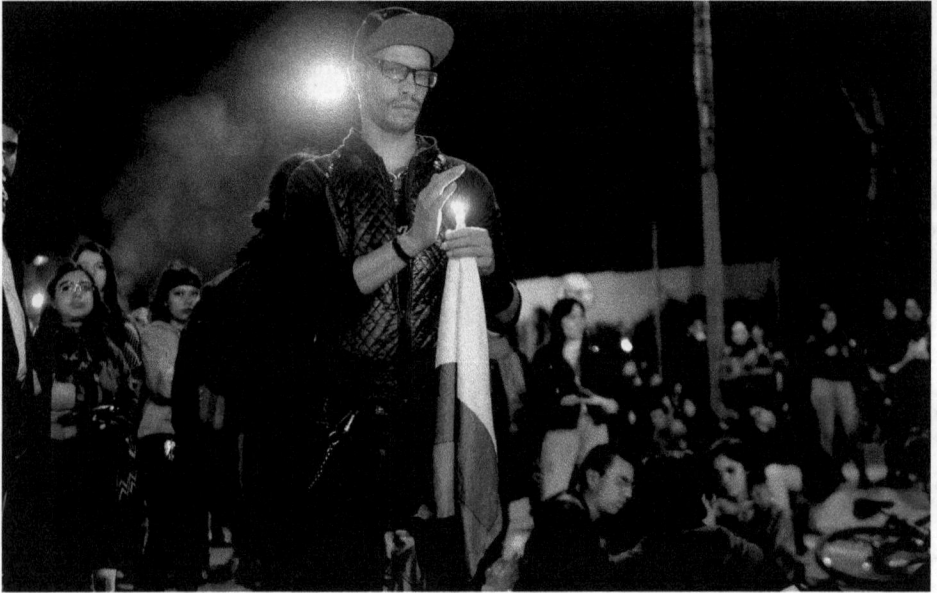

FIGURE 7.1. Photo "Velatón por Dilan Cruz, Hospital San Ignacio, Bogotá paro nacional 2019" [Candlelight parade for Dilan Cruz, San Ignacio Hospital, Bogotá national strike 2019]. (Courtesy of Gustavo A. Fernández Vega.)

CHAPTER 7. Learning and Practicing
Medicine in a For-Profit System

This chapter depicts the new business conditions in which medical students learn and recent graduates from medical school or residency programs work in Colombia. The process of replacing a particular set of social practices, such as medical care and medical training, does not occur overnight. It is a long-term process, during which previous generations are phased out and new generations take over.

We have seen how remnants of the past, such as El Materno, are co-opted, reduced to their minimum expression, or eliminated so that new generations do not experience them and cannot fight for what they do not know they are missing. In this chapter, we will see how newer generations receive medical training and work in ill-performing schools and hospitals; consciously or unconsciously, they end up reproducing the system. Aided by the proliferation of medical schools, the Marxist logic of the reserve army of labor applies to physician labor in Colombia; the nonworking labor force serves to regulate salaries since the demand for labor exceeds the supply of jobs. We will read how El Materno workers and professors, and in general the health care labor force, face employers who tell them, "If you don't like the contract, do not sign." There is always someone willing to take the job under whatever conditions are offered.

What we will recount in this chapter is the result of twenty-five years of transformation of medicine in Colombia, after the signing of the privatization law (Law 100) in 1993. Several aspects are particularly notable: the rapid defunding and destruction of the country's public hospital infrastructure and its very long history; the direct attack on the traditions of different escuelas as their university hospitals (both in Bogotá and elsewhere) crumbled or were transformed into profit-seeking health centers under the privatization law; and the transformation of labor, which meant not only lower salaries but also the forceful enculturation of physicians into a for-profit ethos of medical care. So much was destroyed in such a short time; that destruction was necessary for the new model to claim a hegemonic position in the country. Unlike other countries that have suffered the effects of neoliberal reforms in health, Colombia implemented a universal reform that did away with the former public and social security sectors; it forced all Colombians to get individual health insurance and all hospitals to adopt a "for-profit" and billing culture. The absence of alternatives has shifted health ideologies toward a universalizing idea that health is an insurable commodity and "profitability" in medical care is the norm. Oppositional proposals find no space in Colombia's field of medical praxis, and physicians' and patients' political imaginations continue migrating toward for-profit logics.

Fortunately, even processes as violent as the destruction of El Materno can never eliminate all traces of the past. This chapter will show how not only do people like professors and alumni carry the history of La Escuela with them but also the buildings and infrastructure constantly retell the story of what they used to be. El Materno and El San Juan Hospital complexes are ruins in the making and, as such, there are a myriad of political and ideological struggles to determine what they represent and how they fit with the current state of affairs of neoliberal Colombian history. We will see how students, even without receiving training at those emblematic centers, are trained by the same professors who used to work there; they get a taste of what it was like to be part of La Nacional Escuela. In debates, protests, and social movements, they study the history of their university and its hospitals and refuse to accept the market-based system as their new professional horizon. They join professors in arguing that "health and education are rights, not commodities," and they make efforts to keep alive an epistemology of medical care in which love, care, and selflessness are at the core of every interaction with patients and of the strategies for innovative subaltern research and medical praxis.

A Generational Transition

Matheo and his brother Nicolas were born at El Materno. Much of their childhood and adolescence were spent visiting and playing at El Materno, while their mom, Patricia Farías, finished her duties as head of the lactation program and of the Teaching and Service Committee. Both boys came to love the hospital. For them both, the process of its destruction and the ways in which their mom suffered and dealt with the situation affected their perspectives on life. Both knew very well the kinds of destruction that neoliberalism in health had caused in Colombia, and both admired tremendously the fight that their mother and the other El Materno workers maintained.

Matheo took one semester of medicine at a private school that had a very good reputation, in part because many of its professors had been trained at La Nacional. Like many others, he then retook the admission test for La Nacional, hoping to be part of La Nacional Escuela and stop paying expensive private school tuition. He remembered that when he passed the test and started studying at La Nacional in 2008, he was told what many other generations of students had been told ever since San Juan closed: "Very soon, next year, the university hospital will open and the 'problem' of not having a site for clinical training will be finally resolved." These were not outright lies from the professors. It was an optimistic trust that the constant efforts and negotiations between the professors and the directorship bodies would finally succeed in reopening El San Juan, recuperating El Materno, establishing a large agreement with an important clinic, and/or purchasing a building for a new university hospital. But none of these solutions had yet come to fruition.

Matheo sees a shift in how La Nacional's training is regarded by medical students. Traditionally, La Nacional graduates have been known for their excellent clinical skills. But now "[a] lot of people say that we receive more theory because we don't have a hospital. Depending on the subject, the professors give you lectures and literature reviews on the given topic, then you do presentations and all that happens from 7 a.m. to 1 p.m. Then you spend the rest of the time studying." In the absence of intense contact with patients, La Nacional students gain a strong basic and social science foundation in the preclinical years then continue with a lot of theory and independent studying during the years that should be clinically intense.

A large agreement with San Carlos Hospital in 2008 ended up supplying most of La Nacional's placements across specialties, although in somewhat undesirable conditions: less autonomy for professors and fewer patients for students to see. Other professors whose areas of expertise were not part of the agreement with San Carlos Hospital needed to find alternative ways to fulfill their professorial responsibilities and make sure students learned their specific areas. In some cases, the professors took the students to their private offices or to the private clinics where they worked. Matheo remembered this happening in ophthalmology. "The professor made some sort of arrangements so that they [the private clinic he worked at] let us in. But we just stood there watching how he did his consultation." Despite his gratitude and his recognition that professors were trying their best considering the difficult circumstances, Matheo remembers this setup as "uncomfortable" for both patient and student. "It was kind of crazy, to be honest. I didn't understand why I was rotating there, nor did I want to go there. First of all, those were not really training sites. Second, you would go there just to watch how the professor or resident did the consultation."

Matheo divides the major areas of intense clinical training into surgery, pediatrics, and gynecology. Surgery, in the absence of El San Juan, is the area where he felt he received the weakest training. Pediatrics maintained its tradition with the children's hospital La Misericordia, an entity that, originally created as a private foundation, could readjust more easily than public hospitals to the new market-based system. Those who don't know its legal status think of La Misericordia as the main center for pediatric care in the country and as part of La Nacional Escuela. In fact, when El Materno closed, the school of medicine's pediatrics department was transferred to La Misericordia; they opened a small neonatal unit there as a way to "replace" some of the care and education offered at El Materno. In terms of gynecology, "I had Engativá [as a placement, where Luis Carlos Méndez also 'migrated'] and [for neonatology I had] Materno. Well, Materno/La Cruz, where we mostly heard professors reminisce about the old Materno."

What it was like for him to go back to El Materno as a student was hard to describe. "It was like a facade without people. There were [the workers' slogans] on the walls, some of the rooms were sealed. The academic area remained. I am not sure how to describe it. It was as if something was missing." The new generation of medical students felt the same ambivalence as did the workers about whether El Materno remained or not after La Cruz. Nonetheless, El Materno's gynecology and neonatology professors' fight to remain at the hospital was very significant for their students' training. According to Matheo,

If you ask alumni from the Nacho [as La Nacional is colloquially referred to], in the last four or five cohorts [that is, 2009–2014], gynecology is the best structured rotation. The conditions are much better in terms of academics, in terms of practice, in terms of interpersonal relations [with professors and among students, interns and residents]. It is the best in terms of both theory and practice. You can do things there. It is where I delivered a baby. And that didn't happen just to me. Depending on what came up during the shift, some classmates would volunteer, "I could suture, I could do this and that" [a situation that was drastically different to the other rotations at city hospitals].

Matheo said that after all the changes from La Cruz's takeover, El Materno "still felt like home, [but] things were a little different. I guess it is the place where you still feel la escuela, or what they call the pedagogy of teaching, being able to be with the professor. You feel that more [at El Materno]." But the interdisciplinary training of the past was definitely lost since many of the experts had left. For example, until 2003 medical students and residents at El Materno learned craniofacial development from Astrid Olivar Bonilla, a pediatric dentist and professor at the School of Dentistry who dedicated her career to the care of pregnant women and neonates. Up until 2006 medical students and residents learned lactation from the country's expert, Matheo's mother, Patricia Farías, who received special training in the United States thanks to a UNICEF training grant. Furthermore, the lack of a general hospital that could offer an adequate learning environment for rotations in surgery, general medicine, and other specialties did cause serious problems in their training.

In addition to the closure of San Juan, however, students and residents from La Nacional faced the additional challenge of an overproliferation of private medical schools around the country.[1] A "market" of placements for medical students and residents was created, and universities started to bid for training spots at city hospitals. Not surprisingly, private universities with more resources began to find placements in better hospitals. For example, students from the country's most expensive medical school, which opened in 2004, not only established an agreement with the largest private clinic in the city but also started to rotate, among other city hospitals, at El Materno under La Cruz's administration. Public universities like La Nacional were unable to justify spending any resources on these placements. One private university that allowed La Nacional students to rotate at its university hospital asked if some of the tuition from La Nacional students could be diverted to its medical school.[2] Neoliberal policies in education had aggravated the university's own economic crisis, which progressively moved toward self-sustainability.[3]

The situation was so critical that in 2011, when Matheo was in his fourth year, the medical school residents and students went on a strike. One of the student movement's representatives used a simile to explain: "A swimmer cannot learn how to swim without a pool. We cannot learn how to become physicians without a hospital." Matheo participated in the protests but was not a movement leader. He remembered the students discussing how other medical schools that still had [an affiliated] hospital did provide hospital-based training. For Matheo, this movement was not really representative of a leftist political platform, as was the distinctive mark of public university students of the past. "The movement was about building a hospital for La Nacional so that there were better clinical training sites and the university could produce high-quality physicians, just like before [in times of El San Juan]."

Some students did discuss the implications of the lack of a university hospital within a context of the increasingly hegemonic neoliberal idea that health and education should be handled as commodities. The slogan "health is a right, not a commodity" was already circulating widely across the country. For these students, who were more critical and more clearly affiliated with leftist politics, having a hospital for the university was not merely a matter of training: it was essential for advancing a political agenda around health and education that countered the market ideology. Government support for private sectors in health and education since the 1980s made public hospitals and public institutions less central to the country's political agenda than they were before. If before the 1960s Ministers of Health were usually affiliated with La Nacional's medical school, during the recent neoliberal decades, they came increasingly from private elite universities—and many have been economists.

Interestingly, however, in the same year as the medical school strike, the government presented to Congress a new bill for higher education. The bill, among other fraught intentions, threatened public higher education funding even more by promoting a "leveled" market competition of educational institutions and created legal grounds for for-profit higher education institutions.[4] There was a massive reaction from university students, who found support in many social sectors. This led to the creation of a new nationwide student movement, many of whose leaders came from La Nacional. The country's main teachers' unions and other social groups joined in nationwide protests; public universities went on strike. Finally, the government withdrew the bill from Congress and promised to start a process to create a new law built on participation rather than imposition. The medical school strike, however, was never integrated into this larger educational social movement platform. As medical school students maintained their strike, the dean remained unsympathetic to their protest and demands. He warned that if they maintained their strike, the semester would have to be canceled; he claimed that this would cost taxpayers a lot of money. The media reported on both the alarming situation of the students and the cost of canceling the semester. The semester was eventually canceled, but calls to help the university resulted in a new agreement with the health care secretariat of Bogotá, which offered more placements for clinical rotations and better conditions in the city hospitals. The new agreements partially solved the problem of having too few rotation sites, but it did not solve the structural problem: the overabundance of medical schools and the absence of a university hospital were hampering student training at the country's most important public university.

Students returned and attended their new rotation sites, but, according to Matheo, "there were [still] many limitations to [the clinical training of medical students] at the public hospitals. For example, Felipe [a friend of his] and I are both from La Nacional, but Felipe and I are different when it comes to clinical practice. That is because he did his internship at Amazonas and I did mine in Cali and Bogotá. I got trained at fourth-level and third-level centers, and he got trained at a second-level center." Matheo is describing how students end up with drastic differences in their clinical training depending on where they were assigned within the new options. El San Juan and El Materno were fourth-level referral centers—the highest level of specialty care where the most complex patients were treated. In contrast, second-level centers received less complex patients; the lack of exposure and of highly trained specialists and university professors resulted in different levels of clinical exposure and expertise for the students placed there. Graduates from La Nacional now represent a wider range of expertise—all of which pale in comparison to the former El San Juan and former El Materno.

The training, however, is not random, nor is it limited to existing agreements. Students, who are well aware of the limitations in their clinical training, think seriously about getting as much exposure as they can and making things happen for themselves. Matheo remembers that, at a certain point during medical school, "in your fifth year, or even before, certain 'profes' tell you, 'Well, it is better if you go to such and such place [for your internship.]' For instance, for surgery [rotation], tons of people try to [find a placement] elsewhere because our [assigned] rotation sites are [four city hospitals,] Samaritana or Tunal or Engativá or San Carlos, but the rotation is very limited and professors are not concentrated in just one place." Too, the hospitals with existing agreements "get way too many people. They are always full of private university students. And our professors [are not there reliably]. There is one professor assigned to us but he stays only a short while, and then leaves." So it is up to the students, especially once they are in their internships, to develop relationships with the residents and get as much clinical exposure as possible. Matheo sees that residents are still very dedicated, but he also knows that they are limited and lost, both because of the health care system and because the academic environment is damaged by the absence of professors.

Matheo explained,

> You meet with the *profe* in charge of the whole curriculum, in our case he was an anesthesiologist. He met with us and told us, "Well, you have these options but definitely the best thing for you is to leave [Bogotá], you need to set yourselves free. You will learn more." And indeed, many students would go outside [of Bogotá for the internship]. And [outside Bogotá] they don't have the same kind of pressure they experience here. As interns, they are allowed to do more things. Depending on the physician in charge, for example, he might tell [the intern], "You can do the whole consultation and then I'll come in and you tell me." Here, in contrast, the physician or the resident does the consultation, and you are just standing there, watching. That has important implications because you don't feel any responsibility for the patient and that [does not bring] confidence when you have to start working [as a physician]. It is learning at a distance; you just see them doing it. So, when you go outside, you have to do it yourself and gain experience.

Like the missing professors, Matheo comments, health care workers' "partial contracts and agreements [between the university and the hospitals] significantly limit medical students' and residents' activities. Compared to what [the professors] tell us the limitations are indeed much bigger than before." Unquestionably, the lack of experience, exposure, comprehensive care, direct instruction by professors, and a third- and fourth-level university hospital have resulted in a significant destruction of La Nacional Escuela. In order to get around the situation, Matheo found an internship placement at the Hospital Universitario del Valle (HUV). Even though it is in a different escuela (called "del Valle" after this department, which is located in the country's southwest region), its hospital has been able to survive within the market-based system in part through a large, cruel administrative adjustment, in which many workers were laid off, and in part because, as Matheo commented, "the students live and work at the hospital. A student works as a physician [and receives no payment]"—a strategy that the hospital has used to reduce health care costs. This is even better for the hospital's bottom line than "free labor," because medical students and residents pay tuition for the training opportunities as physicians and specialists.[5] But it also brings another set of opportunities. "The students there have more freedom and are very good. They have more confidence, you can tell. And they would help me. When I had doubts about what to do or how to do something, they would come and help me." Even though Matheo received more and better training at HUV, he didn't learn certain traditional surgical skills commonly known to all physicians who were going to work in rural areas, such as C-sections and appendectomies. He knows he is limited. During his mandatory social service, in a rural area with a sizable indigenous population and serious geographic barriers to accessing health care services, he depended on referrals or the availability of the other general physicians who could do these procedures. He remembered a patient "who had appendicitis and I didn't know how to do the surgery. I had to refer her to surgery and it took about five days for her to finally get the surgery done, can you imagine?"

It was not just the remoteness of the area that led to this compromised care. Matheo is noting how the system's overall infrastructure had created so many administrative and economic access barriers that patients frequently faced denials in coverage or delayed services. The insurance companies that run the system not only try to block payments to hospital bills, as we saw in chapter 4, but actively deny care to patients, even covered care. Patients have been forced to bring legal suits demanding the protection of their constitutional right to health care. The writ (known as Tutela in Colombia) started as an important legal protection mechanism, but it quickly became an epidemic that overwhelmed the courts.[6] Every year, thousands of Colombians sue the insurance companies (around 100,000), and the judiciary system usually grants their petitions. The chaos of denied care grew to such heights that the constitutional court produced a 2008 decision that became emblematic across the world in terms of judicial protection of the right to health care.[7] With this decision, the Colombian constitutional court elevated health to a fundamental human right, whereas before it was just considered a service. The court also ordered the government to fix the many structural and systemic malfunctions that were infringing on this right.

In spite of the judiciary's efforts and the significant step forward that this decision represented, insurance companies have continued making a mockery of the judiciary and profiting from the health care system. Not only do insurance companies disregard judicial orders and continue denying services to patients and payments to hospitals, but they also divert resources. They have stolen billions of dollars in money designated for health. The government has allowed the consolidation of oligopolies and the reconfiguration and purchasing of some failed insurers by other insurance groups. The same groups that profited by mishandling resources and failing to comply with their contracted obligations were allowed, under new legal and institutional names, to continue managing the health policies of their affiliated bases. In a public outcry, journalists and professors have demonstrated that, under these new names, the groups are exempt from any of the "former" companies' debt obligations.[8] Every few years, a new scandal arises, new debates occur, and a new "corrective law" is passed. But none of these laws, *obviously*, have proposed dismantling the business structure of the system.[9]

ALSO INSPIRED AND AFFECTED by his mother's struggle at El Materno, Nicolás, Matheo's younger brother, wanted to better understand how social problems and conflicts connected to the country's history and to intellectual traditions in critical theory. He found that high school was not offering him what he was looking for. He dropped out and decided to continue studying on his own while his mom, Patricia, worried and wondered to what extent the hospital crisis was affecting Nicolás's important decisions. He found in Marxist and psychoanalytic texts important explanations of society's malfunctions and its impacts on individuals. Medicine was not necessarily part of his career interest, but thanks to Mario Hernández—a physician, historian, well-known scholar, and activist of social medicine in Latin America and professor at the School of Medicine at La Nacional who allowed him and Matheo to participate in his study group—he started to see how medicine really explained many structural social malfunctions and how it could do a lot to confront injustices and inequalities. Nicolás took the national high school exam to receive his diploma and the admission tests for medical school at both La Nacional and El Valle. He passed the test at El Valle. Even though Nicolás had not yet started his clinical training at HUV in 2015, when we talked about his experience as a student, he was glad to be part of that escuela, which was also public and had a good reputation; in fact, its graduates were getting the highest scores in the medical school exit exam.[10]

Given his critical perspective, however, he was very analytical about the hospital's situation. At El Valle, he said, "you see the same division between the academics and the clinicians"—those more inclined to think about social medicine as part of politics and those who maintain an apolitical kind of clinical medicine. About the Hospital Universitario del Valle, Nicolás seemed to retell a very similar tale of what El Materno went through. Ironically, he said, it was under a leftist government that the HUV was closed down for restructuring to meet the newly competitive market demands.[11] HUV did many of the things El Materno refused to do. "What he [the director of HUV] did was terrible. He [brought] the third-party contract system to the hospital and transformed it into an ESE [Empresa de Salud del Estado, or State's Health Company—the restructuring name that hospitals received to be able to compete and bill within the new system]. In other words, he adapted the hospital to the new system."

Later, during 2013, the residents and interns of HUV went on strike to protest the mishandling and mismanagement of the hospital's new director, Marta Lucía Urriago.[12] During her administration, Nicolás recalled, "the hospital went into a terrible crisis. There was no gauze, no bandages. There were not even the basic items necessary for seeing patients. The students started to strike after the workers had already been striking for one month. [The workers alone] had not been able to create a strong enough impact [to win any of their demands], but once the residents and interns joined in, the situation was different because the hospital's clinical services rely on them." It was very difficult to understand the hospital's precarious situation, even with unpaid physicians and highly exploited health care workers and paramedical personnel. Finally, Nicolás remembered, "the director was forced to quit." Then, the governor of the state appointed Professor Jaime Rubiano as new director. But, according to Nicolás, "his mentality is absolutely managerial. He wants the hospital to be self-sustainable and he wants to give away clinical services to private groups. He already handed out angiology and dialysis, meaning that they are no longer part of the hospital."

While Nicolás leaned more toward social medicine and psychiatry, he was very aware of the importance of high-quality regional and university hospitals. For Nicolás, medicine should be a dual strategy that combines high-quality clinical care with work on the social conditions that cause disease: that is, the social *determination* of diseases.[13] "For instance, violence is the first cause of death in Cali and Medellín [the third and second largest Colombian cities, respectively]; obviously, we need to address the economic, social, and cultural causes, don't we? That, however, is only possible through a political transformation of the country. Meantime, we have to suture, close up [the injured], and so on. We have to respond to the emergency cases, don't we? In that sense, the training at the hospital is very good; the hospital offers an excellent kind of medicine for the war context we live in." At the hospital, Nicolás continued, "you see the youth, the gangs, the *sicarios*. But you also see workers, street children, just like at El San Juan, and they can also stay at the hospital for months. So, the hospital is very important, and we will defend it to the end." Continuing his critical analysis, he sees the contradictions that the business model imposes on health and labor. "I just heard that they bought a new MRI at the hospital [HUV]. Who knows where that money came from. So, they bought the MRI, and that is good for us in the sense that we can now learn tons about imaging. But the hospital owes workers half their salaries, so, as Karl Marx said, 'The labor, not the machine, is the substance.' So that sums up our big problem right now [in regard to the HUV]. We want to avoid its continuing privatization. We want it to be public, and we want the insurance companies to pay their debts to the hospital."

Nicolás has been a very active participant in the students' movements. He participated in the nationwide movement against the educational reform in 2011,[14] and he participated in another movement against the further entrenchment of market principles in health in 2014. In 2015 he said that the movement continues. "We [continue] studying. Now we are a small group [of students getting together to discuss those topics] but at the time [2014] the whole medical school was participating in the protest and strike activities, everybody supported [the protest]."

Nicolás agrees that social protest in Colombia around education and health has changed. Nonetheless, these movements were very important because "these moments represent a peak in the cycle of protest. [Despite the end of the peak,] positive things have come from them."[15] His use of specialized terminology, such as "peaks in cycles of protest," come from his studies—particularly the work by Yadira Borrero explaining that 2011 and 2014 could be analyzed as "a peak in the cycles of protest around health," but that there is also movement between peaks. Yadira Borrero, an alumna from La Nacional/El San Juan Escuela, conducted a study about social protests in health as part of her doctorate in public health at the National School of Public Health at the University of Antioquia, another public and highly reputed university. She has presented to students in Cali "about twenty times," according to Nicolás; her work has been very influential around the country in illuminating what social protest looks like in health and what it can accomplish in Colombia.[16]

Not only were public hospitals forced to change their administrative structure and institutional culture to become market competitors,[17] but their legal standing also shifted; once recognized as part of state budgets, they became "private entities" under commercial law. In spite of all the promarket transformations Nicolás recounted, the HUV invoked the bankruptcy law at the end of 2016. Besides managerial problems, the biggest obstacle to the hospital's financial solvency was, as at El Materno, insurers' accumulated debt in the form of glosses and "approved but unpaid bills." There are constant corruption scandals and ongoing legal suits against most insurers, including, in 2011, the "largest embezzlement scandal in the country's history" by the country's largest health insurer, Saludcoop. The legal process against Saludcoop resulted in its president's incarceration and the company's liquidation. But the process was a bit of a sham; the same financial groups that had been part of Saludcoop received the company's 4.6 million affiliates and became the largest insurer in its place. After some years, this other insurance company, also accused of corruption and poor care to its affiliated base, was sold to a consortium in an untransparent and expensive process.[18] By 2017 Saludcoop's ongoing liquidation indicated that most of its pending bills were not going to be paid. It has been estimated that 90 percent of total hospital bills, including but not only Saludcoop's, remained unpaid; the missing money comes from taxes or people's contributions to the system.[19] In all these years, from the late 1990s until 2019, bankrupt and defunded hospitals have gone the same way as their patients—some of whom died on infamous "death trips," during which they traveled from institution to institution looking for care, finally dying between hospitals or at one's door.[20]

The situations of the Hospital Universitario del Valle, El San Juan, and El Materno are far from anecdotal; many other legendary and regional hospitals have entered economic crises or been shut down in the wake of the reform. By 2016, 250 of the country's 947 remaining "public hospitals" were considered at medium to high financial risk.[21] HUV and many public hospitals continue facing liquidation threats. According to the Ministry of Finance, 22 percent of the country's public hospitals are at high financial risk.[22] The executive director of the Colombian association of public hospitals and other health-care-providing institutions, Olga Lucía Zuluaga, said in 2018, "It is sad to see that there are apparently resources to end the public hospitals, but there never were resources to save them."[23]

HEAD NURSE SONIA PARRA acknowledged that "health has become a business, like any other business. It is a production-based industry. We were sold on the idea that it is a business and that if a business does not produce money then you won't receive your salary. So, we started to lose the idea that the important part was to keep the patient healthy, to help her recover, to offer good quality of care." It is not that quality of care is considered unimportant for the new system but that the indicators for standards of care have changed.[24] Sonia explained that "under the pressure of money," quality is measured in "complaints from the patient. If a patient complains because she feels she was not treated adequately, then you [the worker] are gone." The care standards have shifted so that "you are forced to do many things, not because you want to do them but because you are forced to do them." She sees a big difference between people who were trained and worked under the previous system and the new generation, "because they were made under this system and with these kinds of contracts [temporary and poorly paid]. For us, we complain that these kinds of contracts are miserable, [but] young people don't because they were born into this system." In her analysis, it becomes clear how younger people are highly exploitable and malleable to the system's profit conditions. "The problem is for us who lived otherwise," she concludes. Depending on their hierarchy, workers claim that they can just change jobs. Speaking primarily of nursing assistants, Sonia says that "they just say if they are to be fired, they will just find another job, that all places are paying the same, and that they see no problem in that. For them it is very clear, they have a three-month contract; if it is not renewed, they find another three-month contract at a different institution."

Other domains of quality of care resonate with the experiences related by Nicolás and Matheo but contrast with Luis Carlos Mendez's historical perspective. During his internship in the late 1980s, "an internship was really an internship. You lived, slept, ate at the hospital. You were there at all times." Even as a medical student at the Universidad del Quindío, and then as an intern and resident at El Materno, he felt that the experience was intense in terms of training and wonderful in terms of how much he learned and the relationships that he established with peers, professors, workers, and patients. "But all that got lost," he said. "Nowadays, the internship is not an internship, it is an 'externship.' They [the interns] just watch the clock." Then, he repeats what he has heard the interns say to him over and over: "Doctor, it is 5 p.m., I am leaving, I have finished my shift. And they leave no matter what remains to be done, no matter the possibilities [for learning]." For many of the professors, it is painful to see this new generation of physicians who have lost the opportunity to become part of the escuelas, who show no signs of the commitments and ethos that characterized the pre-reform generations. True, there are many students like Nicolás and Matheo, who still demonstrate the desire to take advantage of all the available possibilities, but the hospital and teaching conditions create inhospitable environments that limit how much they can do and learn.

The levels of specialized care and the kinds of multispecialty interactions that characterized referral hospitals before the reform were all lost. For example, when El Materno closed, neonatal units mushroomed around the city, but, according to many at El Materno, "it was a joke to call those places neonatal units." There are new, additional restrictions to clinical practice; the system covers some things and not others, and hospitals offer and insurers contract for a reduced number of services. In the new guidelines for "humanized delivery," for example, Sonia explains that epidural anesthesia is indicated even with a three-centimeter-dilated cervix. "The epidural is included in the health package [meaning that the state or the insurance should pay for it when the bill comes], but that means that the institution needs an anesthesiologist. We are lucky because we inherited that [practice] from El Materno [and El Materno even under La Cruz administration does have an anesthesiologist given the constant surgical demand]." Sonia signals that many other institutions do not pay for an anesthesiologist, which makes the epidural, in practice, not the standard of care. "This is not to say that in El Materno epidural anesthesia is always and readily available; there is just one anesthesiologist at the hospital, covering the operating and delivery rooms. And they are not going to hire an anesthesiologist just to do epidurals, right?" Jokingly, she concludes that in the new conception of "humanized delivery" the only thing missing is pain control.

The poor functioning of the medical system can be seen through its poorly functioning training system. At the Hospital Engativá, to which Luis Carlos brought a piece of El Materno, interns and residents from different universities are suffering from extreme disorganization and neglect from their medical schools. "A [resident] came to me and told me that he was in his last year of residency in pediatrics. 'I graduate in three months and they [the university where he was doing his residency] told me to come and talk to you, that it is up to you [whether to accept him for the rotation]. But I do want to rotate with you. You can tell me to do anything. I can bring you the exams, the X-rays, I can do rounds with you, take notes and type them afterwards.' So," Luis Carlos muses, "the university sent someone who in three or four months was going to become a specialist in pediatrics to see what I could do for him and I wasn't even aware of that arrangement." Luis Carlos told the student that he thought that what the university was doing to him was intolerable. "At least let me ask them what this is about, what kinds of programs they have, what kind of organization [for their residency training], the structure that supports your coming here." He also asked himself and the student, attempting to demonstrate the absurdity and precariousness of the student's situation and how the university was at fault, "How is it that I am qualified [to be his mentor], has the university validated my credentials?"

He is pained to see how the residents that do remain at Engativá "stay to the side of the rooms, by the door, watching, listening, alone, without a professor. . . . It is so sad, what kind of educational model in health is that? It is part of the new business model," he concludes. In the contracts that general practitioners and specialists sign with the hospitals, like the one he signed with Engativá, their teaching responsibilities are in the fine print. That means that nonacademic physicians without official affiliations to any universities end up "teaching" students like Matheo at the hospitals. "And it is the same in both public and private [medical schools]. Students arrive and wait until someone takes pity on them and asks them, 'And what about you? What do you want to see?' That is the business model," Luis Carlos asserts. "And they continue mistreating you [the physician] and not giving you any recognition because you work and teach, both for the same salary. If you [the worker] don't want it that way, then [they tell you, you shouldn't have] sign[ed the contract]."

NICOLÁS SEES THE WORKING conditions of residents and interns as inhumane. They have to pay to work—a condition made legal by calling itself "clinical training." Their labor conditions are slave-like. "They have to do whatever the chief of the department tells them to do, and the chief of the department is appointed by the hospital director." In the new market-based system ruled by the powerful insurance companies, the labor conditions of new graduates, whether general physicians or specialists, are as dire as for interns and residents.

In addition, research is out of the question. There was a shift from clinical-based research to basic sciences or epidemiologic studies, usually with the participation of foreign interests. The absence of strong clinical research has been devastating, according to Elena Fino, the alumna of La Nacional/ El Materno introduced in chapter 1. She specialized in gynecology and epidemiology and completed a master's degree in education. She has carried El Materno with her in her desire to prevent maternal deaths and complications. But the situation is dire. Before, El Materno, based on its clinical research and in partnership with medical societies, produced national guidelines in gynecology and neonatology. This knowledge, according to Elena Fino, "was not imposed. It was offered as part of a philosophy that knowledge should be free and available." Elena noticed "the influence of El Materno" when she began traveling around the country, offering training in epidemiologic surveillance, assessments of pregnancy complications, and evaluations of maternal deaths, "Outside [of Bogotá] people paid close attention to the developments coming out of El Materno. When a professor lectured at a conference [in a different city], the shared knowledge was very valuable." The situation in the new system, according to Elena, "is one of great practical confusion. There are guidelines but there is not any kind of support [for people to adopt the guidelines]. Very few people have continued to work hard on maternal health." Unlike the "access to free knowledge" dictum of the past, Elena noticed that most of the current trainings happen within sizable "training contracts," when health care institutions from rural or remote areas manage to pay someone to come and train them.

Not surprisingly, the lack of medical autonomy has been accompanied by the overexploitation and proletarianization of medical labor. The labor conditions of general physicians and specialists are critically precarious. Nurses and physicians have both seen a significant drop in their salaries over the last thirty years. Lida Pinzón asked a relative who is a gynecologist how much she was getting paid per C-section—one of the most important income-generating procedures in gynecology but also one with many associated risks. The relative told her 40,000 pesos, around US$15. Small salaries result in workers trying to take on more than one job to make ends meet. Not surprisingly, then, people have to rush from one workplace to the next, and that has important implications. El Materno professors, nurses, workers, and alumni report that the system does not allow them to develop any sense of belonging to any institution. Lida said, "You just work where you get paid and for what you get paid for. If your shift ends at 5:00, you finish at 5:00." This impediment to belonging also damages any possibility of building close relationships with coworkers and developing the special dedication that patients deserve. Lida explains that it works both ways: "Physicians are less committed to the institutions and the institutions are less committed to them." As institutions use the "contract renewal" strategy to keep people in line with institutional demands, workers make their own calculations and change institutions whenever they have a better opportunity.

"Better opportunities," however, might come with higher pay but can also include more exploitation. Physicians are being asked to fulfill many administrative tasks, are limited to what billing protocols dictate, and have been made into a proletariat class: unsatisfied with their labor and insecure about their economic future and their chances of providing for their families. Adriana Ardila, an alumna from La Nacional School of Medicine, conducted a doctoral thesis in public health to understand the transformation of medical labor as a result of neoliberal reform. As part of El Materno's story, she was enthusiastic about contributing her data to this book. Her exemplary thesis, which received the highest university honors by the jury, allows us to answer this question: What is it like to work as a general practitioner in Colombia after twenty-five years of neoliberal health care reform?[25]

Speaking about productivity, sustainability, cost-efficiency, and the ways in which the logic of production has made its way into clinical practice, one of Adriana's interviewees commented that to be productive or profitable means "to see eighteen patients a day, to not prescribe more than 85 percent [of the patients], to not refer more than 10 percent [of the patients], to not order diagnostic images to more than 10 percent [of the patients], and to not order more than 32 percent in labs. A physician who goes over those limits is not cost-effective for the institution." In Adriana's analysis, "productivity" is measured in terms of spending caps. The hospital administrators pressure with emails or letters those who exceed the caps and praise those with "better results"—those who are more cost effective. Those who go over the expense quotas do not get their contracts renewed. Institutions reward physicians who have good "resolution capacities," those who can manage patients without medical orders or referrals, even if that means not providing the treatment the patient needs. Another physician told Adriana how institutions rank physicians in class A, B, and C types. "If you are class A [the institution tells them], then you are a good physician for us and we will continue hiring you because you don't prescribe too much, you don't ask for many things, and you string patients along, asking them to come to more appointments and such. If you are a class C physician, then you are more of an academic physician who does what people need. But for the EPS [insurance company], this is the kind of physician who spends too much, who represents too much money, and for that reason you can easily be out [of a job]."[26]

Another physician explained that insurers and hospital administrators force doctors to implement treatment guidelines as a way of delaying more expensive care, regardless of the patients' needs or clinical parameters, indicating that the first line of care is not effective. One general physician, discussing dermatologic patients who need to be referred to the specialist for adequate treatment, said, "If a patient arrives with a lesion that clearly needs to be handled by the dermatologist, what do you need to do? Register everything [in the medical record] then prescribe Betamethasona [a steroid-based cream], or any other [ineffective] thing, then I must see [the patient] two more times, and then I can refer him. Why do I have to do all that? So that IT IS REGISTERED in the medical record [emphasis in the physician's voice] that you prescribed first; that is, that you TRIED to do something [cheaper] and that it didn't work." The paper trail in the medical record is not intended as an adequate treatment. But from the physician's perspective, it justifies referrals and keeps the doctor out of trouble with the quota limits, saving the physician from being deemed unprofitable and not having a contract renewed.

This practice of delaying necessary medical care began to emblematize the health care system. It began to be recognized as the cause of "death trips" and "bureaucratic itineraries."[27] The delay in medical care, such as a proper evaluation by a dermatologist, can result in a worsening of the patient's condition, which can have serious consequences. Indeed, in a doctoral study that used the bureaucratic itineraries framework to understand skin cancer, Guillermo Sánchez discovered the patients' version of Adriana's physicians' narratives. Patients reported that physicians only prescribed ineffective creams while their cancerous lesions grew bigger. While the national guidelines establish that the maximum time from first visit to a confirmed diagnosis with biopsy should be ninety-five days, prompt diagnosis occurred only in 32.5 percent of Guillermo's sample, which consisted of people seen at a main dermatologic referral center.[28] Not only was diagnosis delayed, but 28 percent of the people with skin cancer diagnoses reported that the required referrals or treatment (biopsies and surgery) were denied by their insurers, which forced them to resort to the courts and initiate a legal suit.

Adriana's work further allows us to connect the bureaucratic itineraries that patients experience with the ways in which the health care system forces physicians to deny and delay care. She shows how physicians internalize pressure from the health care system to spend less and end up reformulating clinical protocols in their minds and in their practice to match the profit needs of insurers and hospital administrators. Adriana calls these new protocols "clinical itineraries." Over time, physicians end up following health care protocols that automatically include the different steps demanded by the insurers and hospital administrators; they stop fighting the system. Even more worrisomely, some insurers have built their own medical schools with their own affiliated clinics, leading to debates about whether students are truly learning medicine or just practicing it within the limits of Colombia's for-profit insurance-based model. However, this sort of training is not restricted exclusively to insurance-owned clinics; most hospitals where students "learn medicine" already practice medicine under for-profit administration and reduced standards of care.

Over the decades, even as early as the 1970s, physicians' incomes started to fall. With the advent of neoliberal labor reforms, their work also became "flexible"—based on temporary contracts, and without benefits. While official data show that physicians' salaries increased after the health care reform, Adriana's data demonstrate that if we consider salary, labor time, and type of contract, we can better understand current working conditions and how physicians' real income changed after the neoliberal health and labor reforms. One physician told Adriana, "We work by the hour and we get paid by the hour. Physicians who work full time have to work between 220 and 240 hours per month. Those who work half-time work between 90 and 140 hours a month. This includes nights and holidays . . . we have to do at least seven nights a month and, well, [that leaves] just one free weekend." These calculations result in weekly labor times between forty-seven and fifty-seven hours—a number that supports other national studies indicating that physicians are holding multiple jobs as a way to make up for the ongoing loss of income that, for instance, El Materno workers experienced with their new contracts.

Some job offers are advertised as offering higher salaries. Adriana found several advertisements for contracts for physicians. For example, a 4-hour day (i.e., part time) is advertised as paying 2.2 minimum monthly wages, an 8-hour day (i.e., full time, based on the official 40 hour/week jobs) paid 5.9 minimum monthly wages, and a 220 hours a month job (i.e., over the official full time) paid 9.7 minimum monthly wages. Some higher-paid jobs are for remote areas. What these job descriptions don't say is that in each kind of contract, there are many hidden deductions that are taken directly from the physician's salary; also obscured is the fact that, though some contracts include benefits like vacations, many others do not. Once we factor in all the deductions, the net wages are much lower, which begins to explain why physicians need to maintain several jobs.

The rates of physician labor exploitation start to make sense when we understand that the health care system has tariffs per medical consultation. In the boss's mind, the less money that goes to the physician's salary, the more they can keep. So the neoliberal reform is not only about restricting clinical activities, referrals, and treatments to keep money in the institution's pockets[29] but it is also about paying physicians as little as possible. Adriana discovered that the rate of exploitation is increased through several mechanisms, including scheduling patients more frequently, which reduces clinical time and increases the total number of patients one physician sees during any given day. The physician gets paid the same, but the institution gets to charge for more patients. Some physicians were unaware that a higher rate of exploitation meant that they were in fact being paid less as the hospital was making more money. Physicians report "trainings," in which they are taught how to save time and move things more rapidly to increase their "productivity," even if that means doing two things at the same time, like conducting a clinical exam while doing counseling. Insurers and clinics prefer newer physicians, "who are more malleable and complain less," according to another of Adriana's interviewees. Older physicians still resist the parameters imposed by the system, while newer physicians don't know any better and accept the impositions more passively. Two very lucrative strategies for the administrators of health as a business are "intensification" and "densification"—getting physicians to do things more rapidly and to do more things in the same period of time, respectively.[30]

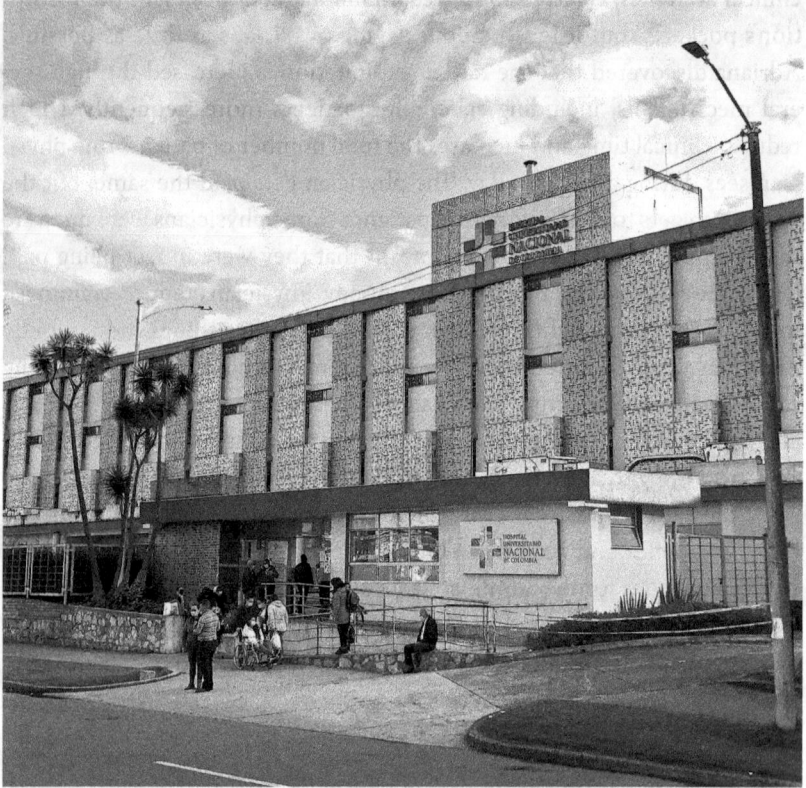

FIGURE F.1. Hospital Universitario Nacional (HUN) [National University Hospital]. (Courtesy of Levinson Niño.)

FINAL REMARKS. Medicine as Political Imagination

Thanks in part to the efforts of workers, patient associations, and human rights organizations, a ten-year process behind a class action lawsuit granted judicial protection to El San Juan and El Materno hospitals. The 2017 ruling reiterated that these university hospitals are a national patrimony destined to treat the poorest populations in Colombia. Despite this ruling, it is unclear when and how the hospitals will reopen.[1] In parallel efforts and as a way to find a definitive solution to the closing of El San Juan, La Nacional purchased an abandoned hospital building that had also succumbed to neoliberal reforms. Resources needed for renovations and needed equipment came only after Congress approved the creation of a university postage stamp. The independent administration was made possible with the creation of a public-private corporation, whose members are La Nacional and AEXMUN (the alumnae association of the university's School of Medicine). The first outpatient services of the *Hospital Universitario Nacional de Colombia* (HUN) opened in November 2015, with the hopes of other services being progressively opened until reaching a fully functioning fourth-level hospital.[2] Aware of the new for-profit context and in trying to blind the hospital from legal battles, the manager acknowledged that this hospital "enters the free market: we will compete for patients with the quality, service, and characteristics of the National University of Colombia."[3] Over time, rather than thinking of it as a single building, the project to rebuild a university hospital for La Nacional is intended to more closely resemble an integrated network of health care facilities, ideally including El Materno and a future reopening of El San Juan.

Even though the new hospital is much smaller than El San Juan and lacks an emergency department and obstetrics, HUN still offers 230 hospital beds, including intensive care units, and 8 operating rooms to professors and students, is closer to the university campus, and does not have any legal problems. Furthermore, the independent administrative figure of the corporation ensures the financial feasibility of the hospital, even if that means, at least initially, contracting only with the insurers of the contributory regime that are known to pay their bills. Indeed, by February 2018 HUN generated small profits.[4] The greatest challenge, however, is to rebuild the interdisciplinarity and larger sense of excellence in training and "clinical social medicine" that characterized the La Nacional Escuela. This rebuilding, with projections to increase the hospital's infrastructure, is not intended as a return to an idyllic past. Learning and practicing medicine now occur in the context of the tension between adapting to the new conditions imposed by the for-profit system and revamping and updating the critical perspectives needed for practicing a kind of medicine that responds to the needs of Colombians. Importantly, the new hospital, along with La Misericordia (the children's hospital), whatever remains of El Materno, and the prospect of a future reopening of El San Juan, allows the La Nacional Escuela to keep on building from the past, shaping the present, and imagining the future. In this process, the history of glory, collapse, and resistance of El San Juan and El Materno continues to haunt the epistemology of medical care of not only La Nacional Escuela but also the whole country.

Then we can argue that health and medical care are a dynamic political field in which violent actions such as the defunding, closure, and privatization of public hospitals lead to undeniable physical, symbolic, and emotional destruction, but also in which committed professors, students, and health care workers fight for decommodifying health and work to rally enough social support to change the for-profit and insurance-based system. This is not to say that a new system without insurance companies would be perfect, but in Colombia's current political environment as related to health care, this idea is seen as the first and most important step toward advancing the rights to health and medical education.

EL MATERNO IS UNIQUE in its high-quality care provided to poor populations, subaltern health innovations, epistemology of care, and ways in which professors, workers, and students confront the advances of health care markets on health. Nonetheless, as Khiara M. Bridges argued for Alpha Hospital in New York, "The hospital ought not to be understood as singular."[5] In her case, Alpha Hospital's dependence "upon public dollars to deliver health care to uninsured, marginalized persons" connects its history to other public hospitals in the United States.[6] Likewise, El Materno is not the product of a peculiar quality of the institution but a product of how health institutions, both in Colombia and across the world, are confronting the new configurations in the political economy of health. While the financial sector via insurance companies dictates more and more how health is governed,[7] the intercapitalist alliance between the financial sector and the medical industrial complex has commodified health so dramatically that the mission of health care institutions is no longer patient care but capital accumulation.[8]

Colombia's privatization law and the incredible role the private insurance sector played in shaping its implementation and regulations allowed the financial sector to transform the country's entire system of health services into a market of insurance. In other countries, different regulations (both market control mechanisms and overseeing institutions) have been more effective at controlling insurance companies' influence on health care and protecting the safety net provided by public institutions. In other countries, there have been decisive efforts to defend public health care networks and the role of university hospitals as the backbone of public medical education. In some Latin American countries, for instance, financial sectors' advances in global health came alongside newly elected progressive governments, which made incredible attempts to reduce the national impact of neoliberalism, sometimes by formulating and implementing integral, public, and unified health care systems.[9] In many aspects, then, El Materno is an exceptional case, both as an ethnographic example and as a lens through which to observe how financialized capital took over social security in Colombia. And yet, financialized capital is advancing all over the world by dispossessing public health, health care, and medical education communities and publicly oriented countries more broadly.

Let us consider just a handful of examples from other countries in which the financialized economy is taking over health, whether by implementing individual insurance schemes or by attacking public health care institutions and workers—two schemas that, as El Materno showed, usually go hand in hand. Many countries in the world are implementing some sort of privatizing health care reform; the trend includes European countries that once epitomized the welfare state, where social security and single-payer health care systems were both administered by the state. After years of strikes and mobilizations, nurses and care workers at the Charitè Hospital in Berlin, the largest university hospital in the city and one of the largest in Europe, achieved an agreement on working conditions. Alongside striking workers at other important hospitals, workers at Charitè were fighting their precarious labor conditions and denouncing the profit-based health care market that has advanced in Germany. Cuts in public expenditure have come hand in hand with a profit-oriented health care management; the outsourcing of workers' contracts has encouraged bigger workloads and lower wages. The success of the workers' struggle under the slogan "more of us is better for all" is a promise to reverse "the financialization of welfare cuts across national borders."[10]

If periods of "economic crisis" in Latin America were used to force the implementation of the neoliberal policies known as Structural Adjustment,[11] they have also been used elsewhere to push neoliberal reforms. In Madrid, medical workers and their supporters marched in the last decade denouncing government cuts to health care that they see as "setting the stage for full privatization."[12] The European Commission has told the Spanish government to reduce public spending significantly—the same way that privatization started in Latin America. Even though the economic "crisis" of 2008 was controlled, theoretically recuperative strategies like further cuts to public spending on health, a progressive worsening of working conditions, and lowered salaries have kept physicians across Spain marching and protesting well into 2018.[13] In Greece we can see a similar pattern. On top of the severe cuts in public spending required to be eligible for the loans that would avoid default, more social spending cuts are constantly being announced—and denounced. In 2013 physicians protested the first waves of cuts, which harmed access to health care services and served as a first step to defunding the country's public health care infrastructure. Like in Spain, doctors continue marching in 2018, still denouncing the drastic situation of public hospitals and new attacks on their labor contracts. The Greek government announced their goal of suspending on partial pay twenty-five thousand public-sector workers by the end of 2018 and making four thousand redundant.[14] Mirroring the reconfigured Colombian class struggle in which some physicians are finally understanding that they must join forces with others who have been dispossessed by the neoliberal reconfiguration of capital, a Greek physician said in the news: "Our only option is to join forces with the rest of the society and fight back."[15]

Outside of Europe, the profit-seeking administration of Seoul National University Hospital in South Korea's capital has seen health care workers' strikes since 2013.[16] Years of protests against poor working conditions, salary freezes, and, as at El Materno, several months of unpaid salaries forced women health care workers in Lahore, Pakistan, to stage a sit-in before the Assembly in March 2018.[17] A mix of neoliberal labor policies, with government relying on contract labor rather than salaried employees with full benefits and pensions, and Kashmir's exceptionalism as an occupied territory, resulted in junior doctors going on an indefinite strike in October 2009. "The state government had been unresponsive to months of lobbying by [the Junior Doctor's Association (JDA)]," who were underpaid in comparison to other Indian states. "Because junior doctors provide the bulk of hospital care, many patient services ground to a standstill."[18]

Health care privatization has also been pushed in Africa since the 1990s. Given the continent's colonially induced lack and precarity of health care infrastructure and social security, privatization in many African countries comes through the transnational funding of health care and the delegation of service provisions to transnational nongovernmental organizations (NGOs), which charge user fees and push for "unregulated" pharmaceutical markets.[19] In Mozambique and Tanzania, doctors went on strike, demanding higher wages and better working conditions.[20] Privatization has also been launched in affluent countries without economic crises—without a neoliberal economic justification for austerity reforms. Saudi Arabia announced a plan for "full foreign ownership in the health sector," with the ministry becoming the regulator rather than the service provider.[21] The plan includes the privatization of 290 hospitals and 2,300 primary health centers by 2030.[22] Outsourcing of hospitals to private hospitals has also been announced in Australia.[23]

In Latin America, the process of confronting neoliberalism in health continues to see progress, challenges, and setbacks. Until recently, Brazil was a regional leader, showing progress in fulfilling the citizen's right to health through a unified health care system supported by a robust public health infrastructure and public programs. Even during the years when neoliberal doctrines in health were hard to challenge, Brazil demonstrated that providing free health care services to its citizens, and thereby fulfilling its constitutional mandate, was a better strategy than charging people or denying treatments altogether. During the AIDS epidemic, Brazil became a world example by integrating the national AIDS program into the Unified Health Care System (SUS), thereby challenging the pharmaceutical industry and even transforming World Trade Organization international agreements about patent protection laws.[24] However, the institutional coup that impeached president Dilma Rouseff and jailed former president Lula has signified a worrisome rise in right-wing Brazilian politics. The racist, misogynist, and xenophobic speeches of Bolsonaro's government resemble those of authoritarian governments and parties around the world, which are on the rise. The 2018 government and Congress, which attacked the leftist presidents from the Workers Party, are also defunding and dismantling the public health care sector, which has been called by academics a "health catastrophe in the making."[25] Something similar is happening in Argentina, where major hospitals are going bankrupt, leftist leaders are being prosecuted, a neoliberal ideology in regard to health care is on the rise, and massive social mobilizations are attempting to defend the accomplishments of progressive administrations.

In El Salvador, the 1992 peace accords that ended the war came at the same time as heavy enforcement of neoliberal reforms. A large social movement, led by physicians marching in the streets, managed to stop health privatization efforts.[26] With their own challenges, inconsistencies, and incongruences, efforts at nationally funded health care systems had moved forward in Bolivia and Ecuador with intercultural health and a respect for nature as fundamentals. Cuba, of course, continues to be the regional example of a noncommodified understanding of the right to health. But it has not escaped the rising inequalities between those with access to remittances and private health—a system mostly geared to the tourism industry—and those who rely for their health care needs on the national health system.[27] At least in Latin America, regional associations of scholars, activists, and health care professionals, such as ALAMES, play a key role in cross-fertilizing denunciations and resistance strategies within and across countries.

THERE ARE MANY MORE examples around the world. To that end, we can think of El Materno's history as one among many. El Materno's history and the others briefly mentioned here demonstrate that each story contains both the devastation caused by capitalism in health and the incredible, ongoing resistance to it. Privatization efforts around the world are similar in their defunding of public health care infrastructures, their attacks on health care workers' rights, their outsourcing of services and workers, and their introduction of private and speculative capital, particularly insurance companies. While these are all different strategies for moving forward with capitalist accumulation processes, El Materno's history shows us how all these transformations amount to a larger shift in the ideological domain around health.

Looking back at the roughly sixty years of health in Colombia presented in this book, we see a slow but radical transformation in how workers, students, professors, and patients experience and think about health. This transformation in the "political imagination" about health is necessary for the capitalist ideology of health as an insurable individual commodity to become hegemonic. To attain hegemony, changes in political imagination must cut across all population groups of a given sector: in our case, the health sector. Patients have to imagine that insurance companies are the only institutions capable of managing their health needs and that they must choose among them in a "free market" competition scenario. Health care professionals have to shift from a public employee or liberal professional perspective to seeing themselves as workers or contractors at institutions that bill for services. All patient-doctor interactions must be imagined within profit and productivity quotas. As professors, recent graduates, and students fail to find alternatives, they adapt their learning and practice of medicine to the constraints of the market. While they can discuss and imagine a different practice of medicine, primarily by resorting to past experiences, the material conditions that they find at hospitals and clinics force them to make clinical decisions within the system's confines.

Medicine as political imagination is, therefore, not a purely rational or intellectual exercise of ideas. The way we politically imagine health is the result of a particular epistemology of care resulting from merged and socially constructed theories and praxes; it depends on people's shared experiences, history, and materiality.[28] What this book has shown is twofold: how the epistemology of care and medicine as political imagination are coproduced, and how they are changing in Colombia.

But we also know that to see a given ideology as hegemonic means understanding it as an always-contested process.[29] In El Materno's case, the force of historical consciousness is constantly reshaping the ruination of health care and medical education. History is not only embodied in peoples and institutions. El Materno workers, students, professors, and patients show that history is also used, reframed, reformulated, retold, and revamped in a way that is useful to counterhegemonic struggles. As history is made tangible, one can experience a sense of loss—which, as we have seen, is important to the political debates of the new generation of students and health care professionals that is refuting the restriction of their careers to a market of health insurance and health institutions privileging profit. As generations meet within groups of patients, workers, professors, and students, their communication helps maintain the escuela—and simultaneously helps promote continuous contestations to also-dynamic capitalist logics in health. If during the previous welfare regimes, it was harder to see the state as "possessed" by corporate capital,[30] this relationship has become clearer in neoliberal times. The counterhegemonic struggles that we are beginning to witness decisively confront corporate governance in health, opening up new dimensions in how social groups might imagine different alternatives and struggle to achieve them.

The fight, then, is against the progressive destructive transformation of health by capitalist forces and actors, including the developmental and econometric narrative of capitalism during its neoliberal phase, in which universal coverage, productivity, and measurables constitute the goals and premises of health progress.[31] El Materno history shows that the fight also consists of not letting insurance companies and biomedicine with its related market of technologies dictate what we imagine a mother, a family, or a newborn baby to need. While the importance of biomedical knowledge and biotechnology can be acknowledged, the importance of other domains of existence, like the bodily love we and other species exert through our bodies to protect our offspring, should not be disregarded. When love, warmth, breast milk, and a respected umbilical cord, among others, are understood as better medically, emotionally, and economically, this southern epistemology of care opens up the "political imagination" around medicine and health. Alternatives to medicine need not, as KMC illustrates, be "anti-medicine."[32] They are about acknowledging other ways of healing and promoting life that might replace or complement Western biomedicine. This radical shift relies on the acknowledgment that medicine has been taken over by capitalist interests to the point that we no longer trust it to be about helping people but raising profits.[33] We hope that El Materno's history helps other groups around the world in their fight against the capitalist takeover of health and in their imagining of different alternatives.

Introduction

1. See Appadurai (1995) for the formulation of studying "the social life of things." For neoliberal legislation in postcolonial settings and the concept of lawfare, see, in particular, Comaroff and Comaroff (2006). For discussion of the law as a technology of power, see Coutin and Yngvesson (2008).

2. This initially happened in Latin America and was later exported to other geographic areas in both the Global North and South. Significant restructuring occurred more around pension funds than health (Stocker, Waitzkin, and Iriart 1999; Iriart, Merhy, and Waitzkin 2001). The Colombian case is particularly interesting because it was the country where the most comprehensive market-based health care reform took place. For original work by academic neoliberals on this subject, see Londoño and Frenk (1997). For its original expression in international financial institutions' documents, see The World Bank (1993).

3. Why this book uses "we" to signal collective authorship will be explained shortly.

4. (Santos 2018).

5. (Santos 2018, 2).

6. Santos, as other postcolonial and decolonial scholars, draws from the understanding of a colonial matrix of power, as originally discussed by Quijano (2000).

7. (C. Giraldo 2007).

8. We use quotation marks here to indicate that several scholars disagree with the idea advanced by some government officers, international institutions, and academics that neoliberalism is a completely deregulated "free market" resulting from the total dismantling of the state. In contrast, neoliberalism advances new roles of the state and of state actors in the reconfiguration of a global class (Jasso-Aguilar and Waitzkin 2007; Robinson 2007). In health, these thinkers argue against the idea that the market

regulates itself through competition and that the government plays a crucial role in regulating the market through specific legislation, even including incentives, and finer mechanisms of regulation such as accounting (J. Mulligan 2016).

9. Health is but one aspect of neoliberal reforms, privatization, deregulation, and financialization that happened in virtually all sectors of the economy (Harvey 2007; Klein 2007).

10. (Harvey 2007; Kim et al. 2000; Klein 2007).

11. Such fragmented welfare systems were common in other Latin American countries as well (C. Giraldo 2007; Hernández Alvarez 2004). They were characterized by three sectors: a public sector, a social insurance sector for private and public employees, and a private sector. These systems frequently suffered from inequality and a lack of articulation. With the election of progressive governments and constitutional reforms in the 1980s and 1990s, several countries made advances in unifying their health care infrastructures and strengthening their public orientations. Colombia stands in this history as an opposite example given that it moved toward full privatization.

12. Mulligan's ethnography in Puerto Rico offers important insights into the financial and administrative logics of market-based health care reform (Mulligan 2014, 2016).

13. For a historical analysis of the competing intercapitalist sectors in health and the alliance between the medical industrial complex and financial sectors during neoliberalism, see Iriart and Merhy (2017). See Waitzkin and Working Group for Health Beyond Capitalism (2018), Rosenthal (2017), and Bugbee (2019) for a description and analysis of the competing interests of several capitalist players in a U.S. context.

14. The transnational insurance sector that dealt with health insurance and pension funds began to face problems of overaccumulation; that is, insurance companies had been such successful capitalists that they saturated all their markets and could not inject their profits back into the market. In other words, there was a halt in the necessary circulation cycle of capital, which threatens with stagnation of the economy, or worse, recession. Thus, insurance companies followed what David Harvey called "accumulation by dispossession" (2007) seeking market expansion to areas, like health care, that were not previously within their reach. See Stocker, Waitzkin, and Iriart (1999); Iriart, Merhy, and Waitzkin (2001).

15. Initially, health insurance companies threatened the profits of the medical industrial complex (Iriart, Franco, and Merhy 2011). Currently, the medical industrial financial complex (MIFC) represents an alliance of capitalist sectors in health in which profits are ensured for all sectors as medical care bills and insurance become more expensive (Iriart and Merhy 2017).

16. (Fischer 2009).

17. Here, we follow Sunder Rajan when he states that the ways in which our very ability to comprehend "life" and "economy" in their modernist guises are shaped by particular epistemologies that are simultaneously enabled by, and in turn enable, particular forms of institutional structures (Sunder Rajan 2006, 13–14).

18. (Cooper and Waldby 2014; Street 2012, 2014).

19. (Wendland 2010).

20. (McKay 2018, chap. 2).

21. See Fraser (2016) for a feminist Marxist approach to social reproduction. See Smith-Morris (2018), Strong (2020), and Arango et al. (2018) for several discussions on care and caring, including feminist perspectives.

22. (Martin 2001).

23. (Shepard 2006, ix).

24. Also seen in other Global South settings. See Strong (2020) for her ethnography at a maternity ward in Tanzania and the powerful 2017 documentary *Motherland*, based on the Philippines. Nonetheless, "Global South" should not be homogenized. It is clear that regarding child and maternal health, the conditions in hospitals and even the conditions of poverty in which women and families live vary enormously among regions and within regions and countries.

25. The racial domain appears as "autonomous" or "innate" thinking that connects medical care and the human body with nature. This knowledge and respect for "mother nature" is rooted in indigenous cosmogonies. See chapter 2.

26. In a way similar to indigenous feminist proposals in Latin America that speak about the messiness and intersectionality of their struggle and stand in contrast to the hegemonic liberal feminist tradition from the Global North (Duarte 2012).

27. (Hernández and Upton 2018; Martin 2001; Strong 2020; Vallana Sala 2019). Strong offers examples of the complex maneuvering between abuse and "fierce care" in Tanzania, whereby nurses and doctors yelling at and hitting women in labor can be expected as caring practices given that they can avoid complications or even save the baby and mother's lives. Under a reproductive justice framework, however, these practices are always condoned in light of the structural elements that should always stand as unacceptable.

28. (Gilligan 2000).

29. (Martin 2001, p. xxii). Rather, they acknowledged that each birth and each woman's and child's body is unique and wonderfully powerful, hence is each delivery, or celebration of a new life as they called it.

30. As argued by midwifery proposals that demedicalize the birthing process (Davis-Floyd et al. 2009).

31. Arguably, a fully feminist practice within a larger patriarchal, racist, and capitalist global and national order would be impossible to realize.

32. Research in sociocultural anthropology rebuffs the idea of ruins as "archaeological," reminding us that remnants of the past have important contemporary meanings, which themselves affect our sense of the connections between the past and the present. Colonial histories and histories of violence experience a dual historical process of material and human interaction. Ruins speak to those histories as, over generations, people tell what happened. Ruins, rubble, debris, and so on, serve as powerful historical reminders and, as such, become material history that is itself re-created in contemporary symbols, political struggles, and interpretations. See Gordillo (2014); Stoler (2013).

33. Anne Stoler emphasizes that "ruin" is both a noun and a verb, "the claim about the state of a thing and a process affecting it" (2013, 11). She complicates ruin as a conceptual element for anthropological inquiry by linking things to their imperial history. "Imperial projects," she continues, "are themselves processes of ongoing ruination, processes that 'bring ruin upon,' exerting material and social force in the present. By

definition, *ruination* is an ambiguous term, being an act of ruining, a condition of being ruined, and a cause of it. Ruination is an *act* perpetrated, a *condition* to which one is subject, and a cause of loss."

34. See Povinelli (2011) for the concept of carnality and the role of time in late capitalist destruction.

35. What is important here is the relationship between symbol and value. Value can take many forms; anthropologists can detect these many forms and show how they overlap. Graeber (2016) suggests that value in anthropology can adopt different symbolic, material, and economic forms, which usually coalesce. In his research about an ecotourism project in Q'eqchi'-speaking communities in the Guatemalan forests, Kockelman (2016) elegantly shows how use value (function), exchange value (price), semantic value (meaning), and deontic value (morality) constantly influence each other and how specific approaches give specific values meaning at the expense of other possible interpretations. Value can travel from one domain to another (e.g., from a commercial value to a semantic value), but Kockelman demonstrates that not everything contained within a given value can be translated into the other domain. Some of this value incommensurability will be relevant in the analysis of epistemologies of care at El Materno, when we show that not all health care can be translated into economic forms.

36. Artifacts in this case can take many forms: for example, legal documents. See Góngora et al. (2013) for a discussion of legal documents as artifacts in El San Juan. The idea of thinking of documents as artifacts open to ethnographic inquiry as examples of social practices and actors' actions comes from the work of Riles (2006).

37. Even regarding race as Bridges (2011) discusses for the Women's Health Clinic at Alpha Hospital in New York. See also Strong (2020).

38. (Benjamin 2013).

39. For some of the most relevant ethnographies from medical anthropology, see Adams (2016); Bridges (2011); Cooper (2008); Cooper and Waldby (2014); Dumit (2012); Han (2012); Keshavjee (2014); Knight (2015); Livingston (2012); McKay (2018); Mulligan (2014); Peterson (2014); Povinelli (2011); Smith-Nonini (2010); Street (2014); Sunder Rajan (2006, 2017); Wendland (2010).

40. There is, in other words, no "neoliberal culture" or "culture of neoliberalism."

41. We position ourselves here against a reading of capital as supreme and victorious in the wake of socialism's collapse in Europe. Instead, we join critical scholars who read the defeat of socialist European states and the rise of neoliberalism as a new capitalist phase that brings more social contradictions and conflicts.

42. Waitzkin and other scholars insist on the need to decommodify health care (Waitzkin and Working Group for Health Beyond Capitalism 2018). With the advent of market-based health care reform in Colombia, debates abound around the decommodification of health and the need to advance a concept of health in other terms. For debates in Colombia see, among many others, Franco Agudelo (2003); M. Hernández (2003); Useche (2007).

43. (Ortner 2006, 7). See also Butler, Laclau, and Žižek (2000); Crehan (2002).

44. Here, Ortner draws on Raymond Williams' elaboration of Gramscian notions in order to connect Marxism with literary theory (Williams 2009). Crehan (2002)

adequately signals the limitations of Williams' proposal for anthropologists. Nonetheless, Williams' explanations of hegemonic configurations in history are helpful in that they help us understand the incompleteness of hegemony as emphasized by Gramsci. Hegemony is also a useful lens through which to consider the conflicts between colonial epistemologies and epistemologies of the south.

45. (Crehan 2002, 99).

46. [Hegemony] rejects any simple base-superstructure hierarchy (Crehan 2002, 200).

47. (Crehan 2002, 101). Discussing the role of the intellectuals as subalterns to the world of production, for example, Gramsci speaks of the social hegemony achieved through "spontaneous consent" and the state domination or coercive power achieved through "legal" channels (Gramsci and Hoare 1985, 12–13). As part of his view on political praxis, Gramsci notes that critical consciousness (i.e., critical understanding of self) requires the worker to be aware of the hegemonic force that has influenced his moral and political passivity. Then, the first step for a revolutionary praxis is "working out at a higher level of one's own conception of reality," a progressive self-consciousness in which "theory and practice will finally be one" (Gramsci and Hoare 1985, 333). While Crehan speaks to the dominant position of those in power, Guha (1998) reiterates that regarding hegemony full dominance is never accomplished.

48. (Butler 2000, 14).

49. (Butler 2000, 12).

50. Including the work of Paulo Freire, Liberation Theology intellectuals, and Orlando Fals Borda (Rincón Diaz 2015; Santofimio-Ortiz 2018; Vivero-Arriagada 2014).

51. (Santofimio-Ortiz 2018).

52. Following the original formulation of Coloniality of Power by Quijano (2000). See also Grosfoguel (2011). For the original critique about the intertwining of race and gender, see Lugones (2008). For colonial configurations around race, gender, and labor see Moraña, Dussel, and Jáuregui (2008, 11).

53. (Crehan 2002). Sunder Rajan also finds the Gramscian notion of hegemony useful for understanding how the pharmaceutical industry is dominating the political field of global health (Sunder Rajan 2017).

54. The system was far from perfect; see, for example, Hernández and Obregón (2002). In later chapters, we will explore the former health care system's problems through the lens of El Materno. For now, we present it as, generally, functional in order to advance our discussion of hegemony. For a general overview of the welfare state and its transformation by neoliberalism, see Giraldo (2007).

55. (Ramos 2008). See also the World Anthropology Network (WAN). See also DaMatta (1994); Escobar (2000); Victoria et al. (2004).

56. (Jimeno 2005; 2006, 72).

57. (Bourgois 1990; Victoria et al. 2004).

58. See also Hale (2006) and our own analysis of how we conducted this ethnography (Abadía-Barrero et al., "Etnografía como acción política," 2018).

59. As is the title of our edited volume, *Salud, Normalización y Capitalismo en Colombia* (Abadía-Barrero et al. 2013).

60. (Abadía-Barrero et al., "Etnografía como acción política," 2018).

61. This is evident in, for example, a collaborative and coauthored ethnography with El San Juan workers, in which the expertise of the workers is emphasized by their description as "native historians" (Góngora et al. 2013).

62. See Rappaport's work on the legacy of Orlando Fals Borda, which both clarifies and complicates the definition and praxis of PAR (Rappaport 2008, 2018, 2020). Gramscian legacy on the thinking-feeling epistemology that Fals Borda advanced is evident in Gramsci's argument that the intellectual's error "consists in believing that one can know without understanding and even more without feeling and being impassioned . . . [about] the elementary passions of the people, understanding them and therefore explaining and justifying them in the particular historical situation and connecting them dialectically to the laws of history and to a superior conception of the world, scientifically and coherently elaborated—i.e. knowledge" (Gramsci and Hoare 1985, 418). See also Vasco Uribe (2007).

63. (Ramos 2008).

64. See Jimeno, Varela Corredor, and Castillo Ardila (2015) and Macleod and de Marinis (2017) for an edited volume that expands the concept of emotional communities to other Latin American contexts. The volume expands and complicates Jimeno's original proposal.

65. In addition to Haraway's original article (1988), see also Lamphere, Ragoné, and Zavella (1997). From a Latin American perspective, see the classic work by acclaimed anthropologist Rosana Guber (2001), and the edited volume *Trabajo de Campo En América Latina: Experiencias Antropológicas Regionales En Etnografía. Tomo 2* [Fieldwork in Latin America. Regional anthropological experiences in ethnography, vol. 2] (2019).

66. Charles Hale offers important critiques of this idea (2006). He also explains the high stakes of activist-oriented anthropology, which must be accountable to the differing standards and demands of the subject and the academic communities.

67. In Sunder Rajan's original formulation (2006), *biocapital* refers to the historical coproduction of life sciences and capitalism. Here, we use it to think about the coproduction of health care and capitalism, in particular as it relates to the MIFC.

68. Throughout the book, short quotes and long passages come from conversations or interviews. The speaker is identified within the context of the paragraph.

1. The National University Escuela

1. This understanding is, of course, inspired by Rudolph Virchow's famous dictum: "Medicine is a social science and politics is nothing else but medicine on a large scale." Virchow, the father of social medicine, and all the scholars, clinicians, and activists who followed him, emphasized not only the political domain of medicine but also the fact that health is the result of politics. For the Latin American social medicine tradition see, among other reviews, Waitzkin et al. (2001). See also the association's main web page ALAMES (www.alames.org) and major journal, *Social Medicine/Medicina Social*. Our discussion here, however, takes a different approach. We want to stress how medicine

is politicized; we see that relationship between power and health as a historical process that changes as biocapital evolves.

2. Recent debates about southern epistemologies are also expressed by Arturo Escobar, Mario Blaser, and Marisol de la Cadena as "political ontology." According to Escobar, every ontology or worldview creates a particular way of seeing and enacting politics. On the other hand, political conflicts often indicate fundamental ontological premises about the world, life, and reality. These and other authors are emphasizing what Orlando Fals Borda understood long ago, when he proposed Participatory Action Research. People from Colombia and many other global southern contexts do not approach reality and politics as purely rational. Instead, they rely on *el sentipensamiento* (the deep conflation between thought and feeling) as a mode of understanding reality (ontology) and the shifts in that reality (epistemology). Experience, rather than any separate scientific neutrality, commands both knowledge and action. According to southern epistemologies, the attempt to separate the ontological domain from its epistemology is nothing but a modern Western fiction. See Escobar (2014, 2018).

3. There are important differences between El Materno's "subaltern health practices/ subaltern health innovations" (Abadía-Barrero 2018) and the kinds of medical care in, for instance, Botswana (Livingston 2012) or Haiti (Maternowska 2006), where lack of resources is all encompassing. There are also differences with medical praxes in the United States, where medical ethics are subordinated to profit and professional medical associations have been co-opted as part of a system of capitalist alliances (Waitzkin and Working Group for Health Beyond Capitalism 2018; Rosenthal 2017). It is these sorts of political historical differences that we argue are important for understanding the role of medicine and medical training in promoting or contesting the kind of medicine that furthers emancipatory political struggles. For wonderful ethnographies of the role of medicine and health care professionals in revolutionary contexts, see Smith-Nonini (2010) and Adams (1998). From these ethnographies, we learn the importance of emphasizing, as we do in our conclusion, that the political imagination of medicine (or medicine as political imagination) depends on the material conditions in which medicine is practiced. These material conditions include the larger context of political struggles.

4. For debates about the impact of neoliberalism on the right to health, see Chapman (2016). For the transformation of citizenship demands through technological interventions and neoliberal politics, see Von Schnitzler (2016).

5. The Universidad Nacional de Colombia was founded in 1867. Since its origin, its national character has been evident in the composition of the student body. In its first decade, the university admitted students from nine departments, including students from the United States, England, and France (Ruiz and Forero Niño 2017, 210). The state funding of the Universidad Nacional, as a percentage of the university's total income, shows a progressive reduction from the 1970s, when it was over 90 percent, to the 2000–2018 period, in which it was barely 50 percent. This indicates that the university has had to fund itself through increased tuition and business maneuvers. According to Bonilla Sebá and González Borrero (2017), the university stopped being a priority for the Colombian government. As we will see, the reduction of student welfare, such as

the elimination of university dorms and cafeterias that benefited students like Carlos, and the progressive increase in tuition impacted the accessibility of La Nacional for many low-income students.

6. For the specific history of the National University of Colombia, see Restrepo Zea, Sánchez, and Silva Carrero (2017). In health, the promotion of national science in Latin America at the end of the nineteenth and beginning of the twentieth centuries was part of national projects to demonstrate to the world independent thinking, the possibility for scientific development and, importantly, to contest eugenic ideas about racial inferiority and the tropics as a natural habitat for infectious diseases. Scientific projects were also a way to connect science and state politics regarding class, region, disease, religion, sex, and race. See Armus (2003), Cueto and Palmer (2015).

7. Dolly Montoya, the first female *rectora* (president) of the university, took office on May 1, 2018. Of her time as a university student in the late 1960s and early 1970s, she remembers that "all student[s] from La Nacional were revolutionaries. We received offers to enlist with the guerrillas" (Granja 2018).

8. (Castro 2009).

9. In Colombia, on June 8 and 9 we commemorate the day of the fallen student (*día del estudiante caído*) paying tribute to the students who were murdered during social protests in 1929, 1954, and 1973 (Anadolu 2020; Falcón Prasca 2020).

10. The superior council composed by the university president (called *rector*), former university presidents, and several delegates from the country's president.

11. (Castro 2009).

12. In 1938 the rural population was 69 percent; the urban population was 31 percent. In 1973 the percentages were completely reversed (Universidad Externado de Colombia and United Nations Population Fund 2007). By 2018 the rural population was estimated to be only 22.9 percent (Semana Rural 2019).

13. Facultad Nacional de Salud Pública Héctor Abad Gómez.

14. Héctor Abad Gómez and Leonardo Betancourt were murdered on their way to the funeral services of professor and union leader Luis Felipe Vélez. Their murder was part of a larger plan to eliminate human right activists, union and civil society leaders, and members of leftist political parties and organizations. The plan was orchestrated by an association of right-wing political and paramilitary organizations in Colombia (Padilla 2017; Sánchez 2018). For more on the life of Héctor Abad Gómez, see his son's memoir (Abad Faciolince 2013); for the "political genocide" against members of the political party Unión Patriótica, see Campos Zornosa (2003).

15. (Bochetti, Arteaga, and Palacio 2005, 178).

16. At very high interest rates through the ICETEX (*Instituto Colombiano de Crédito Educativo y Estudios Técnicos en el Exterior,* or Colombian Institute for Educational Credit and Foreign Technical Studies).

17. Alfredo Rubiano (1932–2008) was an emblematic and distinguished professor of the School of Medicine. He received many teaching awards, including the university's most prestigious, the Orden Gerardo Molina (Florido Caicedo 2009).

18. A private version of the school was founded in 1826. The public medical school of the National University was officially founded in 1867. Law 66 of 1867 indicated that

the medical school was the academic reagent of the Hospital San Juan de Dios. For a history of the School of Medicine, see Eslava Castañeda, Vega Vargas, and Hernández Alvarez (2017).

19. This religious institution founded many public hospitals in Colombia and Latin America during colonial times. These hospitals have lasted through the colonial, independent, and republican histories of Latin American countries and have been at the center of the state's welfare infrastructures.

20. Bridges' work in Alpha Hospital in New York offers similar descriptions of the high-quality care performed at this "war-zone" hospital (Bridges 2011).

21. We will talk more about the instinctive and emotional aspects of learning and practicing medicine. Importantly, however, this idea differs from what is sometimes called "empathy" or "bedside manners." Rather, what Elena and others constantly described was the need to be emotionally present in all aspects of learning and interacting. This proposal challenges the rational domain at the core of Western knowledge, prioritizing instead a combination of intellect and emotion.

22. This kind of male dominance in medicine imposes particular gender hierarchies. The most common one, evident in most medical settings is, of course, that between male physicians and female nurses. And yet, female medical students, physicians, and professors also had to navigate gendered relationships carefully, even more so when there was no active engagement in gendered debates or gender politics.

23. See B. J. Good (1994).

24. See Bochetti, Arteaga, and Palacio (2005); Restrepo (2011).

25. "Tropics" here refers not only to a type of geographical region in which certain infectious diseases prevail but also to a larger geopolitics of public health. "Tropical medicine" was consolidated as an area of expertise that carried powerful metaphors about the role of former colonies in harboring and transmitting infectious diseases. Both the environments and the people were understood as polluted and prone to disease; this sense of colonial inferiority and contamination had political effects in areas like eugenics. Tropical medicine was consistently politicized, as doctors worked to advance ideas of independence and development. But it also retained important ties with former colonizers, and consistently navigates the new U.S. imperial influence in medicine; these relationships make any clear distinction between colonial and postcolonial medicine impossible. See Cueto and Palmer (2015).

26. Many studies use Bourdieu's concept of habitus to understand clinical medicine.

27. There were also private institutions that treated poor people who couldn't access public institutions or wanted a different kind of care not provided by the public infrastructure. The three tiers also frequently overlapped in complex ways. Nonetheless, for clarity, I use this class and labor breakdown from earlier studies (see, e.g., Hernández Alvarez [2002]). A similar structure of health and social security exists in other Latin American countries; see Hernández Alvarez (2004); Giraldo (2007); Cueto and Palmer (2015). For a different history of public/private health care distinctions in Brazil and the effect of colonial legacies on perceptions of the Brazilian health care system, see Jerome (2016).

28. See Ahumada (2002) and Echeverry López (2002). For an interesting history of the media's treatment of the Seguro Social during the neoliberal reform, including the

effects of its positive treatment of private insurance companies and negative treatment of the public sector, see Mesa Melgarejo (2018). Other health care networks, with a funding scheme similar to El Seguro, were created for public sector workers.

29. This Bismarckian schema is the basis of social security in many European countries. In Colombia, however, the government never contributed its portion; this had an important impact on how El Seguro's crisis unfolded. For a history of El Seguro's economic crisis and the role of the Colombian state and media, see Ariza Ruíz, Abadía-Barrero, and Pinilla Alfonso (2013); Mesa Melgarejo (2018).

2. Clinical Social Medicine

1. The notion of health being subsumed by politics has been advanced by Latin American social medicine scholars. See, in particular, Jaime Breilh's work (1986, 2003, 2013).

2. Iriart and Merhy (2017) explain how the medical industrial complex and the health financial sector shifted, in neoliberal times, from being profit competitors to becoming partners largely by co-opting social justice struggles in health (Birn, Nervi, and Siqueira 2016).

3. Perhaps the best-known example is Pulitzer Prize winner Tracy Kidder's (2009) biography of physician/anthropologist Paul Farmer. See also Singer and Rebecca Allen's (2017) history of another remarkable physician, Bruce Gould.

4. See Bochetti, Arteaga, and Palacio (2005); Pinilla and Abadía (2017). For a description of the tradition of beneficence in the Brazilian health care system, see Jerome (2016).

5. See Restrepo (2011). After independence, beneficence was intended to facilitate a transition from the charitable and religious orientation of colonialism. According to Estela Restrepo (2006), El San Juan transitioned over the nineteenth century from the charity model to the beneficence model and, finally, to a modern hospital characterized by greater professional autonomy and independent institutional financing. Nonetheless, the social dynamics of the charity and beneficence periods remain pervasive. The dependence of the Beneficencia ended in 1979, when a private non profit foundation was established to administer the hospitals. That structure, however, was declared illegal in 2005, and the hospitals were reassigned to the Beneficencia, as we will later describe.

6. Bogotá had several epicenters of commercial, intellectual, and administrative life. Beside the downtown area, Chapinero and Usaquén were the most notable centers. But it took a long time to get to these centers; people from Gabriel's generation see the journey as significant. Chapinero was always considered part of Bogotá. Usaquén was officially annexed to the city in 1954, along with the municipalities of Usme, Bosa, Fontibón, Engativá, and Suba (Saldarriaga, cited in Cortés Díaz 2006, 30). These former municipalities are now part of the city's twenty existing localities (administrative entities). Each locality has a local mayor's office and corresponding administrative offices.

7. (Baker 2000, 321–22).

8. We will say more about the origin of medical ideas and political imagination in the conclusion, but Gabriel's recollection serves as a perfect application of Karl Marx and

Friederich Engels's *The German Ideology* (1968). In a coauthored piece from early in their long friendship and collaboration, they mocked the way philosophers disregard the material basis of thought and helped turn Hegelian dialectics on its head by privileging the material manifestations of reality over its abstract representations. Gabriel's recollections and Marx and Engels' work help us think about the material basis of medical ideas and the transformations in material medical practice and imagination. In Gabriel's case, we see a mix of poverty, incipient technologies, and suffering underlying what we will see next.

9. (Méndez and Ulloque 2006).

10. (IDEASS n.d.; Whitelaw and Sleath 1985).

11. (Pinzón 2006).

12. (Whitelaw and Sleath 1985, 1206).

13. (Méndez and Ulloque 2006).

14. Along with the saliva path that the mother has painted, joeys are apparently guided by their sense of smell and gravity (Nelson and Gemmell 2004).

15. (Méndez and Ulloque 2006).

16. (Martínez and Rey 1983, cited in IDEASS n.d.; Whitelaw and Sleath 1985).

17. (Grant and UNICEF 1984, 48).

18. (Grant and UNICEF 1984, 48).

19. (IDEASS n.d.).

20. See the WHO Sasakawa award page: http://www.who.int/governance/awards /sasakawa/en/.

21. Historically, southern epistemologies have been discredited by what Boaventura de Souza Santos calls the Cognitive Empire (Santos 2018). While southern epistemologies are disregarded in scientific power struggles, southern innovations are often co-opted by transnational companies for profit. KMC was called a "reverse innovation," and efforts to make commercial products out of this natural, zero-cost technology abound. For a critique of El Materno's KMC as a "reverse innovation" see Abadía-Barrero (2018). For other debates about differences in Latin American health epistemologies, see Spiegel, Breilh, and Yassi (2015).

22. (IDEASS n.d.; Pinzón 2006). Finding alternatives in medical care differs from trying to provide good enough or improvised care when resources are lacking (Strong 2020; Livingston 2012). "Intertwined biological, economic, and institutional configurations" (Roberts 2012, 4) can lead to adjusting medical protocols to "nuestra realidad" (Roberts 2012). KMC clarifies that subaltern health innovations are not about substandard parameters or "ethical variability" (Petryna 2009), but alternative epistemologies of care that constitute alternative ethics, whether in direct care or research.

23. See Good (2001).

24. This interaction is a modality of medical syncretism (Law et al. 2014).

25. It is very likely that his paranoia is related to political violence. He mentioned how growing up in Medellín at the height of the Medellín Cartel meant living in a constant state of violence. His narrative suggests that his sense of persecution could be classified as "paranoid schizophrenia," but also that it is deeply entangled with his cultural environment. Medical anthropology has eloquently argued for a cultural interpretation of

severe psychopathology, including schizophrenia, and the role of postcolonial societies in mental health (Good 2008).

26. What Bourdieu has called social capital. There is extensive research on the importance of social capital in health. For the relationship between social capital and access to the health care system in Colombia see, among others, Hurtado, Kawachi, and Sudarsky (2011), Abadía-Barrero and Oviedo (2008).

27. A symbolic homogenization that allows for the repetition of institutional protocols with disregard for the needs of each particular case (Vallana Sala 2019).

28. See Jimeno for the concept of emotional communities (Jimeno, Varela Corredor, and Castillo Ardila 2015; Macleod and de Marinis 2017). Drawing from Williams' work on the structures of sentiment, Jimeno argues that emotional expressions are not exclusive to intimate places like nuclear families but that emotional ties within social sectors result in shared feelings, both affectionate and political.

29. For the experiences of families at NICUS and the emotional aspects of having very sick relatives see, among many others, Seo (2016), Navne, Svendsen, and Gammeltoft (2018).

30. Currea Guerrero at a public presentation at the National University as part of the conference cycle, Memoria Viva del Hospital San Juan de Dios, December 4, 2006.

31. (IDEASS n.d., 1).

32. For a critique of the hegemony of biomedicine and markets in global health, see Abadía Barrero, Crane, and Ruíz (2012). In the introduction to their coedited volume, Metzl (2010) advances the argument that health driven by markets has become a specific moral imperative, imposed as a powerful discourse of power and largely influenced by a consumerist rhetoric. In the case of the United States, he cites physician H. Gilbert Welch at length: "H. Gilbert Welch argues that true health-care reform will only take place when America moves away from definitions of health that profit the 'medical-industrial complex' of health professionals, pharmaceutical companies, biotechnology firms, manufacturers of diagnostic technologies, surgical centers, hospitals, and academic medical centers" (6). Dumit (2012) explains how the health consumer is constructed by pharmaceutical advertisements. Recent studies demonstrate that the growth of for-profit sectors constructing "health as business" under neoliberalism is not only economically unsustainable but also harmful for the health of populations; see Rosenthal (2017) and Waitzkin and Working Group for Health Beyond Capitalism (2018). Importantly, the tensions between health industries and health finance have offered further profits through mergers, acquisitions, corruption, and the manipulation of guidelines, protocols, and legislations (Iriart and Merhy 2017; Birn, Nervi, and Siqueira 2016; Bugbee 2019).

33. (Grant and UNICEF 1984).

34. (Pinzón 2006).

35. For the original formulation of medical hegemony from a Latin American perspective, see Menéndez (1985).

36. This same argument is found in Mol's (2008) *The Logic of Care*.

37. (Currea Guerrero 2004, chap. 4).

38. These unhinged forceps are known as Velasco spatulas. For a history of forceps and their many developments, see Lattus Olmos (2008).

39. See Adams (2016) for an overview of how numbers and statistics became the new parameters in global health and began to trump the individual experience, local interpretations, and local health proposals that this book argues for.

40. (Currea Guerrero 2004, 72).

41. Thinking with nature, trusting nature, and making an effort to re synchronize our senses with the world that surrounds us has parallels with decolonial proposals that propose epistemologies from the south (Vanhulst and Beling 2014; Escobar 2014, 2018). This approach is also consistent with demedicalizing approaches to birthing (Davis-Floyd et al. 2009). El Materno proves that less medicalization is possible even in high-risk pregnancies and severely compromised newborns.

42. For a review of medical vitalism, see Wilson (2004).

43. Meaning that, even though it is impossible to insert these complex clinical and emotional practices in statistical calculations to assess whether they are more or less effective or worse or better than other clinical parameters, their importance cannot be denied. This realm of logics is presented as a way to emphasize the limits of a "rational" approach to medicine, which is what commands biomedicine.

44. See Abadía-Barrero (2018) for this concept as a critique of the global health trend of using business models to think about "reverse innovations."

3. Religion and Caring in a Medical Setting

1. This is different from charismatic healing, as explained by Csordas (1994). But many of the same ideas are applicable in both cases: the importance of a phenomenological interpretation, the emotional aspects, and the guiding role of spiritual figures.

2. There are many unknowns in medicine that speak to the importance of other forces than logic and science in healing. Unlike biomedicine, charismatic healing and indigenous and folk medicine all assume a fundamental role of faith in the healing process.

3. Anthropology has seen many efforts to destabilize anthropocentric and rational-oriented approaches. Alter-ontologies, multispecies ethnography, and decolonial thinking, among others, argue for expanding anthropology to include what has been marginalized by Western scientific thinking.

4. Anthropological discussions on care, care giving, and caring have emerged as powerful moral and intersubjective domains that disrupt philosophical ideals about universal ethics. There is a multiplicity of care and caring practices, which makes caring a polysemic concept; there is also a range of cultural and social domains that influence the ways in which subjects and communities care for one another. Caring can be understood as a deeply moral and personal experience that transforms the subjective and intersubjective domains of medicine (Kleinman 2012). Care can also be seen as a part of the intersections between moral economy and political economy (Han 2012; Mol 2008; Mol, Moser, and Pols 2010; Stevenson 2014; Garcia 2010; Povinelli 2011), in that historical forces (including medicine, political violence, and welfare systems) shape the particular ways in which kin and communities care for one another. The emotional domain is important in care for the self and others (Garcia 2010; Bourgois and Schonberg 2009). Analysis of these different interactions destabilizes idealized constructs of

the ethics behind human action (Strong 2020). Elana Buch offers a review that works "across scales of social life and theoretical approaches to care to highlight connections and fissures between global political-economic transformations and the most intimate aspects of daily life" (2015). More specifically, she addresses the circulation of care among aging bodies and how issues of kindship, morality, and social reproduction intersect. Her work speaks to the importance of feminist theory in politicizing notions of care and caregiving, particularly the unpaid and unrecognized labor that care and caring demands. In El Materno's research, it is important to note how the religious domain of caring, symbolized in the humanization proposal, became an institutional practice that affected all interactions inside the hospital and created special emotional and spiritual bonds that influenced its clinical practice and everyday dynamics.

5. Here, we borrow Jimeno's concept and apply it to a different setting and discussion. See Macleod and de Marinis (2017) for an overview of Jimeno's concept and its usefulness as a conceptual tool for many different contexts.

6. We use "logic of caring" here to differentiate from Mol's concept of "logic of care" (Mol 2008). Several similarities can be found between Mol's concept and what is presented here. Mol explains the dramatic difference between a medical logic of care and the market logic of choice that is becoming dominant in health care interactions. While individual power and responsibility are seen as key Western principles that should be embraced by medicine, solidarity and attentiveness to people's needs offer valuable alternatives. These elements are dwindling as individualism gains more traction, leaving patients with the responsibility for making rational decisions about their own care. Nonetheless, Mol's concept of "logic of care" is meant to inform medical decisions about care. In El Materno, the logic of caring extends further out into many other domains of life. In this regard, medical care is also challenged by larger "epistemologies of care" that conceive of deep relationships between humans and the natural world and between social and political aspects that influence health and are also relevant for people's well-being. This "logic of caring" as part of a larger "epistemology of care" can be understood as belonging to the larger tradition of Latin American social medicine, which is being incorporated into the clinical realm as what we have called "clinical social medicine" in chapter 2.

7. Humanization is different than what now is called "bedside manners." It involves both cordial relationships and paying attention to what people are telling you without a judgmental attitude and with the idea of finding a way to help them. It is about respect, but it is also about creating an environment of empathy and support.

8. Used when there is incompatibility between the Rh blood factor of baby and mother.

9. Including class, gender, and religious hierarchies. Likely, there were also racialized hierarchies in the postcolonial context, made visible in demeanor, clothing, and education.

10. Abortion remained illegal in Colombia until the Constitutional Court promulgated the sentence C-355 on May 10, 2006, which authorizes abortion when there is a danger to the life or health of the woman, in cases of severe fetal malformation that makes the fetus unviable, and in pregnancies that are the result of sexual violence.

11. Accompaniment is an important word among community health workers. Farmer has discussed the importance of accompaniment in his work in Haiti and elsewhere.

Many of his discussions are available online. Accompaniment, however, has a longer tradition in Latin America and it is different to the model advanced by Partners in Health for primary health care. In our context, accompaniment refers to a sense of collective caring in which a person's presence, rather than any specific action, is valued. In can be seen in health, academic, and social movement settings.

12. This scholarship was in fact partial and depended on the performance of the student. Part of the scholarship "debt" was waived, and part had to be paid after graduation. By the time Veronica and Natalia entered the National University, cafeterias and dormitories had been closed down and tuition was on the rise.

13. The relationship between machismo, fatherhood, and conservative views on religion is well known. For a classic anthropological study of families in Colombia, see Gutiérrez de Pineda (1964). For the relationship between Catholicism and the conservative values of machismo and Marianism, see Lagarde and de los Ríos (2015).

14. When the angel Gabriel appears to the Virgin Mary and announces that she has been chosen to bear God's son.

15. For an explanation of church prudence in cases of Marian Apparitions, see Bastero (2011).

16. According to Verónica, she had a "quebranto," an overwhelming emotional experience of a spiritual presence.

17. (Murphy and González Faraco 2011).

18. (Murphy and González Faraco 2011).

19. (Murphy and González Faraco 2011; Bastero 2011).

4. Hospital Budgets before and after Neoliberalism

1. See Sunder Rajan (2006).

2. "Regulated markets" were an idea proposed by neoliberal think tanks (Latin American/World Bank officers) to claim that health was a special commodity that did not belong to a free-market scenario (Londoño and Frenk 1997). Over time, the "regulated markets" came to represent another neoliberal "fallacy" that hid the influence of health markets in shaping health policies and the operating conditions of health care institutions (Hernández 2003).

3. According to Mulligan, "financialization in health care produces new forms of inequality, valuations of deservingness, and forms of profiting from risk. Ultimately, I argue that financial techniques obfuscate how much health care costs, foster widespread gaming of reimbursement systems that drives up price, and 'unspool' risk (Erikson 2012) by devolving financial and moral responsibility for health care onto individual consumers" (Mulligan 2016, 38).

4. For the relationship between "stupid deaths" and structural violence, see Farmer (2003). For analysis of new health care inequalities and the ways in which neoliberal morality has permeated the whole system, including the judiciary, see Abadía-Barrero (2015a), Ewig and Hernández (2009); Hernández Alvarez and Vega (2001).

5. (Mulligan 2016).

6. (Ardila-Sierra and Abadía-Barrero 2020).

7. (Bochetti, Arteaga, and Palacio 2005, 26).

8. See also Eslava Castañeda, Vega Vargas, and Hernández Alvarez (2017).

9. (Bochetti, Arteaga, and Palacio 2005; Restrepo 2006, 2011). See also examples of the pervasiveness of the charity orientation in chapters 2 and 3.

10. El Materno was formally created on May 4, 1944, by *Acuerdo 14* from the *Junta General de Beneficencia de Cundinamarca* as *Instituto de Protección Materno Infantil*. In 1953, as a tribute to the mother of hospital director José del Carmen Acosta Villaveces, El Materno was renamed *Instituto Materno Infantil "Concepción Villaveces de Acosta"* (Redacción El Tiempo 2016).

11. While the conception of welfare did not exist at the time, the Beneficence functioned as the country's main welfare institution.

12. The hospital, however, remains of central importance to the government. In 1964 President Guillermo León Valencia honored the hospital by giving it the country's highest medal, the *Cruz de Boyacá* (Méndez and Ulloque 2006).

13. (Bochetti, Arteaga, and Palacio 2005, 66).

14. (Méndez and Ulloque 2006).

15. (Bochetti, Arteaga, and Palacio 2005, 70).

16. According to a 1971 study (Bochetti, Arteaga, and Palacio 2005, 60).

17. (Bochetti, Arteaga, and Palacio 2005, 70).

18. (Bochetti, Arteaga, and Palacio 2005, 71).

19. (Méndez and Ulloque 2006).

20. The SNS (*Sistema Nacional de Salud*, National Health System) worked across regions and integrated units offering all levels of care. The SNS worked from 1975 until 1993, when it was replaced by market-based health care reform.

21. (Méndez and Ulloque 2006).

22. Decrees 290 and 1374 of 1979 and decree 371 of 1978.

23. Presidential Decree 290, 1979, Republic of Colombia. Previous Beneficence directorship bodies included members of the National University.

24. (Bochetti, Arteaga, and Palacio 2005, 99).

25. (Bochetti, Arteaga, and Palacio 2005, 88).

26. This juridical effort was led by a woman with minimal education, who had begun working in the hospital's general services department in 1984 (Góngora et al. 2013).

27. (Méndez and Ulloque 2006).

28. (Méndez and Ulloque 2006).

29. (Bochetti, Arteaga, and Palacio 2005, 87–88).

30. (Bochetti, Arteaga, and Palacio 2005, 100).

31. For a historical account of the reform, see Jaramillo (1999), Uribe (2009).

32. In Colombia, debates about seeing patients and citizens as customers abound. For the international context, see Mol (2008).

33. (Gaviria, Medina, and Mejia 2006; Yepes et al. 2010; Molina Marín et al. 2010; Molina, Muñóz, and Ramírez 2009).

34. El Materno's 50th anniversary was in 1994. The hospital complex received recognition in 1996 (Bochetti, Arteaga, and Palacio 2005, 109–11). For subaltern health innovations see chapter 2 and Abadía-Barrero (2018).

35. The Chilean model was one of the first neoliberal experiments with health care reform. It was imposed during Augusto Pinochet's dictatorship; this was done violently and in collaboration with the Chicago School of Economics, known as the orchestrator of neoliberal doctrine (Klein 2007).

36. For several years, insurance companies were top ranked economically, alongside the most successful companies in Colombia. Over the years, such economic success would be highly criticized given the horrific stories of hospital closures and patients facing lack of care.

37. (M. Hernández 2003). The percentage each plan covered has been debated and has changed over the years. Initial reports indicate that the subsidiary plan was about 60 percent of the contributory. However, the contributory plan was far from comprehensive, and the system was plagued with exclusions. This legalization of inequality was challenged by the Constitutional Court in 2008 with the sentence T-760, which asked the government to make both health care plans equal. Initially, the government had promised to accomplish this by 2000, but the goal was delayed. Even after making the plans formally equal, inequalities have persisted—the capitation unit remains different between both plans and insurance companies offer a more extensive network of services for the contributory plans. There are also extra-coverage plans, which ensure fewer "bureaucratic itineraries" for patients and more contracts between insurance companies and health care institutions (Abadía-Barrero and Oviedo Manrique 2009; Molina Marín et al. 2010).

38. For issues of inequalities in the health care system, see Hernández Alvarez and Vega (2001).

39. (Molina Marín et al. 2010).

40. Cesantía was a special savings fund based on a percentage of the worker's salary that employers deposited monthly and workers could use for education, for purchasing their first house, or for retirement. Cesantías still exist, but neoliberal labor reforms transformed the ways they work. Now administered by private funds—usually the same funds that administer pensions—cesantías more closely follow the logic of regular savings funds, including penalties, higher administrative charges, and calculation averages that lower the sum that workers receive.

41. (Antunes 2005; Allison 2013). Precarious work is "employment that is uncertain, unpredictable, and risky from the point of view of the worker" (Kalleberg 2009, 2).

42. Allowing the ISS to keep its insured population proved over time to be a strategy for keeping down competing insurers' costs. The ISS managed the most complex patients that required the most expensive care. "High-cost" patients were not received by other insurers. Analyses of the ISS's own crisis report uneven competition and a permanent failure of the government to keep their promised funding (Ariza 2008; Ariza Ruíz, Abadía-Barrero, and Pinilla Alfonso 2013).

43. The "rights verifier" became, in fact, a rights refuser—the first gatekeeper of the system. Over time, this and other administrative barriers to health care became emblematic of the judicialization of the right to health in Colombia. The ombudsman (who reports on the status of the right to health), the general attorney's office, nongovernmental organizations, and academic sectors all denounce the constant violation of the right to health as a result of the system's for-profit structure.

44. The complexity behind billing/tariffs in health care is intentional, because it allows financial institutions to drive up their profits by hiding real costs (Mulligan 2016). In Colombia, there are two tariffs, one for SOAT (mandatory auto insurance) and one for ISS. Depending on when the tariff was updated, insurance companies negotiate a percentage above the tariff. These negotiations, as indicated by Sonia, are done on a case-by-case basis; the negotiating power of any given hospital or clinic is variable. Specialists with a monopoly on their clinical service account for the highest tariffs in the system. Hence, the final cost of a given procedure, and the distribution of that cost between the institution and the professional, are determined by a set of institutional and interpersonal negotiations, including labor contracts (or rates of labor exploitation). We expand on physicians' contracts in chapter 7. When vertical integration—which was first illegal, but later authorized—occurs, the insurance premiums revert to the owners of the insurance companies and clinics. For more on this, see Molina Marín et al. (2010).

45. "Savage capitalism" refers to the current capital accumulation pattern that brings an unprecedented rise in inequality rates and the interrelated destruction of social welfare, human beings, and environments. See, among many, Valqui Cachi and Espinosa Contreras (2009); Graeber (2014); Hogan (2009). See Naomi Klein (2007) for her similar concept of "disaster capitalism."

46. To facilitate international comparisons, all the numbers have been converted to dollars, according to exchange rates of the time.

47. Auditing and accountability became a new norm through which neoliberal economic logics took over the functioning of national and global institutions (Strathern 2000). The neoliberal idea that auditing culture ensures efficient use of resources and intended outcomes has been challenged, both by demonstrating its inefficiencies and the identification of new bureaucratic disruptions in governance and other programs. Jessica Mulligan's analysis of Puerto Rican health care reform shows how the increasing administrative presentation of health care systems in numbers or codes represents "a larger trend in American medicine towards administering health care according to business logics that value efficiency, profit maximization, and performance measurements" (Mulligan 2010, 304). Mulligan's research challenges neoliberal assumptions of auditing and accountability as administrative logics that improve the quality of health care (Mulligan 2016, 2014).

48. (Bochetti, Arteaga, and Palacio 2005, 119–20). A formal liquidation of El San Juan's 1393 workers would have required recognizing all their collective bargaining agreements, including severance payments for ending contracts without justification. The estimated cost of such a formal process was around US$24 million (Bochetti, Arteaga, and Palacio 2005, 129).

49. Different research and art initiatives agree that El San Juan should not be considered "closed." Workers still go to "work" at the hospital; their struggles and the hospital's history suggest imagining the hospital as a "living organism" that continues to resist. Artist Maria Elvira Escallón describes El San Juan as being in a "coma state," waiting to wake up. Several other metaphors have been used to describe this increasingly prolonged liminal state. See, for example, El San Juan "dies standing" (Góngora et al. 2013).

50. The official closing date is September 29, 2001, resolution 1933, but the factual end of patient care was during 1999–2000.

51. Resolution 1933 of September 21, 2001, Supersalud, Ministry of Health, which ordered the full administrative intervention of the Foundation San Juan de Dios and adopted additional measurements in relation to its institutions (López Hooker 2004).

52. (Caracol radio 2005a).

53. For more on the intricate substantive relationship between matter and people, see Povinelli (2011).

5. Violence and Resistance

1. (Adams 1998; Can 2016; Hamdy 2016; Brouwer 2011; Dewachi 2017). See also biographical analyses of social medicine physicians, which show famed physicians' political subjectivities in action (Kidder 2009; Singer and Allen 2017). It is worth noting that the "social determinants approach" favored by the World Health Organization (WHO) and Western medical traditions has been criticized as overly reductionist of the larger political scope of medicine and public health (Navarro 2009). For the Latin American perspective on the social determination of health, see Breilh (2013). In short, the Latin American perspective sees medicine and public health as tools for social transformation, not merely as determinants of health. Furthermore, these perspectives have a clear Marxist orientation that, like other emancipatory traditions, sees inequality as an issue of historical oppression requiring emancipatory efforts.

2. In his work on structural violence, Farmer distinguishes between invisible and visible violence and argues that anthropology's job is to make visible the invisible structures that sustain structural violence (Farmer 2004, 2003). Writing on political trauma, Kleinman (1995) argued that "these techniques of violence are intended to tyrannize through the development of cultural sensibilities and forms of social interaction that keep secret histories of criticism secret and hidden transcripts of resistance hidden. . . . That is, trauma is used systematically to silence people through suffering" (175).

3. Bourgois has clarified that there is a continuum of interrelated violence (political, symbolic, structural, and everyday) (Bourgois 2004).

4. See the original analysis of "psychosocial trauma" produced by Martín-Baró (1996) in the context of war in El Salvador during the 1970s and 1980s.

5. This analysis resonates with what one of the counselors at Kashmir's Mental Health hospital explained to Saiba Varma. In a context of violence, in this case military control, "the hospital is deliberately being kept understaffed and underequipped by the state government. This is collective punishment against the local population who sheltered and supported militants during the armed struggle" (Varma 2020, 80). In El Materno's case, the body politic is less about claims of support to a militant group and more about a militancy with a subaltern epistemology of care.

6. (Comaroff and Comaroff 2006; Allison 2013).

7. According to Pink (2012), everyday life and activism are intricately linked. They form a dynamic entity that is constantly shifting, filled with shifts in perception, feeling, knowledge, and social and sensory environments (Abadía-Barrero and Ruíz-Sánchez 2018).

8. (Caracol radio 2005b, 2005c).

9. For "social risk management" as the technical framework for neoliberal social policy, see Giraldo (2007).

10. For another example of health care burnout, particularly in cases related to HIV, see Raviola et al. (2002).

11. Precarious labor conditions imposed by neoliberalism extend to other experiences of having to live a precarious life (Allison 2013). Allison expands the concept of economic and labor precarity in powerful ways, several of which apply to El Materno's case.

12. Similar to Allison (2013), Epele (2020) explains that to aguantar, to bear the burden of the precarious labor situation imposed by neoliberal policies, is not simply a labor-related phenomenon. Rather, it is when people bear the burden of precarious life through profound verbal, bodily, and emotional experiences.

13. All numbers here are converted into US dollars based on the exchange rate of the time.

14. We use Žižek's idea of systemic violence here, privileging an understanding of the systemic or chronic violence inherent to the capitalist system. This violence controls populations by creating disposable and dispensable subjects and social projects (Žižek 2008, 14). This framework differs from other approaches that conceive of the structural forces of history and economy as forms of oppression. The concept of "structural violence," which helped advance our understanding of long-lasting historical forces producing contemporary suffering, has been critiqued for its lack of specificity and potential emptying out of each of the structural forces at play (see the exchange of Farmer's 2004 article). Systemic violence, on the other hand, allows us to see the implications of specific forms of capitalist-driven violence, such as the process of household economic precarity narrated by Lucía. Clearly, there are specific legislation reforms that favor the economic interests of capitalist sectors. These affect workers directly, as they experience direct losses in salaries and benefits, but they also have indirect effects in that people must resort to (and are then made vulnerable by) loans and debts. It is important to differentiate between "unintended consequences" and the indirect effects of a given policy or act. While loans, debts, losing houses, and forcing families to cut costs at their children's expense are not explicit legal or governmental goals, it would be absurd to label these events "unintended," which implies that such consequences were not imagined or foreseen. A systemic violence framework allows us to see the direct and indirect effects of single aggressive acts like labor reforms or the withering of El Materno workers.

15. Terms like *survival mode* underemphasize the everyday suffering and destruction of lives and life projects, as Povinelli (2011) has explained. Survival mode implies a static state, or at least a state of relative tranquility between less stable moments. A longer historical analysis forces us to unpack the meaning of this term, to put it into dialogue with the conditions of previous and future unstable moments, and to uncover the transformation of life and its value. We must understand that "survival modes" occur as part of the "slow rhythm" of systemic violence (Povinelli 2011, 153).

16. The Minister argued that the government budget should not include significant funding for the hospitals until tax reform was completed (Caracol radio 2005c).

17. (Caracol radio 2006).

18. Head nurse Patricia Farías, like many others, thought of El Materno as the big city's womb, where thousands of people were born. To Patricia, like Luis Carlos in chapter 1, the hospital smells maternal, with scents like breast milk, her area of expertise. She saw the hospital as a place where training and teaching helped generations of talented and caring health professionals. Perhaps it is because of this symbolism that her most significant traumatic memories are related to that specific episode. It is hard to assess exactly how many workers' narratives count as expressions of post-traumatic stress disorder, but the number seems high. However, the kinds of trauma caused by this systemic violence, including outbreaks of physical and emotional violence, invite us to think about trauma differently. For a longer discussion, see Abadía-Barrero (2015b).

19. For the militarization of hospitals, the wider criminalization of health care institutions, and health care workers' participation in revolutionary struggles, see Adams (1998); Can (2016); Hamdy (2016); Brouwer (2011).

20. She continues to be a national expert in this strategy. See Farías-Jiménez et al. (2014).

21. Clara Arteaga, the hospital's pathologist and professor of La Nacional's School of Medicine, who was awarded the 2005 National Prize in Medical Research for her project about the genetics of ectopic pregnancies she conducted at El Materno.

22. Varma's proposal to think about disturbance is helpful and has many parallels to El Materno (Varma 2020). In the contexts of India-controlled Kashmir, unused expensive infrastructures and "deserted inpatient wards" (79) represent a ruined health care system. "Disturbances had unleashed strange irregularities and 'randomness' into the atmosphere" (81).

23. (Redacción El Tiempo 2006a, 2006b).

24. (Redacción El Tiempo 2006c).

25. (Redacción El Tiempo 2006d).

26. Más de 1.400 bebés han nacido en el Materno Infantil desde que el Distrito empezó su administración. http://www.eltiempo.com/bogota/2007-07-17/ARTICULO -WEB-NOTA_INTERIOR-3642730.html Retrieved July 17, 2007. Link no longer available.

27. Más de 1.400 bebés han nacido en el Materno Infantil desde que el Distrito empezó su administración. http://www.eltiempo.com/bogota/2007-07-17/ARTICULO -WEB-NOTA_INTERIOR-3642730.html Retrieved July 17, 2007. Link no longer available.

28. Such technical problems are common and well known. Ironically, the managed-care model ends up personifying the system, attributing to it actions and decisions, often at real people's expense.

29. De facto disentitlements in managed-care systems have been previously described by Lopez (2005).

30. This was clarified by the director of El San Juan, Alvaro Casallas, and by a lawyer familiar with the workers' struggle. See http://radioambulante.org/audio/episodios/el -hospital. Retrieved June 16, 2016.

31. (Consejo de Estado 2012).

32. (Abadía-Barrero, Crane, and Ruíz 2012).

33. Byron Good's productive concept of "hauntology," following Derrida's original formulation, or the value of unspeakable and incomprehensible makers of political violence as contemporary expressions of political subjectivity (B. Good 2012), is helpful in this analysis. Past political violence cannot be spoken directly but is nonetheless expressed in domains of culture and subjectivity. Interestingly, El Materno workers articulate themselves as the future ghosts of the hospital, which indicates the ways in which they are projecting their struggle into the future.

34. http://www.fundacionsanjuandediosenliquidacion.com/ is the original site and is no longer available.

35. (El Espectador 2012).

36. (El Espectador 2012).

37. (Valenzuela 2013).

38. (Redacción El Tiempo 2013).

39. (Redacción El Tiempo 2013).

40. As discussed in the introduction. See also Abadía-Barrero et al. (2018); Abadía-Barrero and Ruíz-Sánchez (2018).

41. (Abadía-Barrero and Ruíz-Sánchez 2018).

42. (Redacción El Tiempo 2015a).

43. (Redacción El Tiempo 2015b).

44. (Redacción El Tiempo 2015c).

45. (Redacción Bogotá 2015a).

46. One of the last pieces of news they were able to publish explained their situation: http://www.desdeabajo.info/ediciones/item/27284-no-nos-han-reconocido-nuestras-acreencias-laborales-ni-pensionales.html. Retrieved October 10, 2015

47. (Redacción Bogotá 2019).

6. Remaining amid Destruction

1. (Gramsci and Hoare 1985, 235).

2. Job insecurity and job precariousness have become standards of labor under neoliberalism. Not only has the reserve army increased but neoliberal labor laws have largely rendered outdated full contracts with benefits. Most workers now contract for some number of months in a given year and remain unemployed in between contracts. Some contracts are product based, intensifying workers' self-exploitation as their hours extend significantly into evenings and weekends. The end of benefits has meant that workers are forced to pay for social security benefits out of their meager incomes. Self-employment has also become a new facet of job insecurity. For Latin America and most of the Global South, self-employment means meager income from several informal activities like selling small objects or food on the street. Survival labor has been euphemistically described in neoliberal statistics as self-employment and entrepreneurship. For a Latin American perspective on labor changes under neoliberalism, see Antunes (2005, 2003, 2018).

3. Labor flexibility and insecurity have indeed increased the rate of worker exploitation and, hence, augmented companies' profit rates.

4. Biobureaucratic expansion came about with the new accounting impositions of for-profit systems. Strong (2020, 53) shows a similar process in Tanzania, where global metrics for maternal health produced a scarcity of time for clinical patient care. "It also produced a scarcity of emotional reserves for affective caring as nurses had to engage with petulant gatekeepers and as physical time away from the ward prevented additional intersubjective care exchanges."

5. This ethnographic fragment demonstrates how administration of individual insurance-based systems is more expensive than the simpler administrative schemes offered by social insurance or single-payer systems.

6. See C. V. Giraldo and Ceballos (2011); Molina, Muñóz, and Ramírez (2009); Yepes et al. (2010).

7. Contracts between insurers and health care institutions is the most important factor contributing to this insufficiency of appointments and continuity of care. For commercial reasons, insurers have different contracts with different health care institutions; often, contracts end or fragment the care in such a way that patients cannot receive all the care they need at any single institution (Molina Marín et al. 2010).

8. Quality of care has been compromised. Even though programs continue to exist, it is evident that they no longer run at the same level of comprehensiveness and care they did before the reform. Hence, historical analyses of policies must take into account these descriptions of quality, which usually escape quantitative analysis.

9. This is a clear case of work harassment. Discussions about the possibility of suing indicated that the university's fragile status prevented people from filling legal suits, because they didn't want to increase the tension between the university and La Cruz directorship. Interestingly, we see how work harassment and the capitalist-driven violence in health merge, not only by transforming the interactions between patients and doctors at the hospital but also (see chapter 5) by targeting the workers who embodied an epistemology of care defying the system's for-profit structure. This proves that different types of violence act in tandem (Bourgois 2004) and can be identified in the workplace and in the context of the transformation of capital accumulation patterns.

10. The ongoing presence of history indicates the inescapability of the past. As we saw in earlier discussions of ruins and ruination, the past haunts the present and can never be eliminated; its narrative and imaginative force keeps appearing in people's knowledge and their perceptions of places (Stoler 2013; Gordillo 2014). Interestingly, Santiago acknowledges that it is this historical presence that allows La Nacional Escuela to keep existing, even if the conditions are not the same. This process of ruination also speaks to the intricate relationship between self and matter, which Povinelli describes as carnality (as opposed to embodiment) (2011). For Povinelli, both ontologies—objects and persons—co-define existence. This discussion is important to theories of active destruction through violence, or attempts to ruin or get rid of the past, because both the hospital and its people (professors, patients, and students) co-define the meaning of health at El Materno. In a way, as long as the hospital exists, even if in ruins, and as long as its people continue existing, even if their labor and teaching conditions are ruined, the epistemology of care of El Materno will continue fighting for recognition and for hegemony over the country's health.

11. This situation is exemplary of a kind of excessive violence that, rather than killing directly, produces slow deaths through the "weakening of the will" (Povinelli 2011, 132)—this violence is "inherent to the social conditions of global capitalism" (Žižek 2008,14).

7. Learning and Practicing Medicine in a For-Profit System

1. The number of medical schools in Colombia went from seven in 1960 to fifty-eight in 2011. The growth of primarily private medical schools is linked to neoliberal education policies and has received great criticism both for its lack of planning and coordination in regard to public health needs and for the economic interests behind the new and mostly for-profit programs. Graduates, as we will see, find a job market characterized by overexploitation and inadequate conditions for practicing medicine. Furthermore, many newly trained physicians "learn" medicine within the context of the neoliberal reforms and its new kinds of hospital exposure; this training has raised serious doubts about the quality of medical education and medical care in the country (Fernández Ávila et al. 2011).

2. (Facultad de Medicina 2010).

3. (Bonilla Sebá and González Borrero 2017).

4. (Cruz Rodríguez 2012).

5. After another lengthy battle, medical associations got Congress to pass Law 1917, a law that regulates the system of medical residences, on July 12, 2018. This law grants residents the status of health care system workers with standing formal contracts and a monthly wage that should not be less than three minimum monthly wages. If free labor was once considered slave labor, the idea of paying to work has now grown common. Migrant smugglers and the agricultural, construction, and industrial business owners hold migrants' passports and force them to work for years, supposedly to cover the costs of their journey. In the Indian software industry, Xiang (2007) describes information technology workers who pay institutions for "training," during which they produce software; workers are forced to accept this "benching," which is an important analytical category for understanding contemporary labor exploitation.

6. This process is known as judicialization of human rights, which represents "that zone where medicine and law intersect in unexpected and deeply personal ways, and where our notions of how medicalization and biopolitics operate from the bottom up" (Biehl 2013, 421) and where the patient-citizen-consumer is configured (Biehl and Petryna 2013). Notably, while judicialization in Brazil speaks to how the judiciary deals with the malfunctioning of the public Unified Health Care system (Biehl, Socal, and Amon 2016), in Colombia it is about the co-optation of the judiciary by the for-profit structure of the system and the impossibility of a privatized health care system to comply with the right to health in Colombia (Abadía-Barrero 2015a). Besides the reports from the Defensoría del Pueblo, which compile the new Tutela cases, see Abadía-Barrero and Oviedo Manrique (2009); Everaldo Lamprea (2017).

7. (Eduardo Lamprea 2014; Yamin 2016; Chapman 2016; Echeverry López and Arango Castrillón 2013).

8. Insurance companies illegally established vertical integration with clinics owned by their same financial and commercial groups, thereby establishing highly inefficient monopolies and oligopolies that provide poor quality health care (Bejarano-Daza and Hernández-Losada 2017). For an analysis of how the "new" laws are simply an iteration of the same neoliberal logic with minor "adjustments," see Hernández and Tovar (2010); Useche (2015). Social mobilizations achieved the passage of a statutory health law in 2015, which elevated health to a human right and has an important language intended to limit the interference of the market in the right to health. Unfortunately, this law was not able to eliminate insurance companies, which raises serious concerns about its effectiveness (Useche 2015).

9. We stress "obviously" here to emphasize the logical consequences of an analysis deeply informed by history and critical political economy. This method allows us to assess the ideological domains sustaining the state, its legislation, and the status of confrontation between contradictory forces. The economic interests in the health care system in Colombia are such that dismantling the market-based system is unthinkable without a larger force advancing deeper structural changes. This is not, of course, economic determinism, but an analysis informed by the state of the balance of power forces at play.

10. (Fernández Ávila et al. 2011).

11. This is unsurprising, since many leftist Latin American governments end up instituting reforms intended to ameliorate the neoliberal crisis but do not significantly alter the course of neoliberal reforms. These sorts of neoliberal reforms under more progressive governments have been called postneoliberal reforms (Stolowicz 2011; Rodas and Regalado 2009). Most governments, if not all, are unable to implement drastic changes, primarily due to the United States' continued influence in regional affairs and the alliance between corporate sectors and governments (an alliance known as corporate governance). Recent cases of "Congress[ional]/insitutional coups" and the prosecution of progressive leaders indicate the new forms of democracy instability in the region and the lack of progress on the right to health; consider, for instance, the case of Brazil (Doniec, Dall'Alba, and King 2018), or Bolivia, which passed a new public unified health care system before Evo Morales was forced to resign.

12. Nicolás remembered that she "was affiliated with the senator recently incarcerated and so-called physician, Dilian Francisca Toro." Not surprisingly in a Colombian context, the senator was released, and in 2016 was elected as the governor of the state. At the beginning of 2018, the supreme court filed away the preliminary investigation against Dilian Francisca Toro for her alleged relationship with paramilitary groups. For many politicians, investigations against Alvaro Uribe's political circle fail through technicalities or the direct murder of witnesses (González 2018; Redacción Juicial 2018; and Segura 2018).

13. This is different from the Eurocentric concept of social determinants of health. One of the important aspects of this difference that we want to highlight is that the social *determination* of the "health-disease-treatment" process is a Latin American perspective on social medicine that has been fundamental to the regional training of health professionals. Hence, El Materno's particular epistemology of care is part of a larger conception of health within politics (chapter 1) that can be found in other places

both in and beyond Colombia. Of course, escuelas vary across Colombia and within the Latin American region, but all of them share a critical lens that accounts for social *and* historical forces of oppression and domination, and that plays a fundamental role in how power and health are conceptualized (Navarro 2009; Breilh 2013, 2020). Although the social *determination* of health paradigm comes from social medicine, as we argued in chapter 2 and as Nicolas's narrative conveys, the political approach to health in clinical medicine produces a particular "clinical social medicine" approach.

14. The movement, known as MANE (Mesa Amplia Nacional Estudiantil), has been fundamental to advancing discussions about the right to education in Colombia. As we saw in the first chapters, students' social mobilization has been fundamental to shaping the university system. MANE joined a long history of student struggle and proved fundamental in forcing the government to negotiate a new educational law (López Rendón 2015; Cruz Rodríguez 2012). A new nationwide mobilization of public institutions of higher education in 2018 forced the government to add important funds to these institutions and to start a plan for a steady increase in funds.

15. López Rendón (2015) and Cruz Rodríguez (2012) offer a similar conceptual framework for understanding MANE. The student organization was facilitated by the political opportunity presented by the regressive and for-profit education law presented by the government and by the electoral climate that signaled the end of Uribe's term. Another nationwide student protest happened in 2018. Students were more successful than the presidents of public higher educational institutions in challenging many of the government's neoliberal proposals and forcing it to commit important resources for public higher education (Alarcón 2018).

16. Yadira Borrero's research offers an innovative framework for the analysis of collective action and social movements in health. She integrates the theoretical approaches of Charles Tilly's contentious politics, Melucci's constructionism, theories from resistance and critical feminism, and frames of meaning (Borrero 2014). In her research, she identified 1,399 collective actions for health in the country between 1994 and 2010. Besides the waves of protests and peaks, she highlights the correspondence between social protests in health and crucial moments in labor rights history, hospital crises, new health care legislation, and patients' access problems—aspects that were also identified in her coauthored piece with Maria Esperanza Echeverry (Echeverry López and Borrero-Ramírez 2015). In her thesis, later published as a book, Yadira Borrero identified places, actors, and adversaries, illuminating who protests, where, why, and when. She retells the important story of how a national movement for health has responded to privatization efforts in the country. Over time, the movement has innovated its repertoire of political strategies and has understood that the main adversary is not necessarily the government, as an emblematic unit, but that both the government and the private insurers are major local adversaries representing larger global trends in capital financialization. She identified differences and tensions between regions and among actors in terms of how they think political demands can be met; she also explored how the country's political violence affected health care union members and activists and how the capitalist system's advances in health in the country have shaped the political subjectivity of social movement actors (Borrero 2014).

17. (Valdés 2008; García 2007; Molina Marín et al. 2010).

18. (Hernández 2017a, 2017b). Mergers, acquisitions, and corruption are not extraordinary; they are an ingrained part of capitalist logics and intercapitalist maneuvers in health and other sectors (Waitzkin and Working Group for Health Beyond Capitalism 2018; Rosenthal 2017; Bugbee 2019).

19. This confirms that in David Harvey's "accumulation by dispossession" (2003), there is a direct transfer of public taxes and individual patrimonies to private sectors. (ACESI, n.d.)

20. Thousands of citizens resort to the judiciary annually to demand that their right to health be granted (this process is known as judicialization). See note 6.

21. ("Editorial," 2016).

22. (Gossain 2018).

23. (ACESI 2018).

24. There is a significant and ongoing debate about "quality-of-care" indicators. These indicators used to be intended to ensure the coverage of patients' comprehensive medical needs at a high standard of care; under neoliberalism, they have more to do with commercial ideas of patient satisfaction, the "free choice" of neoliberal citizenship, the transformation of clinical standards of care in response to the medical industrial financial complex's handling of evidence, and the imposition of economic terminology like the "value-based chain." Most importantly, health care facilities are evaluated based on whether their numbers show "healthy" balances, rather than on how well their patients are doing. For discussions of the quality of health care under neoliberalism see, among many, Martínez (2008); Iriart and Merhy (2017); Mulligan (2010).

25. (Ardila 2016). The situation explored by Adriana only applies to general practitioners. Specialists' labor situation is different; certain specialties have established monopolies of care which assure very high incomes.

26. Adriana's analysis doesn't stop at presenting the narratives describing physicians' new working conditions. She goes on to demonstrate that such destruction of medical labor is profitable. Drawing on Arouca's approach to medical labor (2008) and linking physicians' work with profit and exploitation, Adriana argues that one now needs to demonstrate the economic "productivity" of physicians' work: that is, that surplus value is generated by exploiting physicians. Treating health as a commodity, however, is challenging. In addition to medical industrial complex commodities like pharmaceuticals, tests, equipment, therapeutics, and so on, we must consider physicians' labor during medical consultations as part of the profit-generating activities of capitalist sectors. Unlike industrial commodities, Adriana clarifies that the "health" produced during a medical consultation is an intangible commodity—one that, to add more complexity—is consumed even as it is being produced. At the time of Arouca's original writing (1975), it was even more difficult to conceive of a medical consultation as part of the capitalist engine. Adriana offers six theses based on Arouca's original work: (1) Medical consultations include the consumption of tools and equipment but the addition of the physician's knowledge adds value to what is consumed. (2) The patient-doctor encounter allows money to circulate. (3) Physicians' income places them in high-consumption sector. (4) Medical labor cares for the workforce and keeps it in productive condition. (5) Medicine has a role in maintaining the reserve army of labor via child and maternal health and prevention

activities. (6) Medicine plays a role in collective work processes during the selection of personnel (Ardila 2016, 41). The main conclusion of Adriana's work was that medical labor as part of the capitalist system in Colombia was indirectly productive (as noted in most of Arouca's categories) and also unproductive; that is, it only produced sustenance rents for physicians. Under neoliberalism, medical labor has been transformed to a directly productive and exploited form of labor through a formal and real subsumption to capital (Ardila-Sierra and Abadia-Barrero 2020).

27. Bureaucratic itineraries are the administrative and legal procedures patients are forced to complete in order to access medical appointments, medications, supplies, or treatments (Abadía-Barrero and Oviedo Manrique 2009).

28. The health care system is not the only factor leading to delayed diagnoses. There are also geographic, cultural, and socioeconomic barriers. It is, however, clear that the health care system has imposed new barriers to care (Sánchez Vanegas 2012).

29. Insurance companies refer to this as the "medical-lost ratio." With the financialization of health care, there are disputes between the financial sector (the insurers), the clinics (which charge the insurers, as we see in El Materno's case), and the medical industrial complex. Such intercapitalist disputes have been described by Iriart and Merhy (2017) as an alliance, in that all players push for higher health care costs.

30. Importantly, with the financialization of the economy, it is not owners but administrators who end up imposing labor practices that increase rates of labor exploitation; these practices can also translate into better organizational finances and improved speculative outcomes.

Final Remarks

1. (Abadía-Barrero et al. 2018). As of December 2020, when this book was going to press, there was a heated debate in the Bogotá city congress after the announcement that the main hospital tower of El San Juan was going to be demolished rather than reinforced and rehabilitated, as technical studies indicated. According to leftist congresswomen, senators, and other defenders of the hospital, this is another proof of the desire to destroy the legacy of the hospital.

2. (Barragán 2008; Redacción Bogotá 2015b).

3. (Barragán 2008). Also from interview with Raúl Sastre on July 30, 2019.

4. Interview with Raúl Sastre on July 30, 2019. Raúl Sastre is one of the professors who knows more about the history of HSJD and defended it. He served as Dean of the School of Medicine from 2012 until 2014 and was behind many of the efforts behind the University Hospital, including HUN.

5. (Bridges 2011, 24).

6. (Bridges 2011, 24).

7. Corporate governance is a useful construct for considering corporations' influence on the government. Working in a Marxist tradition, Waitzkin and Jasso-Aguilar have clarified that we should not think of the state and the market as separate domains, or as the state exerting control over the market (as liberal analysis suggests). Rather, it is becoming increasingly clear that government is subservient to the needs of capital

accumulation and that legislation, regulations, and state institutions accommodate the historical demands of capital. See Breilh (1986); Jasso-Aguilar and Waitzkin (2007); Waitzkin (2011). This book has shown how Law 100 of 1993, which privatized health and social security in Colombia by incorporating individual insurance into the financial sector as system administrator, was, in El Materno's case, a powerful legal technique of corporate governance. Much of what this book describes results directly from this technique, which has also shifted the moral landscape of health and justice to the right (Abadía-Barrero 2015a).

8. While health, or the health domain, has often been centered in histories of capital accumulation, the financialized accumulation of capitalism during neoliberalism represents a powerful ideological shift in the relationship between health and capitalism (Iriart and Merhy 2017). If, during the regulated accumulation of the welfare state dominating the world during much of the first part of the twentieth century, health was seen as a necessary social investment in the health of a productive national workforce, health was transformed, during neoliberalism, from a social contract to an individual responsibility (Metzl and Kirkland 2010; Mol 2008; Waitzkin 2011). Given the assumption of individual responsibility, health risks are no longer seen as related to a social pact in which we all take care of one another; in which, in times of sickness, a social welfare scheme helps individuals avoid catastrophic expenses caused by sickness, disability, or death. This further individualization of risk, which created a new kind of neoliberal subjectivity (Rose 2007), forced people not only to manage their own risk but also to pay individually to cover those risks through personal insurance. The ideological domain materialized in individual insurance plans, individual pension funds, individual disability insurance, and individual savings accounts, all of which imply a direct contract between the citizen and the financial sector, so that the speculative aspects of the economy come to dominate social life (Buitrago Echeverri, Abadía-Barrero, and Granja Palacios 2017).

9. While neoliberal governance has remained the backbone of a good deal of Latin American politics, some countries with progressive governments have encountered local and national strategies designed to "interrupt" neoliberalism, open alternatives, and offer regional resistance (Goodale and Postero 2013). Some health-specific examples of these interruptions can be seen in Nicaragua, El Salvador, Brazil, Bolivia, Venezuela, Ecuador, Argentina, and Uruguay, where legislation defending the public orientation of health came hand in hand with efforts to revitalize primary health care and intercultural health—all of which are effective obstacles to the interests of financial capital. And yet, the recent history of some progressive countries shows a painful mixture of allegations of corruption (pervasive in the whole region) and a reaccommodation of elites through the removal of progressive governments by electoral scandals or congressional coups. The United States continues, worrisomely, to influence regional affairs by destabilizing democratically elected governments, manipulating elections, and helping right-wing politicians come to power and criminalize the progressive governments that dare to contest for-profit interests—consider, for instance, Venezuela, Honduras, Brazil, Bolivia, and Argentina. Noam Chomsky has described former Brazilian president Dilma Rouseff as having experienced a "soft coup" that gave a seal of legal approval to corrupt right-wing politicians dismantling prior right-to-health gains

advanced under Workers Party presidencies. Before his release, Chomsky considered former president Lula "the world's most prominent political prisoner," suffering a "virtual life imprisonment" in solitary confinement, without access to the press and limited visits one day a week (Chomsky 2018). Hence, theories of empire continue to be fundamental to understand the shifting landscape of health and capitalism in the region (Waitzkin 2011).

10. (Reeck 2017). The third-party employer that created Charité Facility Management was founded in 2006 "as part of massive cuts to wages in Berlin's public sector" (Flakin 2017). Since then, health care workers' strikes have been constant.

11. Rather than indicating a concern about citizens' well-being, the regional economic crisis led international financial institutions to worry that countries might default on their financial obligations.

12. (Day 2013).

13. (Agencia EFE 2018; Kehr 2019).

14. (Guillot 2013).

15. (Guillot 2013; Edgar 2017).

16. (Min-sik, Yoon [윤민식] 2013).

17. (Express Tribune 2018; Farwa 2018).

18. (Varma 2020, 82–83).

19. The joint WHO/UNICEF Bamako initiative launched in 1987 is perhaps the first neoliberal attack on Africa's health. See Chapman (2016); Mukherjee (2018, chap. 1); Turshen (1999). For the efforts of the pharmaceutical industry to control African markets and the role of neoliberal policies in dismantling locally produced pharmaceuticals, see Peterson (2014).

20. (McKay 2018; Strong 2020).

21. https://www.imtj.com/news/saudi-arabia-launches-healthcare-privatisation -programme/ Retrieved October 3, 2018.

22. (IMTJ Team 2018).

23. (Duckett 2013).

24. See, among others, Galvão (2001, 2002).

25. (Doniec, Dall'Alba, and King 2018).

26. (Smith-Nonini 1999).

27. (Brotherton 2012; Andaya 2014). Also worrisome is the role Cuba can play in the reconfiguration of its internal government and its new role in global health. For example, Howard Waitzkin has signaled how *The Lancet* has partnered with "Medical Education Cooperation with Cuba (MEDICC), a non-governmental organization based in the United States, to produce a Spanish-language translation of *The Lancet*'s series on UHC in Latin America." Waitzkin wonders why Cuba is being used as an epicenter for furthering neoliberal UH*Coverage* plans in the region, and warns about the incredible difficulty of thinking of Cuba's "health care for all" under a UH*Coverage* model. Waitzkin speculates on whether Cuba is moving toward health care privatization, and on how we are to read this partnership (Waitzkin 2015).

28. We are advancing the idea of "medicine as political imagination," building upon Marxist critiques of idealistic imaginations of reality and proposals for linking theory

and praxis through the material conditions of existence (Marx and Engels 1968). We are also contributing to the ongoing rescue of epistemology as "ways of knowing," including ways of imagining that are not Eurocentric, anthropocentric, or driven primarily by reason.

29. Sunder Rajan explains hegemony in global health as an interplay of power, value, and knowledge (2017).

30. (Jasso-Aguilar and Waitzkin 2007; Jasso-Aguilar, Waitzkin, and Landwehr 2004).

31. For how market-oriented approaches that shift and shape numbers in global health and force countries to abandon certain metrics and replace them with others, see Adams (2016). One of the most telling examples in shifts in the political imagination in health at a global level is the push for universal health coverage (UHC). At first glance, the proposal to achieve UHC around the world, as established in the Sustainable Development Goals (SDGs), seems like a sound strategy to promote the right to health that we should all embrace and support. However, critical scholars clarify that the proposal co-opts social justice struggles over health through the problematic replacement of universal health *care* with universal health *coverage. Coverage* inherently and symbolically supports the individual risk paradigm, with its many limitations, including the market co-optation that defines current global health policies and interventions. Presenting universal health coverage as a goal could easily make the indicators imposed on all countries those of the financialized economy—for instance, the number of people insured through individual, market-based coverage. The Astana declaration on primary health care and the WHO 2019 assembly postulated UHCoverage as the goal and co-opted PHC (primary health care) as a strategy to achieve UHCoverage. Denunciations of this inadequacy have proliferated, including the Latin American Social Medicine Association (ALAMES) statement at the October 2018 conference. See also Abadía-Barrero and Bugbee (2019), Birn et al. (2016).

32. (Abadía-Barrero 2018). See also the interesting discussion of Varma around psychiatric care in Kashmir, "a counterhegemonic approach to psychiatric and psychological care, emphasizing its relational and empathetic capacities," in which the idea would be, similar to El Materno, to expand on accepted guidelines (Varma 2020, 95–96). In Varma's case, the DSM-IV; in El Materno's case, the guidelines around pregnancy, delivery, and neonatal care.

33. A discussion advanced in Metzl and Kirkland (2010). Sunder Rajan describes the critical relationship between health and capital, and the impossibility of separating the two domains (2006, 2012). The U.S. scenario is presented in Waitzkin and Working Group for Health Beyond Capitalism (2018).

Abad Faciolince, Héctor Joaquín. 2013. *El olvido que seremos* [Forgotten we'll be].
15th ed. Biblioteca Breve. Barcelona: Seix Barral.

Abadía-Barrero, César Ernesto. 2015a. "Neoliberal Justice and the Transformation of the
Moral: The Privatization of the Right to Health Care in Colombia." *Medical Anthropology Quarterly* 30 (1): 62–79. https://doi.org/10.1111/maq.12161.

Abadía-Barrero, César E. 2015b. "The Transformation of the Value of Life: Dispossession as Torture." *Medical Anthropology* 34 (5): 389–406. https://doi.org/10.1080
/01459740.2015.1048859.

Abadía-Barrero, César Ernesto. 2018. "Kangaroo Mother Care in Colombia: A Subaltern
Health Innovation against For-Profit Biomedicine." *Medical Anthropology Quarterly*
32 (3): 384–403. https://doi.org/10.1111/maq.12430.

Abadía-Barrero, César Ernesto, and Mary Bugbee. 2019. "Primary Health Care for Universal Health Coverage? Contributions for a Critical Anthropological Agenda." *Medical Anthropology* 38 (5): 427–35. https://doi.org/10.1080/01459740.2019.1620744.

Abadía-Barrero, César Ernesto, Emma Shaw Crane, and Camilo Ruíz. 2012. "Defending
the Right to Health in Colombia." *NACLA Report on the Americas* 45: 70–73.

Abadía-Barrero, César, and Diana Oviedo. 2008. "Intersubjetividades Estructuradas:
La Salud En Colombia Como Dilema Epistemológico y Político Para Las Ciencias
Sociales" [Structured Intersubjectivities. Health as a Social Sciences, Political, and
Epistemological Dilemma]. *Universitas Humanística* 66: 57–82.

Abadía-Barrero, César Ernesto, and Diana Goretty Oviedo Manrique. 2009. "Bureaucratic Itineraries in Colombia. A Theoretical and Methodological Tool to Assess
Managed-Care Health Care Systems." *Social Science & Medicine* 68: 1153–60.

Abadía-Barrero, César Ernesto, and Héctor Camilo Ruíz-Sánchez. 2018. "Enfrentando
al Neoliberalismo En Colombia: Arte y Colaboración En Un Hospital En Ruinas"

[Confronting Neoliberalism in Colombia: Art and Collaboration in a Hospital in Ruins]. *Etnográfica* 22 (3): 575–603.

Abadía-Barrero, César Ernesto, Héctor Camilo Ruíz-Sánchez, and Maria Yaneth Pinilla Alfonso. 2018. "Etnografía como acción política: articulación del compromiso antropológico a estrategias contra hegemónicas" [Ethnography as political action: Articulation of the anthropological commitment to counter-hegemonic strategies]. In *Trabajo de Campo en América Latina. Experiencias Antropológicas Regionales en Etnografía* [Fieldwork in Latin America. Regional anthropological experiences in ethnography], edited by Rosana Guber, Cornelia Eckert, Myriam Jimeno, Esteban Krotz, 438–55. Buenos Aires: Editorial SB.

Abadia-Barrero, César, Andrés L. Góngora Sierra, Marco Alejandro Melo Moreno, and Claudia P. Platarrueda Vanegas, eds. 2013. *Salud, Normalización y Capitalismo en Colombia* [Health, Normalization, and Capitalism in Colombia]. Colección CES. Bogotá, Colombia: Universidad Nacional de Colombia, Sede Bogotá, Facultad de Ciencias Humanas, Centro de Estudios Sociales - CES, Grupo de Antropología Médica Crítica: Editorial Universidad del Rosario: Ediciones Desde Abajo.

ACESI (Asociación Colombiana de Empresas Sociales del Estado y Hospitales Públicos). n.d. "Paso definitivo para conducir a la 'quiebra' a prestadores de salud" [Definitive step to drive health providers to "bankruptcy"]. Accessed March 11, 2017. http://acesi.com.co/?p=1484.

ACESI (Asociación Colombiana de Empresas Sociales del Estado y Hospitales Públicos). 2018. Press Report. "En vez de intentar recuperarlos, abre la puerta para acabarlos. Gobierno Santos se despediría con liquidación masiva de hospitales: mejor cerrarlos que salvarlos" [Rather than recuperating them, opens the door to finish them. The Santos government will end its mandate with a massive liquidation of hospitals: it is better to close them than to save them]. Accessed July 26, 2018. https://acesi.com.co/gobierno-santos-se-despediria-con-liquidacion-masiva-de-hospitales-mejor-cerrarlos-que-salvarlos/.

Adams, Vincanne. 1998. *Doctors for Democracy: Health Professionals in the Nepal Revolution*. Cambridge Studies in Medical Anthropology 6. Cambridge, UK: Cambridge University Press.

Adams, Vincanne, ed. 2016. *Metrics: What Counts in Global Health*. Critical Global Health—Evidence, Efficacy, Ethnography. Durham, NC: Duke University Press.

Agencia EFE. 2018. *Cientos de médicos marchan por dignificar su profesión y contra los recortes* [Hundreds of physicians march for dignifying their profession and against cuts]. March 21. https://www.efe.com/efe/espana/sociedad/cientos-de-medicos-marchan-por-dignificar-su-profesion-y-contra-los-recortes/10004-3559784.

Ahumada, Consuelo. 2002. "La Globalización y Su Impacto Sobre La Salud" [Globalization and Its Impact on Health]. In *La Salud Pública Hoy: Enfoques y Dilemas Contemporáneos En Salud Pública* [Public Health Today: Contemporary Approaches and Dilemmas in Public Health], edited by Saúl Franco Agudelo, 19–34. Bogotá, Colombia: Universidad Nacional de Colombia.

Alarcón, Norman. 2018. *Movimiento estudiantil, el personaje del 2018* [The students' movement, the person of 2018]. *Las2Orillas* (December 13). https://www.las2orillas.co/movimiento-estudiantil-el-personaje-del-2018.

Allison, Anne. 2013. *Precarious Japan.* Durham, NC: Duke University Press.

Anadolu. 2020. "¿Por qué se conmemora en Colombia el Día del Estudiante Caído?" [Why Does Colombia Commemorate the Day of the Fallen Student?]. *Semana* (June 10). https://www.semana.com/educacion/articulo/por-que-se-conmemora -en-colombia-el-dia-del-estudiante-caido/678660/.

Andaya, Elise. 2014. *Conceiving Cuba: Reproduction, Women, and the State in the Post-Soviet Era.* New Brunswick, NJ: Rutgers University Press.

Antunes, Ricardo. 2003. *¿Adios al Trabajo? Ensayo Sobre Las Metamorfosis y El Rol Central Del Mundo Del Trabajo* [Goodbye to Labor? Essays about the Metamorphoses and Central Role of the World of Labor]. 2nd ed. Buenos Aires: Herramienta.

Antunes, Ricardo. 2005. *Los Sentidos Del Trabajo: Ensayo Sobre La Afirmación y La Negación Del Trabajo* [The Meanings of Labor: Essays about the Affirmation and Negation of Labor]. Buenos Aires: Herramienta ediciones, Taller de Estudios Laborales.

Antunes, Ricardo. 2018. "The New Service Proletariat." *Monthly Review—An Independent Socialist Magazine* 69 (11). https://monthlyreview.org/2018/04/01/the-new -service-proletariat/.

Appadurai, Arjun. 1995. "Introduction: Commodities and the Politics of Value." In *The Social Life of Things. Commodity in Cultural Perspective,* edited by Arjun Appadurai, 3–63. Cambridge, UK: Cambridge University Press.

Arango, Luz Gabriela, Adira Amaya Urquijo, Tania Pérez-Bustos, and Javier Pineda Duque, eds. 2018. *Género y Cuidado: Teorías, Escenarios y Políticas* [Gender and Care: Theories, Scenarios and Politics]. Colección Academia. Bogotá, Colombia: Universidad Nacional de Colombia, Pontificia Universidad Javeriana, Universidad de los Andes.

Ardila, Adriana. 2016. "Neoliberalismo y Medicina General: De La Profesión Liberal al Trabajo Explotado" [Neoliberalism and General Medicine: From Liberal Profession to Exploited Labor]. PhD diss., Public Health. Bogotá: Universidad Nacional de Colombia.

Ardila-Sierra, Adriana, and César Abadía-Barrero. 2020. "Medical Labour under Neoliberalism: An Ethnographic Study in Colombia." *International Journal of Public Health* 65 (7): 1011–17. https://doi.org/10.1007/s00038-020-01420-4.

Ariza, Katerine. 2008. "Ideología, Privatización y Salud. Del Cierre Del Seguro Social y Su Programa de VIH/SIDA a La 'Nueva EPS'" [Ideology, Privatization and Health. From the Closing of Social Security and Its HIV/AIDS Program to the "New EPS"]. Undergraduate thesis, Anthropology. Bogotá, Colombia: Universidad Nacional de Colombia.

Ariza Ruíz, Katerine, César Ernesto Abadía-Barrero, and María Yaneth Pinilla Alfonso. 2013. "La Praxis Del Estado Colombiano En La Eliminación Del Instituto de Seguros Sociales y Del Instituto Materno Infantil" [The Praxis of the Colombian State in the Elimination of the Institute of Social Security and the Child and Maternity Institute]. In *Salud, Normalización y Capitalismo En Colombia,* 441–73. Bogotá, Colombia: Universidad Nacional de Colombia, Ediciones desde abajo, Universidad del Rosario.

Armus, Diego, ed. 2003. *Disease in the History of Modern Latin America: From Malaria to AIDS.* Durham, NC: Duke University Press.

Arouca, Sergio. 2008. "Medicina Preventiva y Sociedad" [Preventative Medicine and Society]. In *El Dilema Preventivista. Contribuciones a La Comprensión y Crítica de*

La Medicina Preventiva [The Prevantative Dilemma. Contributions to the Understanding and Critique or Preventative Medicine], edited by Sergio Arouca, 207–28.
Buenos Aires: Lugar Editorial.

Baker, J. P. 2000. "The Incubator and the Medical Discovery of the Premature Infant."
Journal of Perinatology 20 (5): 321–28.

Barragán Duarte, José Luis. 2008. Habemus Hospital Universitario [Habemus University Hospital]. *Unperiodico* (May 11). Accessed September 18, 2018. http://historico
.unperiodico.unal.edu.co/ediciones/111/18.html.

Bastero, Juan Luis. 2011. "Apariciones Marianas: Praxis y Teología" [Marian Apparitions: Praxis and Theology]. *Scripta Theologica* 43: 347–65.

Bejarano-Daza, Javier Eduardo, and Diego Fernando Hernández-Losada. 2017. "Fal-
las Del Mercado de Salud Colombiano" [Failures of the Colombian Market in
Health]. *Revista de La Facultad de Medicina* 65 (1): 107–13. https://doi.org/10.15446
/revfacmed.v65n1.57454.

Benjamin, Walter. 2013. *Tesis sobre la historia y otros fragmentos* [Thesis about History and
Other Fragments]. Edited by Bolívar Echeverría. Colombia: Ediciones Desde Abajo.

Biehl, João. 2013. "The Judicialization of Biopolitics: Claiming the Right to Pharmaceuticals in Brazilian Courts: The Judicialization of Biopolitics." *American Ethnologist* 40
(3): 419–36. https://doi.org/10.1111/amet.12030.

Biehl, João, and Adriana Petryna. 2013. "Legal Remedies: Therapeutic Markets and the
Judicialization of the Right to Health." In *When People Come First. Critical Studies in
Global Health*, 325–46. Princeton, NJ: Princeton University Press.

Biehl, João, M. P. Socal, and J. J. Amon. 2016. "The Judicialization of Health and the
Quest for State Accountability: Evidence from 1,262 Lawsuits for Access to Medicines in Southern Brazil." *Health and Human Rights Journal* 18 (1): 209–20.

Birn, Anne-Emanuelle, Laura Nervi, and Eduardo Siqueira. 2016. "Neoliberalism
Redux: The Global Health Policy Agenda and the Politics of Co-optation in Latin
America and Beyond: Debate: The Co-optation of Global Health in Latin America."
Development and Change 47 (4): 734–59. https://doi.org/10.1111/dech.12247.

Bochetti, Carla, Juan Manuel Arteaga, and Marco Palacio. 2005. *Hospital Universitario:
Desde San Juan de Dios Hasta La Construcción de Un Nuevo Proyecto* [University
Hospital: From San Juan de Dios to the Construction of a New Project]. Bogotá,
Colombia: Universidad Nacional de Colombia.

Bonilla Sebá, Edna Cristina, and Jorge Iván González Borrero. 2017. "La Universidad
Nacional de Colombia Ya No Es Prioridad. Analisis de La Evolución de Sus Finanzas
(1867–2015)" [The National University of Colombia is No Longer a Priority. Analysis of the Evolution of Its Finances (1987–2015)]. In *Universidad, Cultura y Estado*,
274–303. Colección Del Sesquicentenario, vol. 1. Bogotá, Colombia: Universidad
Nacional de Colombia.

Borrero, Yadira Eugenia. 2014. *Luchas Por La Salud En Colombia* [Fights for Health in
Colombia]. Cali, Colombia: Pontificia Universidad Javeriana.

Bourgois, Philippe. 1990. "Eticas Antropológicas En Confrontación: Lecciones Etnográ-
ficas de Centro América" [Anthropological Ethics in Confrontation: Ethnographic
Lessons from Central America]. *Estudios Sociales Centroamericanos* 54: 101–17.

Bourgois, Philippe. 2004. "The Continuum of Violence in War and Peace: Post-Cold War Lessons from El Salvador." In *Violence in War and Peace*, edited by Nancy Scheper-Hughes and Philippe Bourgois, 425–34. Malden, MA: Blackwell Publishing.

Bourgois, Philippe, and Jeff Schonberg. 2009. *Righteous Dopefiend*. Berkeley: University of California Press.

Breilh, Jaime. 1986. *Epidemiología: Economía, Medicina y Política* [Epidemiology: Economy, Medicine, and Politics]. México, D.F.: Distribuciones Fontamara, S.A.

Breilh, Jaime. 2003. *Epidemiología Crítica. Ciencia Emancipadora e Interculturalidad* [Critical Epidemiology. Emancipatory Science and Interculturality]. Buenos Aires: Lugar Editorial.

Breilh, Jaime. 2013. "La Determinación Social de La Salud Como Herramienta de Transformación Hacia Una Nueva Salud Pública (Salud Colectiva)" [Social Determination of Health as a Transformation Tool towards a New Public Health (Collective Health)]. *Revista Facultad Nacional de Salud Pública* 31: S13–27.

Breilh, Jaime. 2020. *Critical Epidemiology and the People's Health*. New York: Cambridge University Press.

Bridges, Khiara M. 2011. *Reproducing Race: An Ethnography of Pregnancy as a Site of Racialization*. Berkeley: University of California Press.

Brotherton, Pierre Sean. 2012. *Revolutionary Medicine: Health and the Body in Post-Soviet Cuba*. Durham, NC: Duke University Press.

Brouwer, Steve. 2011. *Revolutionary Doctors: How Venezuela and Cuba Are Changing the World's Conception of Health Care*. New York: Monthly Review Press.

Buch, Elana D. 2015. "Anthropology of Aging and Care." *Annual Review of Anthropology* 44 (1): 277–93. https://doi.org/10.1146/annurev-anthro-102214-014254.

Bugbee, Mary. 2019. "Intercapitalist Maneuvers and the ICD-10 Transition: The Instrumental Role of the State in the Corporate Governance of U.S. Health Care." *International Journal of Health Services* 49 (3): 457–75. https://doi.org/10.1177/0020731419848294.

Buitrago Echeverri, María Teresa, César Ernesto Abadía-Barrero, and Consuelo Granja Palacios. 2017. "Work-Related Illness, Work-Related Accidents, and Lack of Social Security in Colombia." *Social Science & Medicine* 187 (August): 118–25. https://doi.org/10.1016/j.socscimed.2017.06.030.

Butler, Judith. 2000. "Restating the Universal: Hegemony and the Limits of Formalism." In *Contingency, Hegemony, Universality. Contemporary Dialogues on the Left*, edited by Judith Butler, Ernesto Laclau, and Slavoj Žižek, 11–43. New York: Verso.

Butler, Judith, Ernesto Laclau, and Slavoj Žižek. 2000. *Contingency, Hegemony, Universality: Contemporary Dialogues on the Left*. London: Verso.

Campos Zornosa, Yezid. 2003. *Memoria de Los Silenciados: El Baile Rojo: Relatos* [Memory of the Silenced: The Red Dance: Stories]. Bogotá, Colombia: Ceicos.

Can, Başak. 2016. "The Criminalization of Physicians and the Delegitimization of Violence in Turkey." *Medical Anthropology* 35 (6): 477–88. https://doi.org/10.1080/01459740.2016.1207641.

Caracol radio. 2005a. "Gobernación de Cundinamarca liquidará el hospital San Juan de Dios y el Instituto Materno Infantil" [Cundinamarca's Governor's Office will liquidate the hospital San Juan de Dios and the Instituto Materno Infantil]. *Caracol radio* (June 7). https://caracol.com.co/radio/2005/07/06/nacional/1120650660 _185515.html.

Caracol radio. 2005b. "Procurador notifica al gobernador de Cundinamarca para que frene al proceso del liquidación del Materno" [The Attorney General notifies the Governor of Cundinamarca to stop the liquidation process of El Materno]. *Caracol radio* (August 8). https://caracol.com.co/radio/2005/08/08/nacional/1123505640 _192767.html.

Caracol radio. 2005c. "El gobierno nacional afirmó que salvará al Instituto materno Infantil, más no el hospital San Juan de Dios" [The National Government affirmed that it will save the Instituto Materno Infantil but not the hospital San Juan de Dios]. *Caracol radio* (August 24). https://caracol.com.co/radio/2005/08/24/nacional /1124879340_196635.html.

Caracol radio. 2006. "En firme acuerdo que salva el hospital Materno Infantil" [In firm agreement that saves the hospital Materno Infantil]. *Caracol radio* (June 16). http:// caracol.com.co/radio/2006/06/16/nacional/1150484940_299183.html.

Cardoso de Oliveira, Roberto. 2004. "O Mal-Estar Da Ética Na Antropología Prática" [The Ill-Being of Ethics in Anthropological Practice]. In *Antropología e Ética. O Debate Atual No Brasil* [Anthropology and Ethics. Current Debate in Brazil], edited by Ceres Victora, Ruben George Oliven, Maria Eunice Maciel, and Ari Pedro Oro, 21–32. Niteroi: Editora da Universidade Federal Fluminense.

Castro, Felipe. 2009. "Universidad Nacional, Tiempos Turbulentos" [National University, Turbulent Times]. *Desde Abajo* (May 21). http://www.desdeabajo.info /ediciones/item/4521-universidad-nacional-tiempos-turbulentos.html.

Chapman, Audrey R. 2016. *Global Health, Human Rights and the Challenge of Neoliberal Policies*. Cambridge, UK: Cambridge University Press.

Chomsky, Noam. 2018. "I Just Visited Lula, the World's Most Prominent Political Prisoner. A 'Soft Coup' in Brazil's Election Will Have Global Consequences." *The Intercept* (October 2). https://theintercept.com/2018/10/02/lula-brazil-election -noam-chomsky/.

Comaroff, John L., and Jean Comaroff. 2006. "Law and Disorder in the Postcolony: An Introduction." In *Law and Disorder in the Postcolony*, edited by Jean Comaroff and John L. Comaroff, 1–56. Chicago: University of Chicago Press.

Consejo de Estado. 2012. Sala de Consulta y Servicio Civil. Radicación 2076, 9 de Agosto de 2012. Consejero Ponente: William Zambrano Cetina.

Cooper, Melinda. 2008. *Life as Surplus: Biotechnology and Capitalism in the Neoliberal Era*. Seattle: University of Washington Press.

Cooper, Melinda, and Cathy Waldby. 2014. *Clinical Labor: Tissue Donors and Research Subjects in the Global Bioeconomy*. Durham, NC: Duke University Press.

Corte Constitucional, Colombia. 2008. *Sentencia SU.484/08*. May 15.

Cortés Díaz, Marco E. 2006. *La Anexión de Los 6 Municipios Vecinos a Bogotá En 1954* [The Annexation of the 6 Neighboring Municipalities to Bogotá in 1954]. Punto Aparte. Bogotá, Colombia: Universidad Nacional de Colombia, Sede Bogotá.

Coutin, Susan, and Barbara Yngvesson. 2008. "Technologies of Knowledge Production: Law, Ethnography, and the Limits of Explanation." *PoLAR Political and Legal Anthropology Review* 31 (1): 1–7. https://doi.org/10.1111/j.1555-2934.2008.00006.x.

Crehan, Kate. 2002. *Gramsci, Culture and Anthropology*. Berkeley: University of California Press.

Cruz Rodríguez, Edwin. 2012. "La MANE y El Paro Nacional Universitario de 2011 En Colombia" [The MANE and the National University Strike of 2011 in Colombia]. *Ciencia Política*, Otras Investigaciones, 14 (Julio-Diciembre): 140–93.

Csordas, Thomas. 1994. *The Sacred Self. A Cultural Phenomenology of Charismatic Healing*. Berkeley: University of California Press.

Cueto, Marcos, and Steven Paul Palmer. 2015. *Medicine and Public Health in Latin America: A History*. New Approaches to the Americas. New York: Cambridge University Press.

Currea Guerrero, Santiago. 2004. *La adaptación neonatal inmediata: la reanimación neonatal* [Immediate neonatal adaptation: Neonatal reanimation]. Bogotá, Colombia: Universidad Nacional de Colombia, Sede Bogotá.

Currea Guerrero, Santiago. 2006. Instituto Materno Infantil—El día después [Instituto Materno Infantil—The day after]. Public presentation at the National University as part of the conference cicle "Memoria Viva del Hospital San Juan de Dios. (December 4).

DaMatta, Roberto. 1994. "Some Biased Remarks on Interpretivism: A View from Brazil." In *Assessing Cultural Anthropology*, edited by Robert Borofsky, 119–32. Hawaii: Pacific University.

Davis-Floyd, Robbie, Lesley Barclay, Jan Tritten, and Betty-Anne Daviss, eds. 2009. *Birth Models That Work*. Berkeley: University of California Press.

Day, Paul. 2013. "Madrid's Health Workers Strike over Hospital Privatization. *Reuters* (May 7). https://www.reuters.com/article/us-spain-austerity-health-idUSBRE9460PW20130507.

Dewachi, Omar. 2017. *Ungovernable Life: Mandatory Medicine and Statecraft in Iraq*. Stanford, CA: Stanford University Press.

Doniec, Katarzyna, Rafael Dall'Alba, and Lawrence King. 2018. "Brazil's Health Catastrophe in the Making." *The Lancet* 392 (10149): 731–32. https://doi.org/10.1016/S0140-6736(18)30853-5.

Duarte, Angela Ixkic. 2012. "From the Margins of Latin American Feminism: Indigenous and Lesbian Feminisms." *Journal of Women in Culture and Society* 38 (1): 153–78.

Duckett, Stephen. 2013. "Public-Private Hospital Partnerships Are Risky Business." *The Conversation* (July 30). https://theconversation.com/public-private-hospital-partnerships-are-risky-business-16421.

Dumit, Joseph. 2012. *Drugs for Life: How Pharmaceutical Companies Define Our Health*. Durham, NC: Duke University Press.

Echeverry López, María Esperanza. 2002. "La Situación de Salud En Colombia" [The Situation of Health in Colombia]. In *La Salud Pública Hoy: Enfoques y Dilemas Contemporáneos En Salud Pública*, edited by Saúl Franco Agudelo, 345–70. Bogotá, Colombia: Universidad Nacional de Colombia.

Echeverry López, María Esperanza, and Alejandro Arango Castrillón, eds. 2013. *Indignación Justa: Estudios Sobre La Acción de Tutela En Salud En Medellín* [Just Indignation: Studies about the Writ in Health in Medellín]. Medellín: Hombre Nuevo Editores; Universidad de Antioquia.

Echeverry López, María Esperanza, and Yadira Eugenia Borrero Ramírez. 2015. "Protestas Sociales Por La Salud En Colombia: La Lucha Por El Derecho Fundamental a La Salud, 1994–2010" [Social Protests for Health in Colombia: Struggles for the Fundamental Right to Health, 1994–2010]. *Cadernos de Saúde Pública* 31 (2): 354–64. https://doi.org/10.1590/0102-311X00030714.

Edgar, James. 2017. "Doctors Walk Out in Greece." *Euronews* (March 2). https://www.euronews.com/2017/03/02/doctors-walk-out-in-greece.

"Editorial: Otra vez la crisis hospitalaria" [Editorial: Once again the hospital crisis]. 2016. *El Tiempo* (November 24). http://www.eltiempo.com/opinion/editorial/otra-vez-la-crisis-hospitalaria-editorial-el-tiempo-25-de-noviembre-de-2016/16758414.

El Espectador. 2012. "Secretario de Salud cuestionó proceso de liquidación del San Juan de Dios" [Health Secretariat questioned liquidation process of San Juan de Dios]. *El Espectador* (February 28). https://www.elespectador.com/judicial/secretario-de-salud-cuestiono-proceso-de-liquidacion-del-san-juan-de-dios-article-329322.

Epele, María E. 2020. "When Life Becomes a Burden at the Urban Margins of Buenos Aires." *Medical Anthropology* 39 (2): 153–66. https://doi.org/10.1080/01459740.2019.1667993.

Erikson, Susan L. 2012. "Global Health Business: The Production and Performativity of Statistics in Sierra Leone and Germany." *Medical Anthropology* 31 (4) (July): 367–84. https://doi.org/10.1080/01459740.2011.621908.

Escobar, Arturo. 2000. "El Lugar de La Naturaleza y La Naturaleza Del Lugar: ¿globalización o postdesarrollo?" [The Place of Nature and the Nature of Place: Globalization or Post-Development?]. In *La Colonialidad Del Saber*, edited by Enrique Dussel, 113–43. Buenos Aires: CLACSO.

Escobar, Arturo. 2014. *Sentipensar Con La Tierra: Nuevas Lecturas Sobre Desarrollo, Territorio y Diferencia* [Feelthinking with the Earth: New Readings about Development, Territory and Difference]. Colección Pensamiento Vivo. Medellín, Colombia: Ediciones Unaula.

Escobar, Arturo. 2018. *Designs for the Pluriverse: Radical Interdependence, Autonomy, and the Making of Worlds*. New Ecologies for the Twenty-First Century. Durham, NC: Duke University Press.

Eslava Castañeda, Juan Carlos, Manuel Vega Vargas, and Mario Hernández Alvarez. 2017. *Facultad de Medicina. Su Historia. Tomo I* [School of Medicine. Its History. Vol. I]. Bogotá, Colombia: Centro Editorial, Facultad de Medicina, Sede Bogotá. Universidad Nacional de Colombia.

Ewig, Christina, and Amparo Hernández. 2009. "Gender Equity and Health Sector Reform in Colombia: Mixed State-Market Model Yields Mixed Results." *Social Science & Medicine* 68: 1145–52.

Express Tribune. 2018. "Lady Health Workers' Protest Continues." *The Express Tribune* (March 29). https://tribune.com.pk/story/1671744/1-lady-health-workers-protest -continues/.

Facultad de Medicina. 2010. *Informe académico. Informe al Consejo de Facultad* [Academic report. Report to the School's council]. (June).

Falcón Prasca, Gil Alberto. 2020. "Día del estudiante caído" [Day of the Fallen Student]. *El Universal* (June 12). https://www.eluniversal.com.co/opinion/columna/dia-del -estudiante-caido-AN2960460.

Farías-Jiménez, Patricia, Gina Paola Arocha-Zuluaga, Kenny Margarita Trujillo-Ramírez, and Inés Botero-Uribe. 2014. "Estrategia Instituciones Amigas de la Mujer y la Infancia, con enfoque integral en Colombia" [Women and Children Friendly Institutions Strategy, with Integral Approach in Colombia]. *Gaceta Sanitaria* 28 (4): 326–29. https://doi.org/10.1016/j.gaceta.2014.02.008.

Farmer, Paul. 2003. *Pathologies of Power: Health, Human Rights, and the New War on the Poor.* Berkeley: University of California Press.

Farmer, Paul. 2004. "An Anthropology of Structural Violence." *Current Anthropology* 45: 305–26.

Farwa, Ummay. 2018. "Lady Health Workers End Lahore Protest after Demands Met." *Geo News* (March 30). https://www.geo.tv/latest/188637-lady-health-workers-end -lahore-protest-after-demands-met.

Fernández Ávila, Daniel G., Liliana Carolina Mancipe García, Diana C. Fernández Ávila, Elsa Reyes Sanmiguel, Maria Claudia Díaz, and Juan Martín Gutiérrez. 2011. "Análisis de La Oferta de Programas de Pregrado En Medicina En Colombia Durante Los Últimos 30 Años (1980–2010)" [Analysis about the Offer of Medicine Undergraduate Programs in Colombia during the Last 30 years (1980–2010)]. *Revista Colombiana de Reumatología* 18 (2): 109–20.

Fischer, Michael M. J. 2009. *Anthropological Futures.* Durham, NC: Duke University Press.

Flakin, Nathaniel. 2017. "Strike at Berlin's Largest Hospital." *LeftVoice* (May 16). http://www.leftvoice.org/Strike-at-Berlin-s-Largest-Hospital.

Florido Caicedo, Carlos Arturo. 2009. "Semblanza Del Profesor Alfredo Rubiano Caballero" [Biography of Professor Alfredo Rubiano Caballero]. *Morfolia* 1 (2): 1–7.

Franco Agudelo, Saúl. 2003. "Para Que La Salud Sea Pública: Algunas Lecciones de La Reforma de Salud y Seguridad Social En Colombia" [In Order for Health to Be Public: Some Lessons about the Health and Social Security Reform in Colombia]. *Revista Gerencia y Políticas de Salud* 4: 59–69.

Fraser, Nancy. 2016. "Contradictions on Capital and Care." *New Left Review* 100 (July–August): 99–117.

Galvão, Jane. 2001. "Access to Antiretroviral Drugs in Brazil." *The Lancet* 360: 1862–65.

Galvão, Jane. 2002. "Brazilian Policy for the Distribution and Production of Antiretroviral Drugs: A Privilege or a Right?" *Cadernos de Saúde Publica* 18: 213–19.

Garcia, Angela. 2010. *The Pastoral Clinic: Addiction and Dispossession along the Rio Grande.* Berkeley: University of California Press.

García, Claudia. 2007. "El Hospital Como Empresa: Nuevas Prácticas, Nuevos Traba-jadores" [The Hospital as a Company: New Practices, New Workers]. *Universitas Psychologica* 6: 143–54.

Gaviria, Alejandro, Carlos Medina, and Carolina Mejia. 2006. *Evaluating the Impact of Health Care Reform in Colombia: From Theory to Practice*. Documento CEDE. Bogotá, Colombia: Universidad de los Andes.

Gilligan, Carol. 2000. *La ética del cuidado* [Ethics of Care]. Cuadernos de la Fundació Víctor Grífols I Lucas, 30. Barcelona: Fundació Víctor Grífols i Lucas.

Giraldo, Cesar. 2007. *¿Protección o Desprotección Social?* [Social Protection or Lack of Protection?]. Bogotá, Colombia: Ediciones Desde Abajo.

Giraldo, Clara Victoria, and Grey Yuliet Ceballos. 2011. "Acostumbrarse a Las Barreras: Estudio Cualitativo de Las Barreras Del Sistema de Salud Colombiano Para El Di-agnóstico y Tratamiento Oportuno de Cáncer de Mama" [Getting Used to Barriers: Qualitative Study of Barriers of the Colombian Health Care System for the Oppor-tune Diagnosis and Treatment of Breast Cancer]. *Forum Qualitative Sozialforschung / Forum: Qualitative Social Research*, 12.

Góngora, Andrés, Susana Fergusson, Ramiro Borja, Margarita Castro, and Edelmira Arias. 2013. "El San Juan Muere de Pie: la vida social de un hospital y la construcción de una causa" [San Juan Dies Standing: the social life of a hospital and the construc-tion of a cause]. Report. Facultad de Medicina, Universidad Nacional de Colombia.

González, Guillermo. 2018. "Similitudes en el asesinato de testigos que han hablado contra Álvaro Uribe o sus cercanos" [Similarities in the murdering of witnesses that have spoken against Álvaro Uribe or his close people]. *El Espectador* (May 8). https://www.elespectador.com/noticias/nacional/similitudes-en-el-asesinato-de -testigos-que-han-hablado-contra-alvaro-uribe-o-sus-cercanos-articulo-754080.

Good, Byron J. 1994. *Medicine, Rationality, and Experience: An Anthropological Perspec-tive*. Cambridge, UK: Cambridge University Press.

Good, Byron. 2012. "Phenomenology, Psychoanalysis, and Subjectivity in Java." *Ethos* 40 (1): 24–36. https://doi.org/10.1111/j.1548-1352.2011.01229.x.

Good, Mary-Jo DelVecchio. 2001. "The Biotechnical Embrace." *Culture, Medicine and Psychiatry* 25: 395–410.

Good, Mary-Jo DelVecchio, ed. 2008. *Postcolonial Disorders*. Berkeley: University of California Press.

Goodale, Mark, and Nancy Grey Postero, eds. 2013. *Neoliberalism, Interrupted: Social Change and Contested Governance in Contemporary Latin America*. Stanford, CA: Stanford University Press.

Gordillo, Gastón. 2014. *Rubble: The Afterlife of Destruction*. Durham, NC: Duke Univer-sity Press.

Gossain, Juan. 2018. La verdadera historia de hospitals y clínicas al borde de la quiebra" [The true story of hospitals and clinics on the verge of bankruptcy]. *El Tiempo* (July 25). http://m.eltiempo.com/vida/salud/la-verdadera-historia-de-hospitales-y -clinicas-al-borde-de-la-quiebra-247988.

Graeber, David. 2014. "Savage Capitalism Is Back—and It Will Not Tame Itself." *The Guardian* (May 30). https://www.theguardian.com/commentisfree/2014/may/30 /savage-capitalism-back-radical-challenge.

Graeber, David. 2016. *Toward an Anthropological Theory of Value: The False Coin of Our Own Dreams*. New York: Palgrave.

Gramsci, Antonio, and Quintin Hoare. 1985. *Selections from the Prison Notebooks of Antonio Gramsci*. New York: International Publ.

Granja, Simón. 2018. "La mujer que hace historia al frente de la Universidad Nacional" [The woman who makes history at the head of National University]. *El Tiempo* (March 25). http://www.eltiempo.com/vida/educacion/perfil-de-dolly-montoya-la-mujer-que-hace-historia-al-frente-de-la-universidad-nacional-197780.

Grant, James P., and UNICEF. 1984. *The State of the World's Children*. Oxford: Oxford University Press.

Grosfoguel, Ramón. 2011. "Decolonizing Post-Colonial Studies and Paradigms of Political-Economy." *Transmodernity, Decolonial Thinking, and Global Coloniality* 1 (1): 1–38.

Guber, Rosana. 2001. *La Etnografía. Método, Campo y Reflexividad* [Ethnography. Method, Field, and Reflexivity]. Bogotá, Colombia: Grupo Editorial Norma.

Guber, Rosana, ed. 2019. *Trabajo de Campo En América Latina: Experiencias Antropológicas Regionales En Etnografía. Tomo 2* [Fieldwork in Latin America: Regional Anthropological Experiences in Ethnography. Volume 2]. Paradigma Indicial. Antropología Sociocultural. Buenos Aires: San Benito.

Guha, Ranajit. 1998. *Dominance without Hegemony: History and Power in Colonial India*. Cambridge, MA: Harvard University Press.

Guillot, Adéa. 2013. "Greek Doctors Strike as Government Moves to Tackle Healthcare Debt. *The Guardian* (December 10). https://www.theguardian.com/world/2013/dec/10/greece-doctors-strike-healthcare-reforms.

Gutiérrez de Pineda, V. 1964. *La Familia en Colombia. Volumen I Trasfondo Histórico* [Family in Colombia. Volume I. Historical Background]. Bogotá, Colombia: Editorial Iqueima.

Hale, Charles R. 2006. "Activist Research v. Cultural Critique: Indigenous Land Rights and the Contradictions of Politically Engaged Anthropology." *Cultural Anthropology* 21 (1): 96–120. https://doi.org/10.1525/can.2006.21.1.96.

Hamdy, Sherine. 2016. "All Eyes on Egypt: Islam and the Medical Use of Dead Bodies Amidst Cairo's Political Unrest." *Medical Anthropology* 35 (3): 220–35. https://doi.org/10.1080/01459740.2015.1040879.

Han, Clara. 2012. *Life in Debt: Times of Care and Violence in Neoliberal Chile*. Berkeley: University of California Press.

Haraway, Donna J. 1988. "Situated Knowledges: The Science Question in Feminism and the Privilege of Partial Perspective." *Feminist Studies* 14: 575–99.

Harvey, David. 2003. "The 'New' Imperialism: Accumulation by Dispossession." *The Socialist Register*, 63–87.

Harvey, David. 2007. *Breve Historia Del Neoliberalismo* [Brief History of Neoliberalism]. Madrid: Ediciones Akal.

Hernández, Leandra Hinojosa, and Sarah De Los Santos Upton. 2018. *Challenging Reproductive Control and Gendered Violence in the Americas: Intersectionality, Power, and Struggles for Rights*. Lanham, MD: Lexington Books.

Hernández, Mario. 2003. "Neoliberalismo En Salud: Desarrollos, Supuestos y Alternativas" [Neoliberalism in Health: Developments, Assumptions, and Alternatives]. In

La Falacia Neoliberal. Crítica y Alternativas, edited by Darío Botero, 347–61. Bogotá, Colombia: Universidad Nacional de Colombia.

Hernández, Mario. 2017a. "La venta de Cafesalud: ¿dónde estuvo el negocio?" [The sale of Cafesalud: Where was the business?]. razonpublica (June 5). https://www.razonpublica .com/index.php/econom-y-sociedad-temas-29/10306-la-venta-de-cafesalud -d%C3%B3nde-estuvo-el-negocio.html.

Hernández, Mario. 2017b. "Medimás: el síntoma de una crisis estructural de la salud" [Medimás: the symptom of a structural health crisis]. razonpublica (September 25). https://razonpublica.com/index.php/econom-y-sociedad-temas-29/10558 -medim%C3%A1s-el-s%C3%ADntoma-de-una-crisis-estructural-de-la-salud.html.

Hernández, Mario, and Diana Obregón. 2002. *La Organización Panamericana de La Salud y El Estado Colombiano: Cien Años de Historia 1902–2002* [The Panamerican Health Organization and the Colombian State. One Hundred Years of History 1902–2002]. Bogotá, Colombia: Organización Panamericana de la Salud.

Hernández, Mario, and Mauricio Tovar. 2010. "Nueva Reforma En El Sector Salud En Colombia: Portarse Bien Para La Salud Financiera Del Sistema" [New Reform of the Health Sector in Colombia: Behaving for the Financial Health of the System]. *Medicina Social* 5: 241–45.

Hernández Alvarez, Mario. 2002. *La Salud Fragmentada En Colombia, 1910–1946* [The Fragmented Health in Colombia, 1910–1946]. Bogotá, Colombia: Universidad Nacional de Colombia.

Hernández Alvarez, Mario. 2004. *La Fragmentación de La Salud En Colombia y Argentina. Una Comparación Sociopolítica, 1880–1950* [The Fragmentation of Health in Colombia and Argentina. A Sociopolitical Comparison, 1880–1950]. Colección Sede. Bogotá, Colombia: Universidad Nacional de Colombia.

Hernández Alvarez, Mario, and Román Vega. 2001. *¿Equidad? El Problema de La Equidad Financiera En Salud* [Equity? The Problem of Financial Equity in Health]. Bogotá, Colombia: Ediciones Antropos Limitada.

Hogan, Michael. 2009. *Savage Capitalism and the Myth of Democracy: Latin America in the Third Millennium*. Trenton, NJ Booklocker.com Incorporated.

Hurtado, David, Ichiro Kawachi, and John Sudarsky. 2011. "Social Capital and Self-Rated Health in Colombia: The Good, the Bad and the Ugly." *Social Science & Medicine* 72: 584–90.

IDEASS (Innovation for Development and South-South Cooperation). n.d. "The Mother Kangaroo Method." https://www.ideassonline.org.

IMTJ Team. 2018. "Saudi Arabia Launches Healthcare Privatisation Programme." IMTJ News (February 21). https://www.imtj.com/news/saudi-arabia-launches-healthcare -privatisation-programme/.

Iriart, Celia, Tulio Franco, and Emerson Elias Merhy. 2011. "The Creation of the Health Consumer: Challenges on Health Sector Regulation after Managed Care Era." *Globalization and Health* 7 (February). https://doi.org/10.1186/1744-8603-7-2.

Iriart, Celia, and Emerson Elias Merhy. 2017. "Disputas Inter-Capitalistas, Biomedicalización y Modelo Médico Hegemónico" [Intercapitalist Disputes, Biomedicalization and the Hegemonic Medical Model]. *Interface - Comunicação, Saúde, Educação* 21 (63): 1005–16. https://doi.org/10.1590/1807-57622016.0808.

Iriart, Celia, Emerson Elías Merhy, and Howard Waitzkin. 2001. "Managed Care in Latin America: The New Common Sense in Health Policy Reform." *Social Science & Medicine* 52: 1243–53.

Jaramillo, Iván. 1999. *El Futuro de La Salud En Colombia. Ley 100 de 1993 Cinco Años Después* [The Future of Health in Colombia. Law 100 of 1993 Five Years Later]. 4th ed. Bogotá, Colombia: Fescol, FES, FRB, Fundación Corona.

Jasso-Aguilar, Rebeca, and Howard Waitzkin. 2007. "El Estado, Las Multinacionales y La Medicina Contemporánea" [The State, The Multinationals and Contemporary Medicine]. *Palimpsestus* 6: 69–82.

Jasso-Aguilar, Rebeca, Howard Waitzkin, and Angela Landwehr. 2004. "Multinational Corporations and Health Care in the United States and Latin America: Strategies, Actions and Effects." *Journal of Health and Social Behavior* 45: 136–57.

Jerome, Jessica Scott. 2016. *Right to Health: Medicine, Marginality, and Health Care Reform in Northeastern Brazil.* Austin: University of Texas Press.

Jimeno, Myriam. 2005. "La Vocación Crítica de La Antropología En Latinoamérica" [The Critical Vocation of Anthropology in Latin America]. *Antípoda* Julio-Diciembre (1): 43–65.

Jimeno, Myriam. 2006. "Citizens and Anthropologists." *Journal of World Anthropology* 1: 59–74.

Jimeno, Myriam, Daniel Varela Corredor, and Ángela Milena Castillo Ardila. 2015. *Después de La Masacre: Emociones y Política En El Cauca Indio* [After the Massacre: Emotions and Politics in the Indigenous Cauca]. Colección CES. Bogotá, Colombia: Instituto Colombiano de Antropología e Historia: Universidad Nacional de Colombia, Sede Bogotá, Facultad de Ciencias Humanas, Centro de Estudios Sociales— CES, Grupo Conflicto Social y Violencia.

Kalleberg, Arne L. 2009. "Precarious Work, Insecure Workers: Employment Relations in Transition." *American Sociological Review* 74 (1): 1–22. https://doi.org/10.1177 /000312240907400101.

Kehr, Janina. 2019. "Complaining about Care in Austerity Spain." *Mouvements* 98 (2): 32.

Keshavjee, Salmaan. 2014. *Blind Spot: How Neoliberalism Infiltrated Global Health.* Oakland: University of California Press.

Kidder, Tracy. 2009. *Mountains beyond Mountains.* New York: Random House Trade Paperbacks.

Kim, Jim Y., Joyce V. Millen, Alec Irwin, and John Gershman. 2000. *Dying for Growth. Global Inequality and the Health of the Poor.* Monroe, ME: Common Courage Press.

Klein, Naomi. 2007. *The Shock Doctrine. The Rise of Disaster Capitalism.* New York: Metropolitan Books.

Kleinman, Arthur. 1995. *Writing at the Margin. Discourses Between Anthropology and Medicine.* Berkeley: University of California Press.

Kleinman, Arthur. 2012. "Caregiving as Moral Experience." *The Lancet* 380 (9853): 1550–51. https://doi.org/10.1016/S0140-6736(12)61870-4.

Knight, Kelly Ray. 2015. *Addicted. Pregnant. Poor.* Critical Global Health: Evidence, Efficacy, Ethnography. Durham, NC: Duke University Press.

Kockelman, Paul. 2016. *The Chicken and the Quetzal: Incommensurate Ontologies and Portable Values in Guatemala's Cloud Forest.* Durham, NC: Duke University Press.

Lagarde y de los Ríos, Marcela. 2015. *Los cautiverios de las mujeres: madresposas, monjas, putas, presas y locas* [The captivities of women: Momwives, nuns, whores, convicts and crazy]. México, D.F.: Siglo XXI.

Lamphere, Louise, Helena Ragoné, and Patricia Zavella, eds. 1997. *Situated Lives: Gender and Culture in Everyday Life*. New York: Routledge.

Lamprea, Everaldo. 2014. "Colombia's Right-to-Health Litigation in a Context of Health Care Reform." In *The Right to Health at the Public/Private Divide: A Global Comparative Study*, edited by Colleen M. Flood and Aeyal M. Gross, 131–58. New York: Cambridge University Press.

Lamprea, Everaldo. 2017. "The Judicialization of Health Care: A Global South Perspective." *Annual Review of Law and Social Science* 13 (1). https://doi.org/10.1146/annurev-lawsocsci-110316-113303.

Lattus Olmos, José. 2008. "El Fórceps, Su Exótica e Interesante Historia" [Forceps, Its Exotic and Interesting History]. *Revista Obstetricia y Ginecología Hospital Santiago Oriente Dr. Luis Tisné Brousse* 3 (2): 155–68.

Law, J., Geir Afdal, Kristin Asdal, Wen-yuan Lin, Ingunn Moser, and Vicky Singleton. 2014. "Modes of Syncretism Notes on Noncoherence." *Common Knowledge* 20 (1): 172–92. https://doi.org/10.1215/0961754X-2374817.

Livingston, Julie. 2012. *Improvising Medicine: An African Oncology Ward in an Emerging Cancer Epidemic*. Durham, NC: Duke University Press.

Londoño, Juan Luis, and Julio Frenk. 1997. "Structured Pluralism: Towards an Innovative Model for Health System Reform in Latin America." *Health Policy* 41: 1–36.

Lopez, Leslie. 2005. "De Facto Disentitlement in an Information Economy: Enrollment Issues in Medicaid Managed Care." *Medical Anthropology Quarterly* 19 (March): 26–46. https://doi.org/10.1525/maq.2005.19.1.026.

López Hooker, Eduardo. 2004. "Materno Infantil: La Supersalud agrava el problema" [Materno Infantil: The supersalud worsens the problem]. *UNPeriódico* (October 3). http://historico.unperiodico.unal.edu.co/ediciones/64/06.htm.

López Rendón, Luisa María. 2015. "Significado de La MANE En La Construcción Del Movimiento Estudiantil En Colombia" [Meaning of MANE in the Construction of the Student Movement in Colombia]. *Folios de Humanidades y Pedagogía* (Jan–Jun): 93–118.

Lugones, Maria. 2008. "The Coloniality of Gender." *Worlds & Knowledges Otherwise* (Spring): 1–17.

Macleod, Morna, and Natalia de Marinis. 2017. *Resisting Violence: Emotional Communities in Latin America*. New York: Springer Science+Business Media.

Martin, Emily. 2001. *The Woman in the Body: A Cultural Analysis of Reproduction: With a New Introduction*. Boston: Beacon Press.

Martín-Baró, Ignacio. 1996. *Writings for a Liberation Psychology*. Cambridge, MA: Harvard University Press.

Martínez, Adriana. 2008. "¿Calidad de La Atención o Atención Con Calidad? Condiciones Laborales y Profesionales de La Salud En El Sistema General de Seguridad Social En Salud?" [Quality of Healthcare or Healthcare with Quality? Labor Conditions and Healthcare Professionals in the General Social Security System in Health]. Master's Thesis in Public Health, Bogotá, Colombia: Universidad Nacional de Colombia.

Marx, Karl, and Friederich Engels. 1968. *The German Ideology*. Progress Publishers.

Maternowska, M. Catherine. 2006. *Reproducing Inequities: Poverty and the Politics of Population in Haiti*. New Brunswick, NJ: Rutgers University Press.

McKay, Ramah. 2018. *Medicine in the Meantime: The Work of Care in Mozambique*. Durham, NC: Duke University Press.

Méndez, Luis Carlos, and Héctor Ulloque. 2006. "El IMI: Una Visión Histórica" [IMI: A Historical Overview]. Facultad de Medicina, Universidad Nacional de Colombia, December 6.

Menéndez, Eduardo. 1985. "El modelo médico dominante y las limitaciones y posibilidades de los modelos antropológicos" [The dominant medical model and the limitations and possibilities of anthropological models]. *Desaecon Desarrollo Económico* 24 (96): 593–604.

Mesa Melgarejo, Lorena del Pilar. 2018. "Configuración del campo de consumo relacionado con la atención en salud en Bogotá, 1980–2014" [Configuration of the consumer field in relationship with health care in Bogotá, 1980–2014]. PhD diss., Bogotá, Colombia: Universidad Nacional de Colombia.

Metzl, Jonathan, and Anna Rutherford Kirkland, eds. 2010. *Against Health: How Health Became the New Morality*. New York: New York University Press.

Min-sik, Yoon (윤민식). 2013. "Top university hospital workers go on strike." *The Korea Herald* (October 23). http://www.koreaherald.com/view.php?ud=20131023000113.

Mol, Annemarie. 2008. *The Logic of Care: Health and the Problem of Patient Choice*. London: Routledge.

Mol, Annemarie, Ingunn Moser, and Jeannette Pols, eds. 2010. *Care in Practice: On Tinkering in Clinics, Homes and Farms*. 1. Aufl. VerKörperungen 8. Bielefeld: Transcript-Verl.

Molina, Gloria, Iván Felipe Muñóz, and Andrés Ramírez. 2009. *Dilemas En Las Decisiones En La Atención En Salud. Etica, Derechos y Deberes Constitucionales Frente a La Rentabilidad Financiera* [Dilemmas in Healthcare Decisions. Ethics, Rights, and Constitutional Duties according to Financial Gains]. Bogotá, Colombia: Universidad de Antioquia, Procuraduría General de la Nación, Insituto de Estudios del Ministerio Público, COLCIENCIAS, Universidad Industrial de Santander.

Molina Marín, G., J. Vargas Jaramillo, A. Berrío Castaño, and D. Muñoz Marín. 2010. "Características de la contratación entre aseguradores y prestadores de servicios de salud" [Characteristics of contracts between insurers and health service providers]. *Revista Gerencia y Politicas de Salud* 9 (18): 103–15.

Moraña, Mabel, Enrique Dussel, and Carlos Jáuregui. 2008. "Colonialism and Its Replicants." In *Coloniality at Large. Latin America and the Postcolonial Debate*, edited by Mabel Moraña, Enrique Dussel, and Carlos A. Jáuregui, 1–20. Durham, NC: Duke University Press.

Mukherjee, Joia. 2018. *An Introduction to Global Health Delivery: Practice, Equity, Human Rights*. Oxford, UK: Oxford University Press.

Mulligan, Jessica. 2010. "It Gets Better If You Do? Measuring Quality Care in Puerto Rico." *Medical Anthropology* 29: 303–29. https://doi.org/10.1080/01459740.2010.488663.

Mulligan, Jessica. 2014. *Unmanageable Care: An Ethnography of Health Care Privatization*. New York: New York University Press.

Mulligan, Jessica. 2016. "Insurance Accounts: The Cultural Logics of Health Care Financing." *Medical Anthropology Quarterly* 30 (1): 37–61. https://doi.org/10.1111/maq.12157.

Murphy, Michael D., and Carlos González Faraco. 2011. "Identifying the Virgin Mary. Disarming Skepticism in European Vision Narratives." *Anthropos* 106: 511–27.

Navarro, Vicente. 2009. "What We Mean by Social Determinants of Health." *International Journal of Health Services* 39 (3): 423–41. https://doi.org/10.2190/HS.39.3.a.

Navne, Laura E., Mette N. Svendsen, and Tine M. Gammeltoft. 2018. "The Attachment Imperative: Parental Experiences of Relation-Making in a Danish Neonatal Intensive Care Unit: The Attachment Imperative." *Medical Anthropology Quarterly* 32 (1): 120–37. https://doi.org/10.1111/maq.12412.

Nelson, John, and Robert Gemmell. 2004. "Implications of Marsupial Births for Our Understanding of Behavioural Development." *International Journal of Comparative Psychology* 17: 53–70.

Ortner, Sherry. 2006. *Anthropology and Social Theory: Culture, Power, and the Acting Subject*. Durham, NC: Duke University Press.

Padilla, Nelson. 2017. "A 30 años de su muerte, así pensaba Héctor Abad Gómez" [30 years after his death, this is how Héctor Abad Gómez thought]. *El Espectador* (August 24). https://www.elespectador.com/colombia-20/paz-y-memoria/a-30-anos-de-su-muerte-asi-pensaba-hector-abad-gomez-article/.

Peterson, Kristin. 2014. *Speculative Markets: Drug Circuits and Derivative Life in Nigeria*. Durham, NC: Duke University Press.

Petryna, Adriana. 2009. *When Experiments Travel: Clinical Trials and the Global Search for Human Subjects*. Princeton, NJ: Princeton University Press.

Pinilla, María Y., and César E. Abadía. 2017. "Hospital San Juan de Dios: Actor y Víctima de Las Políticas Públicas En Colombia" [Hospital San Juan de Dios: Actor and Victim of Public Policies in Colombia]. *Revista Peruana de Medicina Experimental y Salud Pública* 34 (2): 287–92. https://doi.org/10.17843/rpmesp.2017.342.2888.

Pink, Sarah. 2012. *Situating Everyday Life: Practices and Places*. Los Angeles: SAGE.

Pinzón, Lida. 2006. "La Trascendencia Del Programa Madre Canguro En El Mundo" [The Predominance of the Kangaroo Mother Program around the World]. Facultad de Medicina, Universidad Nacional de Colombia, November 17.

Povinelli, Elizabeth A. 2011. *Economies of Abandonment: Social Belonging and Endurance in Late Liberalism*. Durham, NC: Duke University Press.

Quijano, Anibal. 2000. "Colonialidad Del Poder, Eurocentrismo y América Latina" [Coloniality of Power, Eurocentrism and Latin America]. In *La Colonialidad Del Saber: Eurocentrismo y Ciencias Sociales. Perspectivas Latinoamericanas*, edited by Edgardo Lander, 201–46. Buenos Aires: CLACSO.

Ramos, Alícida Rita. 2008. "Anthropologist as Political Actor." *Journal of Latin American Anthropology* 4 (2): 172–89. https://doi.org/10.1525/jlca.1999.4.2.172.

Rappaport, Joanne. 2008. "Beyond Participant Observation: Collaborative Ethnography as Theoretical Innovation." *Collaborative Anthropologies* 1 (1): 1–31. https://doi.org/10.1353/cla.0.0014.

Rappaport, Joanne. 2018. "Visualidad y Escritura Como Acción: Investigación Acción Participativa En La Costa Caribe Colombiana" [Visuality and Writing as Action: Participatory Action Research in the Colombian Caribbean Coast]. *Revista Colombiana de Sociología* 41 (1): 133–56. https://doi.org/10.15446/rcs.v41n1.66272.

Rappaport, Joanne. 2020. *Cowards Don't Make History: Orlando Fals Borda and the Origins of Participatory Action Research*. Durham, NC: Duke University Press.

Raviola, Giuseppe, M'imunya Machoki, Esther Mwaikambo, and Mary-Jo DelVecchio Good. 2002. "HIV, Disease Plague, Demoralization and 'Burnout': Resident Experience of the Medical Profession in Nairobi, Kenya." *Culture, Medicine and Psychiatry* 26: 55–86.

Redacción Bogotá. 2015a. "¿Y los ocupantes del San Juan?" [And the San Juan Occupiers?]. *El Espectador* (July 16). http://www.elespectador.com/noticias/bogota/y-los-ocupantes-del-san-juan-articulo-573155.

Redacción Bogotá. 2015b. "Hospital universitario de la U. Nacional fue inaugurado en Bogotá" [University hospital of the National U. was inaugurated in Bogotá]. *El Espectador* (November 18). https://www.elespectador.com/bogota/hospital-universitario-de-la-u-nacional-fue-inaugurado-en-bogota-article-600072/.

Redacción Bogotá. 2019. "Avanza operativo de desalojo en el hospital San Juan de Dios" [Eviction operation advances in hospital San Juan de Dios]. *El Tiempo* (April 3). https://www.eltiempo.com/bogota/desalojo-en-el-hospital-san-juan-de-dios-en-bogota-344726.

Redacción El Tiempo. 2006a. *Hospital Materno Infantil reabrió la atención de consulta externa y sala de atención de neonatos* [Hospital Materno Infantil reopened outpatient services and the neonatal ward]. (October 25). http://www.eltiempo.com/archivo/documento/CMS-3298254.

Redacción El Tiempo. 2006b. *El Materno Infantil volvió a la vida* [The Materno Infantil came back to life]. (October 25). http://www.eltiempo.com/archivo/documento/MAM-2248966.

Redacción El Tiempo. 2006c. *Materno continúa abierto* [Materno remains open]. (November 23). http://www.eltiempo.com/archivo/documento/MAM-2288301.

Redacción El Tiempo. 2006d. *Instituto Materno Infantil continúa prestando sus servicio a pesar de toma de trabajadores* [Instituto Materno Infantil continues operating despite the workers takeover]. (November 22). http://www.eltiempo.com/archivo/documento/CMS-3337435.

Redacción El Tiempo. 2013. *Piden suspensión de la liquidadora del San Juan de Dios* [Removal of liquidating agent of El San Juan de Dios was asked]. (October 18). https://www.eltiempo.com/archivo/documento/CMS-13132920.

Redacción El Tiempo. 2015a. *Gobernación de Cundinamarca, autorizada para vender San Juan de Dios* [Cundinamarca's Governor's Office authorized to sell San Juan de Dios]. (December 1). https://www.eltiempo.com/archivo/documento/CMS-16445978.

Redacción El Tiempo. 2015b. *Restaurar el San Juan de Dios, más cerca pero incierto* [Restoring San Juan de Dios closer but more uncertain]. (December 21). http://www.eltiempo.com/bogota/san-juan-de-dios-restauracion/16463484.

Redacción El Tiempo. 2015c. *Ministerio de Cultura aprobó plan para restaurar el San Juan de Dios* [Ministry of Culture approved plan to restore San Juan de Dios]. (December 18). http://www.eltiempo.com/bogota/hospital-san-juan-de-dios /16462388.

Redacción El Tiempo. 2016. "What Will Happen to the Maternal and Child Institute?" 2016. *El Tiempo.* Accessed July 11, 2018. http://www.eltiempo.com/vida/salud/el -futuro-del-instituto-materno-infantil-46182.

Redacción Juicial. 2018. "Corte Suprema archivó investigación a Dilian Francisca Toro por parapolítica" [Supreme Court archived Dilian Francisca Toro's investigation for parapolitics]. *El Espectador* (February 26). https://www.elespectador.com/noticias /judicial/corte-suprema-archivo-investigacion-dilian-francisca-toro-por-parapolitica -articulo-741396.

Reeck, Sebastian. 2017. "Strikes at the Charité Hospital—Space of Healthcare or Profit Center?" *Transnational Social Strike* (September 30). https://www.transnational -strike.info/2017/09/30/strikes-at-the-charite-hospital-space-of-healthcare-or-profit -center/.

República de Colombia, Colombian Congress. 1993. *Ley Número 100 de 1993* [Law 100 of 1993]. (December 23).

Restrepo, Estela. 2006. "San Juan de Dios: Institución Insignia de La Medicina y de La Beneficencia Pública En Colombia" [San Juan de Dios: Emblem Institution of Medicine and of Public Beneficence in Colombia]. Facultad de Medicina, Universidad Nacional de Colombia.

Restrepo, Estela. 2011. *El Hospital San Juan de Dios 1635–1895* [Hospital San Juan de Dios 1635–1895]. Bogotá, Colombia: Centro de Estudios Sociales, Universidad Nacional de Colombia.

Restrepo Zea, Estela, Clara Helena Sánchez, and Gustavo Silva Carrero, eds. 2017. *Universidad, Cultura y Estado* [University, Culture, and State]. Colección Del Sesquicentenario, vol. 1. Bogotá, Colombia: Universidad Nacional de Colombia.

Riles, Annelise, ed. 2006. *Documents: Artifacts of Modern Knowledge.* Ann Arbor: University of Michigan Press.

Rincón Diaz, Jonnathan Abdul. 2015. "Pensamiento Crítico En Fals Borda: Hacia Una Filosofía de La Educación En Perspectiva Latinoamericana" [Critical Thinking in Fals Borda: Towards a Philosophy in Education in Latin American Perspective]. *Cuadernos de Filosofía Latinoamericana* 36 (112): 171–203.

Roberts, Elizabeth F. S. 2012. *God's Laboratory: Assisted Reproduction in the Andes.* Berkeley: University of California Press.

Robinson, William I. 2007. *Una Teoría Sobre El Capitalismo Global: Producción, Clases y Estado En Un Mundo Transnacional* [A Theory of Global Capitalism: Production, Class, and State in a Transnational World]. Translated by Rigoberto Moncada. Bogotá, Colombia: Desde Abajo.

Rodas, Germán, and Roberto Regalado. 2009. *América Latina Hoy ¿reforma o Revolución?* [Latin America Today. Reform or revolution?]. México, D.F: Ocean Sur.

Rose, Nikolas. 2007. *The Politics of Life Itself. Biomedicine, Power, and Subjectivity in the Twenty-First Century.* Princeton, NJ: Princeton University Press.

Rosenthal, Elisabeth. 2017. *An American Sickness: How Healthcare Became Big Business and How You Can Take It Back.* New York: Penguin Press.

Ruiz, Nubia Yaneth, and Karen Forero Niño. 2017. "La Evolución Sociodemográfica de Los Estudiantes de Pregrado" [Sociodemographic Evolution of Undergraduate Students]. In *Universidad, Cultura y Estado,* 1. ed, 202–73. Colección Del Sesquicentenario, vol. 1. Bogotá, Colombia: Universidad Nacional de Colombia.

Sánchez, Nicolás. 2018. Luis Felipe Vélez: Un profesor que incomodó a los paramilitares [Luis Felipe Vélez: A professor who made the paramilitaries uncomfortable]. *El Espectador* (May 17). https://www.elespectador.com/colombia-20/paz-y-memoria/luis-felipe-velez-un-profesor-que-incomodo-a-los-paramilitares-article/.

Sánchez Vanegas, Guillermo. 2012. "Cáncer de Piel no Melanoma: Riesgos e Itinerarios" [Non-Melanoma Skin Cancer: Risks and Itineraries]. PhD diss., Bogotá, Colombia: Universidad Nacional de Colombia.

Santofimio-Ortiz, Rodrigo. 2018. "El Pensamiento de Antonio Gramsci En América Latina y Colombia" [Antonio Gramsci's Thought in Latin America and Colombia]. *Revista de Antropología y Sociología: VIRAJES* 20 (1): 177–96.

Santos, Boaventura de Sousa. 2018. *The End of the Cognitive Empire: The Coming of Age of Epistemologies of the South.* Durham, NC: Duke University Press.

Segura, Sergio. 2018. "Nueve testigos contra los Uribe Vélez han sido asesinados" [Nine witnesses against Uribe Vélez have been murdered]. *Marcha* (April 19). http://www.marcha.org.ar/los-ocho-testigos-contra-uribe-que-fueron-asesinados-en-colombia/.

Semana Rural. 2019. "The Countryside, with Fewer People Than Was Believed." *Semana Rural* (July 5). https://semanarural.com/web/articulo/el-censo-2018-revelo-que-hay-menos-gente-viviendo-en-el-campo-/1013.

Seo, Bo Kyeong. 2016. "Caring for Premature Life and Death: The Relational Dynamics of Detachment in a NICU." *Medical Anthropology* 35 (6): 560–71. https://doi.org/10.1080/01459740.2016.1145678.

Shepard, Bonnie. 2006. *Running the Obstacle Course to Sexual and Reproductive Health: Lessons from Latin America.* Westport, CT: Praeger Publishers.

Singer, Merrill, and Rebecca Allen. 2017. *Social Justice and Medical Practice: Life History of a Physician of Social Medicine.* New York: Routledge.

Smith-Morris, Carolyn. 2018. "Care as Virtue, Care as Critical Frame: A Discussion of Four Recent Ethnographies." *Medical Anthropology* 37 (5): 426–32. https://doi.org/10.1080/01459740.2018.1429430.

Smith-Nonini, S. 1999. "The Smoke and Mirrors of Health Reform in El Salvador: Community Health NGOs and the Not-So-Neoliberal State." In *Dying for Growth,* edited by Jim Y. Kim, Joyce V. Millen, Alec Irwin, and John Gershman, 359–81. Monroe, ME: Common Courage Press.

Smith-Nonini, Sandra C. 2010. *Healing the Body Politic: El Salvador's Popular Struggle for Health Rights—from Civil War to Neoliberal Peace.* New Brunswick, NJ: Rutgers University Press.

Spiegel, Jerry M., Jaime Breilh, and Annalee Yassi. 2015. "Why Language Matters: Insights and Challenges in Applying a Social Determination of Health Approach in a North-South Collaborative Research Program." *Global Health* 11: 015–0091.

Stevenson, Lisa. 2014. *Life beside Itself: Imagining Care in the Canadian Arctic*. Oakland: University of California Press.

Stocker, Karen, Howard Waitzkin, and Celia Iriart. 1999. "The Exportation of Managed Care to Latin America." *New England Journal of Medicine* 340: 1131–36.

Stoler, Ann Laura, ed. 2013. *Imperial Debris: On Ruins and Ruination*. Durham, NC: Duke University Press.

Stolowicz, Beatriz. 2011. "América Latina Hoy: La Estrategia Conservadora Posneoliberal Para La Estabilización Capitalista" [Latin America Today: The Posneoliberal Conservative Strategy for Capitalist Stabilization]. *EscenariosXXI* 1: 79–89.

Strathern, Marilyn, ed. 2000. *Audit Cultures: Anthropological Studies in Accountability, Ethics, and the Academy*. London: Routledge.

Street, Alice. 2012. "Affective Infrastructure: Hospital Landscapes of Hope and Failure." *Space and Culture* 15 (1): 44–56. https://doi.org/10.1177/1206331211426061.

Street, Alice. 2014. *Biomedicine in an Unstable Place: Infrastructure and Personhood in a Papua New Guinean Hospital*. Durham, NC: Duke University Press.

Strong, Adrienne E. 2020. *Documenting Death: Maternal Mortality and the Ethics of Care in Tanzania*. Oakland: University of California Press. https://doi.org/10.1525/luminos.93.

Sunder Rajan, Kaushik. 2006. *Biocapital. The Constitution of Postgenomic Life*. Durham, NC: Duke University Press.

Sunder Rajan, Kaushik. 2012. "Introduction: The Capitalization of Life and the Liveliness of Capital." In *Lively Capital. Biotechnologies, Ethics, and Governance in Global Markets*, edited by Kaushik Sunder Rajan, 1–41. Durham, NC: Duke University Press.

Sunder Rajan, Kaushik. 2017. *Pharmocracy: Value, Politics, and Knowledge in Global Biomedicine*. Durham, NC: Duke University Press.

Turshen, Meredeth. 1999. *Privatizing Health Services in Africa*. New Brunswick, NJ: Rutgers University Press.

Universidad Externado de Colombia, and United Nations Population Fund, eds. 2007. *Ciudad, Espacio y Población: El Proceso de Urbanización En Colombia* [City, Space, and Population: The Urbanization Process in Colombia]. Bogotá, Colombia: Fondo de Población de las Naciones Unidas.

Uribe, Mónica. 2009. "La Contienda Por Las Reformas Del Sistema de Salud En Colombia (1990–2006)" [The Contest for the Reforms of the Health System in Colombia (1990–2006)]. México, DF: Universidad Nacional Autónoma de México.

Useche, Bernardo. 2007. "De La Salud Pública a La Salud Privada: Una Perspectiva Global a La Reforma En Salud En Colombia" [From Public to Private Health: A Global Perspective to Health Reform in Colombia]. *Palimpsestus* 6: 123–31.

Useche, Bernardo. 2015. "La Reforma de Salud: Un paso adelante y 100 pasos atrás!" [Health Reform: One step forward and 100 back!]. *Revista Deslinde* 57.

Valdés, Ernesto. 2008. "La Transformación de La Gestión Hospitalaria En El Distrito Capital" [The Transformation of Hospital Management in the Capital District]. *Pre-Til* 6 (June): 64–84.

Valenzuela, Santiago. (2013). "El Misterio del lote del Materno" [The mystery of El Materno's lot]. *El Espectador* (March 13). http://www.elespectador.com/noticias/bogota/articulo-410640-el-misterio-del-lote-del-materno.

Vallana Sala, Viviana Valeria. 2019. "'Es Rico Hacerlos, Pero No Tenerlos': Análisis de La Violencia Obstétrica Durante La Atención Del Parto En Colombia" [It's Fun to Make Them but Not to Birth Them: Analysis of Obstetric Violence during Delivery Care in Colombia]. *Revista Ciencias de La Salud* 17: 128–44. https://doi.org/10.12804/revistas.urosario.edu.co/revsalud/a.8125.

Valqui Cachi, Camilo, and Ramón Espinosa Contreras. 2009. *El capitalismo del siglo XXI: violencias y alternativas* [Capitalism of the XXI century: Violences and alternatives]. Cajamarca: Universidad Privada Antonio Guillermo Urrelo.

Vanhulst, Julien, and Adrian E. Beling. 2014. "Buen Vivir: Emergent Discourse within or beyond Sustainable Development?" *Ecological Economics* 101 (May): 54–63. https://doi.org/10.1016/j.ecolecon.2014.02.017.

Varma, Saiba. 2020. *The Occupied Clinic: Militarism and Care in Kashmir.* Durham, NC: Duke University Press.

Vasco Uribe, Luis Guillermo. 2007. "Así es mi método en etnografía" [This is my ethnographic method]. *Tabula Rasa* 6 (enero–junio): 19–52.

Victoria, Ceres, Ruben George Oliven, Maria Eunice Maciel, and Ari Pedro Oro. 2004. *Antropología e Etica. O Debate Atual No Brasil* [Anthropology and Ethics. Current Debate in Brazil]. Niteroi: EdUFF.

Vivero-Arriagada, Luis A. 2014. "Una Lectura Gramsciana Del Pensamiento de Paulo Freire" [A Gramscian Reading of Paulo Freire's Thought]. *Cinta Moebio* 51: 127–36.

Von Schnitzler, Antina. 2016. *Democracy's Infrastructure: Techno-Politics and Citizenship after Apartheid.* Princeton, NJ: Princeton University Press.

Waitzkin, Howard. 2011. *Medicine and Public Health at the End of Empire.* Boulder, CO: Paradigm Publishers.

Waitzkin, Howard. 2015. "Universal Health Coverage: The Strange Romance of The Lancet, MEDICC, and Cuba." *Social Medicine* 9 (2): 93–97.

Waitzkin, Howard, Celia Iriart, Alfredo Estrada, and Silvia Lamadrid. 2001. "Social Medicine Then and Now: Lessons from Latin America." *American Journal of Public Health* 91: 1592–1601.

Waitzkin, Howard, and Working Group for Health Beyond Capitalism, eds. 2018. *Health Care under the Knife: Moving beyond Capitalism for Our Health.* New York: Monthly Review Press.

Wendland, Claire L. 2010. *A Heart for the Work: Journeys through an African Medical School.* Chicago: University of Chicago Press.

Whitelaw, A., and K. Sleath, 1985. "Myth of the Marsupial Mother: Home Care of Very Low Birth Weight Babies in Bogota, Colombia." *Lancet* 1 (8439): 1206–8.

Williams, Raymond L. 2009. *Marxism and Literature.* Oxford: Oxford University Press.

Wilson, Lindsay. 2004. "Review: A Cultural History of Medical Vitalism in Enlightenment Montpellier." *Social History of Medicine* 17 (3): 534–35. https://doi.org/10.1093/shm/17.3.534.

World Bank. 1993. *World Development Report 1993: Investing in Health.* New York: Oxford University Press.

Xiang, Biao. 2007. *Global "Body Shopping": An Indian Labor System in the Information Technology Industry.* Princeton, NJ: Princeton University Press.

Yamin, Alicia Ely. 2016. *Power, Suffering, and the Struggle for Dignity: Human Rights Frameworks for Health and Why They Matter*. Philadelphia: University of Pennsylvania Press.

Yepes, Francisco J., Manuel Ramírez, Luz H. Sánchez, Marta Lucia Ramírez, and Iván Jaramillo. 2010. *Luces y Sombras de La Reforma de La Salud En Colombia. Ley 100 de 1993* [Lights and Shadows of Health Care Reform in Colombia. Law 100 of 1993]. Bogotá, Colombia: Assalud; Universidad del Rosario, Facultad de Economía; Mayol Ediciones.

Žižek, Slavoj. 2008. *Violence: Six Sideways Reflections*. New York: Picador.

Note: page numbers followed by *f* indicate figures.

neonatology, 7, 19, 161–62, 197; La Cruz and, 152; Fundación Vivir and, 110; El Materno and, 1, 33, 43–44, 51, 54, 82, 84, 124, 142, 144, 182, 202, 215

nuns, 105; at El Materno, 82, 85–86, 88–91, 101, 116

Ortner, Sherry, 12, 232n44

Participatory Action Research, 15, 235n2; Latin American, 16

patriarchy, 3, 6–8

pediatrics, 19, 33, 52, 120, 202

pensionados, 42, 106

pensions, 225, 257n8; insurance companies and, 230n14; El Materno and, 110, 123, 133, 139, 146–47, 156–59, 162, 183, 186; neoliberal reforms and, 5, 15, 118–19, 229n2. *See also cesantías*

perinatology, 43–44, 70, 197

pharmaceutical companies, 71, 132, 240n32

pharmaceutical industry, 4, 45, 225, 233n53, 258n19

Pinzón, Lida, 51–52, 68, 72, 146, 185, 215

politics, 3, 235n2; Brazilian, 226; of care, 19; of caring (for), 79, 81; contentious, 254n16; gender, 237n22; health and, 21, 238n1, 253n13; Latin American public universities and, 24; leftist, 204; El Materno and, 110, 160; medicine and, 45, 234n1; neoliberal, 9, 235n4, 257n9; of participation, 15, 25; radical, 27; resources and, 106; of El San Juan, 114; science and state, 236n6; social medicine and, 209

poverty, 23, 38, 49–51, 65, 239n8; classification schemes, 141; conditions of, 231n24; health and, 28; level, 165; line, 122

praxis, 3, 259n28; medical, 200; of medical care, 21; political, 176, 233n47; social, 12

prima, 143, 186

private clinics, 41–42, 96, 202. See also *pensionados*

privatization, 14, 224, 230n9, 230n11; of health care, 11, 15, 225–26, 254n16, 258n27; Hospital Universitario del Valle (HUV) and, 210; El Materno and, 16; of public health, 2; of public hospitals, 222. *See also* Law 100

protests, 149, 225; social, 210, 236n9, 254n16; student, 27, 30, 200, 204–5; workers', 108, 150

providers (health care), 1, 5, 8; budget deficit and, 107; health care reform and, 119, 121

public health, 25, 31, 45, 247n1; in Brazil, 225; geopolitics of, 237n25; neoliberalism and, 1, 3, 252n1; privatization of, 2, 223

quality of care, 104, 107, 120–22, 126, 136, 188, 212, 251n8; indicators, 255n24

racism, 3, 6, 8

religion, 90, 93, 105, 156, 236n6, 243n13

resistance, 12, 14, 226, 247n2; workers', 139–40, 169, 175, 178, 193–94, 222

Rey Sanabria, Edgar, 52–54, 110. *See also* Kangaroo Care Program (KCP)

right to health, 225–26, 235n4, 245n43, 252n6, 253n8, 253n11, 255n20, 259n31

right to health care, 141, 207

risk paradigm, 45, 259n31

rounds, 35–36, 213

ruination, 9, 231–32n33, 251n10; of health care, 20, 227; of El Materno, 10

rural, 31, 38, 42–44, 83–84, 109

El San Juan (San Juan de Dios Hospital), 1, 23, 30–35, 37–42, 85, 105–7, 121, 173, 205, 237n18; administration of, 132; artifacts in, 232n36; Beneficencia de Cundinamarca and, 48, 238n5; church at, 91; closure of, 109, 133, 221, 246n49; directors of, 112; economic crisis and, 114, 132, 147, 211; liquidation process of, 169, 172, 246n48; market-based health care reforms and, 2; Order of Saint Camillus and, 84; reopening of, 177, 201, 222; as ruins, 9, 200, 256n1; shelters at, 87; workers, 135, 163, 168–69, 234n61, 246n48. *See also* El Materno (Instituto Materno Infantil)

San Pedro Claver clinic (La San Pedro), 40–41, 106

Santos, Boaventura de Souza, 3, 229n6, 239n21

El Seguro (El Instituto de Seguros Sociales [Institute of Social Security (ISS)]), 40–41, 43, 237–38nn28–29; 245n42, 246n44; El Materno and, 125–28, 131–32, 134; San Pedro Claver clinic and, 106. *See also* social security

social medicine, 28, 45, 208–9, 234n1, 253–54n13; clinical, 7, 30, 47, 71, 81, 222, 242n6,

254n13; Latin American, 238n1, 242n6; physicians, 247n1

social security, 12, 23, 40–41, 122, 186, 223, 237n27; in Africa, 225; benefits, 250n2; in European countries, 238n29; privatization of, 257n7; reforms, 118–19, 158, 200; right to, 168–69

Stoler, Anne, 9, 231n33

student movement, 27, 204

subaltern health innovations, 200; El Materno and, 47, 70, 78, 121, 222, 235n3, 244n34. *See also* Kangaroo Mother Care (KMC)

trauma, 37, 249n18; care, 32; political, 247n2; psychosocial, 139, 247n4

Tutela, 207, 252n6

umbilical cord: delayed clamping of, 47; respect of, 72–74, 76, 78, 192, 228

UNICEF (United Nations Children's Fund), 203, 258n19; Kangaroo Mother Care (KMC) and, 53–54, 68

universal health coverage (UHC), 259n31; in Latin America, 258n27

Universidad Nacional de Colombia/La Nacional, 1, 31, 126, 183, 235n5; administration of, 19, 27, 113; economic crisis and, 204; Medical School, 105; residency programs, 109. *See also* La Nacional Escuela

Universidad del Quindío, 31, 39, 212

Uribe, Álvaro, 135, 171, 253n12, 254n15

Vecino, Mother Teresa, 82–85, 88, 116–17

violence, 38, 67, 72, 209, 247n5, 252n11; capitalism and, 2, 4; capitalist, 5, 10, 251n9; chronicity of, 137, 139; histories of, 231n32; men and, 7; neoliberalism and, 13; political, 5, 23, 26, 28, 32, 137, 239n25, 241n4, 250n33, 254n16; ruination and, 9, 251n10; sexual, 242n10; structural, 243n4, 247n2, 248n14; systemic, 145, 248nn14–15, 249n18

La Violencia (The Violence), 25–26, 49

welfare, 26–27, 103, 105, 137, 228, 230n11, 237n19, 241n4; destruction of, 246n45; era, 4, 186; financialization of, 224; policies, 141; state, 4–5, 14, 223, 233n54; student, 235n5. *See also* Beneficencia de Cundinamarca (Beneficence of Cundinamarca Province)

women, 72; health care workers, 225; kangaroo care and, 68; El Materno and, 6–9, 19, 43–44, 49–51, 66, 70, 96, 142, 154, 182, 203; medical abuse of, 231n27; modes of care for, 14; poverty and, 231n24

work harassment, 185, 191, 251n9

9781478018933